Schema Therapy

for Cluster C Personality Disorders

Treating Dependent, Avoidant and Obsessive-Compulsive Clients

Remco van der Wijngaart
and Hannie van Genderen

Schema Therapy Approaches & Resources

Schema Therapy for Cluster C Personality Disorders
Treating Dependent, Avoidant and Obsessive-Compulsive Clients

English translation of *Schematherapie voor cluster C-persoonlijkheidsstoornissen.*

© Pavilion Publishing & Media

The author has asserted his rights in accordance with the Copyright, Designs and Patents Act (1988) to be identified as the author of this work.

Published by:
Pavilion Publishing and Media Ltd
Blue Sky Offices, 25 Cecil Pashley Way
Shoreham by Sea, West Sussex, BN43 5FF

Tel: +44 (0) 1273 434 943
Email: info@pavpub.com
Web: www.pavpub.com

Published 2024

All rights reserved. No part of this publication may be reproduced, stored in a retrieval system, or transmitted in any form or by any means, electronic, mechanical, photocopying, recording or otherwise, without prior permission in writing of the publisher and the copyright owners.

A catalogue record for this book is available from the British Library.

ISBN: 978-1-80388-387-8

Pavilion Publishing and Media is a leading publisher of books, training materials and digital content in mental health, social care and allied fields. Pavilion and its imprints offer must-have knowledge and innovative learning solutions underpinned by sound research and professional values.

First published in Dutch under the title *Schematherapie voor cluster C-persoonlijkheidsstoornissen: Behandeling van afhankelijke, vermijdende en dwangmatige cliënten* by Remco van der Wijngaart, edition: 1
Copyright © Bohn Stafleu van Loghum is een imprint van Springer Media B.V., onderdeel van Springer Nature, 2024
This edition has been translated and published under licence from Springer Media B.V., part of Springer Nature. Springer Media B.V., part of Springer Nature takes no responsibility and shall not be made liable for the accuracy of the translation.

Authors: Remco van der Wijngaart and Hannie van Genderen
Cover design: Emma Dawe, Pavilion Publishing and Media Ltd
Page layout and typesetting: Emma Dawe, Pavilion Publishing and Media Ltd
Printing: Independent Publishers Group

Contents

Schema Therapy for Cluster C Personality Disorders ii

Acknowledgements 1

Foreword 5

Chapter 1: Introduction 7

Chapter 2: Developments in schema therapy – concepts and definitions 21

Chapter 3: Case conceptualization for cluster C disorders 61

Chapter 4: From case conceptualization to treatment 135

Chapter 5: Dependent Personality Disorder 151

Chapter 6: Avoidant Personality Disorder 199

Chapter 7: Obsessive-Compulsive Personality Disorder 223

Chapter 8: The middle phase of therapy 257

Chapter 9: The final phase of therapy 297

Conclusion 333

References 335

Appendix: Modes 339

Acknowledgements

The book you are reading is the result of a process that began ten years ago. At that time, Guido Sijbers and Remco van der Wijngaart travelled to Ukraine on several occasions to teach schema therapy. During those trips, they decided to co-write a book on schema therapy for cluster C personality disorders. This turned out to be a bigger and more complex undertaking than they had thought, and the plan was put on hold. They did create an audio-visual production: 'Schema therapy for the Avoidant-, Dependent- and Obsessive-Compulsive Personality Disorder' (2018). The idea of writing the book remained, however, and in another attempt to achieve it, Remco and Hannie took up the project. However, it took until late 2022 before we actually got started. We are pleased to have found Arnoud Arntz willing to write an overview of the origins of schema therapy for cluster C personality disorder, and of the current scientific knowledge in this field.

We are very grateful to Hélène Bögels, Julie Krans and Marjolein van Wijk-Herbrink who provided immensely valuable feedback in reading over the manuscript. Once again, you have shown that you have tremendous expertise and a keen eye, combined with a pleasant, constructive way of giving feedback. Thank you!

Of course, we would also like to thank other people who made it possible to write this book. BSL, and in particular Yulma Perk and Hester Presburg. Thanks again for your confidence that we could get this job done in the ten months we thought it would take us.

Finally, we would like to thank our clients. They dedicated themselves during therapy and tried all the techniques, even though they might have found them strange or difficult at times. In that collaboration, they taught us a lot and we are immensely grateful for that. This book is intended to help improve treatment for them in the future.

A word of thanks from Remco

Hannie, we've worked together for almost thirty years across all kinds of projects and contexts. Writing a book together has not been one of them, until now. Once again, I've found that working with you is outstanding; we know where we stand, we can be honest and open with each other, and our ideas about the subject match almost seamlessly. I am immensely happy to have been able to do this with you!

Arnoud, of course I want to thank you too, for your part in Chapter 2 and for the Foreword. But I also want to thank you for the years of collaboration, during which I've learned a lot from you and have been given so many great opportunities – including participating as a therapist in the cluster C study that forms the basis of this book.

I also want to explicitly mention my children. They are the best thing in my life and the only downside to writing this book has been that I've spent far too much time working on it instead of spending time with them.

A word of thanks from Hannie

I'm happy that, after a long process of development, Remco and I have managed to complete this book on the treatment of cluster C personality disorders. With our years of productive collaboration in the field of schema therapy, we have a good feel for each other and we quickly agreed on the content of this book. I'm always pleasantly surprised by Remco's creativity in developing new insights about treating clients with schema therapy and integrating the results of scientific research into practice.

I am indebted to my colleagues and friends Marleen Rijkeboer and Arnoud Arntz, both of whom made a major contribution to introducing schema therapy in the Netherlands – and helped develop the innovations in schema therapy that we have incorporated in this book.

I've known Arnoud for almost forty years, since we started working together on treatment, research and education at Riagg Maastricht. With his passion in the field of researching the effectiveness of treatment for clients with a number of disorders and developing education in this field, he has contributed to a significant improvement in psychotherapy for clients. That is part of why he has always been a great inspiration for me.

I got to know Marleen from my training in schema therapy by Jeff Young in 1996. In particular, our collaboration on education in schema therapy was inspiring and innovative. She is also a passionate therapist and researcher who is always developing new insights that improve treatment for clients.

I would also like to thank my children Sacha and Zoë Scheffer, who had patience as children when Mama once again needed time to write a book, and who shared their ideas as adults about schema therapy following my book *Breaking Negative Thinking Patterns*. I would also like to thank my partner Jos Halfens for encouraging me to keep writing, even if it was sometimes at the expense of spending time together.

Foreword

Cluster C personality disorders are very common, and lead to low quality of life and high social costs. Despite this, relatively little research has been carried out on them. This is commonly explained by the fact that this group causes relatively few acute life-threatening crises, and that often only anxiety, mood or burnout issues are seen. The problem with this position is that it contributes either to ignoring the personality issues – which can lead to 'revolving door treatments' of superficial anxiety or mood symptoms – or to treatment that lacks a theoretical framework to understand the problems, provide a foundation for the therapeutic relationship and give a basis for therapeutic techniques. These kinds of informal or 'free' treatments also do not address the social costs, because they are undefined and can be applied in almost infinite variations.

Fortunately, a large-scale study using a schema therapy protocol with a maximum of fifty individual sessions showed it to be highly effective for cluster C personality disorders and accepted by most participants. Like schema therapy for Borderline Personality Disorder, this protocol was based on the mode model of psychopathology, which formed the basis for the case conceptualization and the choice of techniques as well as the timing of their application. We can consider ourselves lucky that the authors of this book have further developed this protocol using the latest theoretical and clinical insights. The theory has been embedded into the reformulated model of schema therapy in order to help give a better understanding of the relationship between schemas and schema modes, and to provide a framework for understanding the different modes – particularly those that are important in cluster C disorders.

Featuring accessible examples and summaries, as well as the latest insights on applying experiential techniques, this long-overdue book addresses an urgent need for a clear methodology to treat these often intractable issues effectively, without the practitioner being tempted to prolong the treatment duration unnecessarily. The clear structure and language are a testament to the vast teaching experience of the authors.

Arnoud Arntz

Chapter 1: Introduction

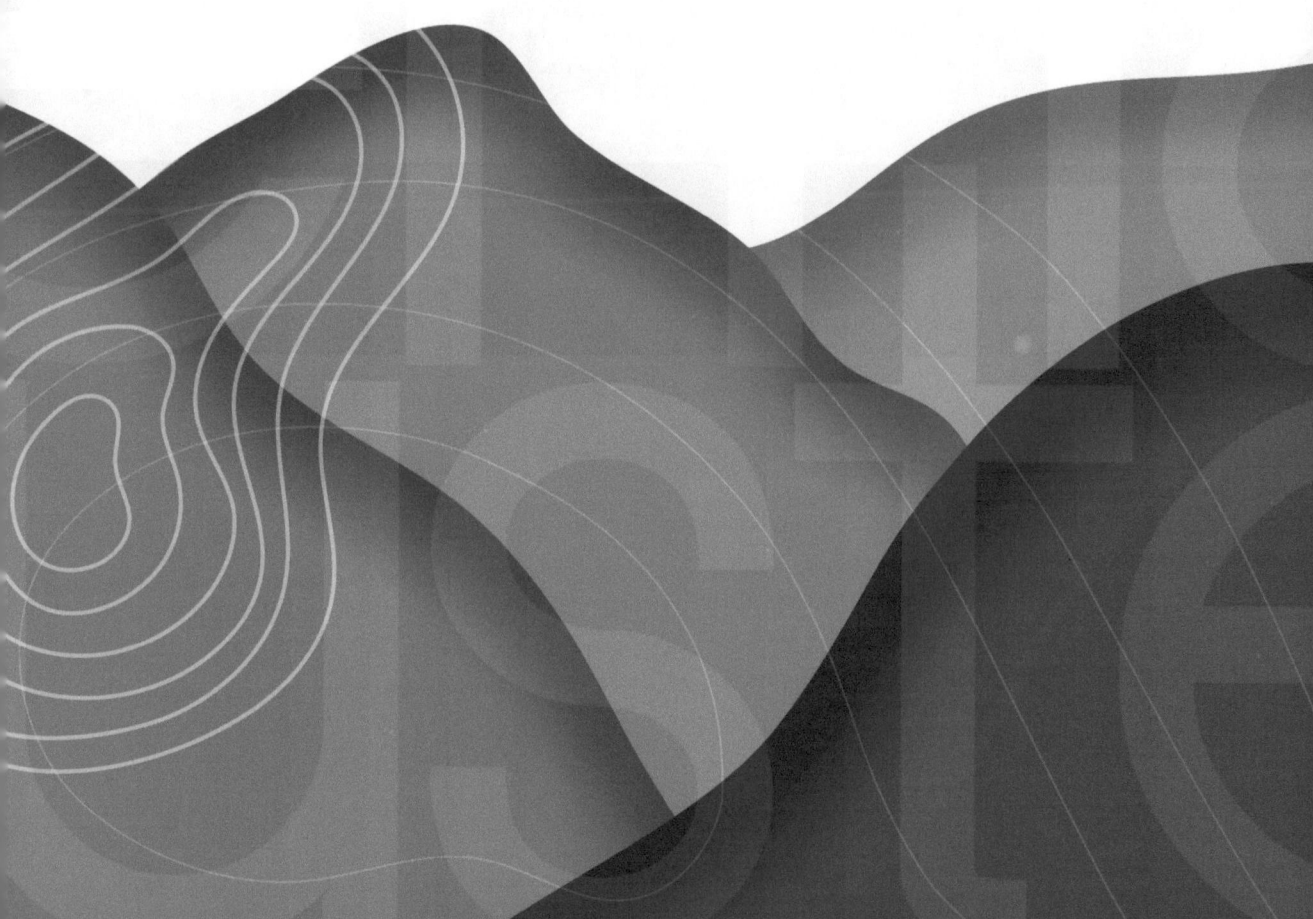

Chapter 1: Introduction

Chapter map	
1.1	Introduction
1.2	The differences between clients with cluster C and cluster B personality disorders
1.3	Dependent Personality Disorder
1.4	Avoidant Personality Disorder
1.5	Obsessive-Compulsive Personality Disorder
1.6	Chapter summary
1.7	A word on terminology

1.1 Introduction

The number of publications and books about schema therapy has grown substantially in the past quarter of a century. Both general and more disorder-focused books have been published; however, we are not aware of any books on the application of schema therapy to cluster C personality disorders in an individual setting. A Dutch manual does exist, but it is largely focused on treatment in a group setting (Tjoa & Muste, 2021). Its authors indicate that the book can also be used for individual treatment, but due to the emphasis on group treatment in thirty sessions, there is inevitably less room for the specific challenges encountered in an individual fifty-session treatment for one of the three cluster C disorders. In addition to which, of course, relatively few people can read Dutch.

Arnoud Arntz took the initiative to conduct the first research on the specific application of schema therapy for clients with a cluster C personality disorder. This began in 2009 and resulted in a new treatment protocol (Bamelis *et al*, 2014). This study found that a number of adjustments were required in the schema therapy treatment of cluster C disorders relative to the treatment of cluster B personality disorders, for which schema therapy was already well-established (see also Section 2.2 on research findings). We have been teaching courses and training programmes based on these experiences and insights since 2011 ('Schematherapie voor Cluster C', Van Genderen Opleidingen B.V.). A specialist audio-visual production has also been developed (Van der Wijngaart & Sijbers, 2018). But until now, there has been no book on how to use this adapted form of schema therapy in the individual treatment of cluster C clients.

In this book, we will begin by examining the characteristic differences between cluster B and cluster C clients. There are clear differences between the two groups, both in the nature and the origin of their issues. These differences have implications for how the therapeutic relationship is approached, how all the techniques are applied, and the duration of treatment. We describe how to structure the therapeutic relationship, and how the methods and techniques can be adapted. We also describe how to design the therapeutic process in a time-limited schema therapy treatment. As such, we think that this book will be a valuable addition to the existing literature on schema therapy.

Each of the three clients used as examples in this book has a single cluster C personality disorder. In clinical practice, there will often be more than one comorbid personality disorder – for instance, a client with Dependent Personality Disorder may also have Avoidant Personality Disorder or avoidant traits. There is also high comorbidity between personality disorders and anxiety (Friborg *et al*, 2013) or mood disorders (Friborg *et al*, 2014). For example, a client with Avoidant Personality Disorder might also have Social Anxiety Disorder and Recurrent Depressive Disorder, a client with Dependent Personality Disorder might also have an anxiety disorder, and a client with Obsessive-Compulsive Personality Disorder might also have recurrent depressive episodes in which exhaustion from hard work is coupled with periods of despondency.

Treatment of these anxiety or mood disorders can be integrated as a component of the personality disorder treatment. Even without adaptation for such disorders, clients in the schema therapy group were found to be less depressed after treatment (Bamelis *et al*, 2014), and as such this book also provides insights and tools for treating clients who have a comorbid anxiety or mood disorder in addition to a cluster C personality disorder. Schema therapy can also be applied specifically to an anxiety or mood disorder without there being a comorbid personality disorder. However, an effort should be made to first treat the depression with a recommended treatment such as CBT; if this is not adequately effective, schema therapy can be considered. Schema therapy specifically for recurrent depressive disorders has been found to be effective (Renner *et al*, 2013; Renner *et al*, 2016), and schema therapy also appears to be promising as a treatment for chronic anxiety, OCD and PTSD (Peeters *et al*, 2021). A review of existing studies on schema therapy for anxiety disorders unfortunately found serious methodological flaws in many studies; for this reason, further research is required on the effectiveness of schema therapy for chronic anxiety, OCD and PTSD (Peeters *et al*, 2021).

Chapter 2 describes the principles of treatment for cluster C disorders. This is based on the treatment protocol used in the research study on cluster C personality disorders (Bamelis *et al*, 2014). It also draws on the latest insights into language and concepts within schema therapy (Arntz *et al*, 2021). We then describe the case conceptualization of the three cluster C disorders in Chapter 3. The conceptualization of anxiety and mood disorders in terms of modes is discussed briefly at the end of this chapter.

Chapter 4 describes how to create a treatment plan for cluster C disorders. We then elaborate on this via case studies of three individuals in Chapters 5, 6 and 7. We have chosen to describe Dependent, Avoidant and Obsessive-Compulsive Personality Disorders separately, as this allows us to clearly demonstrate the specific challenges and adaptations involved in the treatment of each one. In clinical practice, there are of course clients who have a combination of cluster C disorders or have both cluster B and cluster C personality disorders. In the latter case, we recommend focusing on methods and techniques that are appropriate to treat cluster B problems first (van Genderen & Arntz, 2021). The cluster C issues often diminish during the course of this process. If necessary, treatment for the residual cluster C issues can then continue afterwards.

Imagery rescripting, chairwork and empathic confrontation are examples of methods and techniques that will be used in clinical practice with every personality disorder. For the sake of readability, we have decided not to describe these universal methods and techniques and instead to limit ourselves to the specific adaptations and variations for each cluster C disorder. In this way, we have been able to distribute the methods and techniques across many chapters, so that the book as a whole gives a complete overview of what schema therapy can offer in the treatment of cluster C disorders (see Table 1.1).

Table 1.1: Distribution of methods and techniques across chapters

	Chapter 5: Dependent PD	Chapter 6: Avoidant PD	Chapter 7: Obsessive-Compulsive PD
Child Modes	Dependent Child: *Stimulating anger*	Inferior/Shamed Child: *Stimulating self-expression*	Inhibited Child: *Stimulating spontaneity and play*
Coping Mode(s)	Compliant Surrenderer: *Historical roleplay*	Avoidant Protector: *Empathic confrontation*	Perfectionistic Overcontroller: *Chairwork*
Critical Mode(s)	Punitive Mode: *Imagery rescripting*	Blaming Mode: *Imagery rescripting*	Demanding Mode: *Chairwork*
Healthy Adult	Ch. 8: Middle phase Ch. 9: Final phase	Ch. 8: Middle phase Ch. 9: Final phase	Ch. 8: Middle phase Ch. 9: Final phase

In this book, we have chosen to primarily describe experiential techniques, and not to include cognitive and behavioural techniques. This is because these techniques are already well-described in the existing literature on schema therapy (Van Genderen & Arntz, 2021; Brockman *et al*, 2023), and their application for cluster C disorders is not very different from the application of the same techniques for cluster B disorders. For a description of these techniques, please refer to the previously mentioned literature.

1.2 The differences between clients with cluster C and cluster B personality disorders

Broadly speaking, we can say that clients with a cluster C personality disorder have mostly encountered deficiencies in their childhood in the areas of autonomy, competence, identity development, self-expression, spontaneity and play. By contrast, clients with a cluster B personality disorder have mostly encountered deficiencies in the areas of acceptance, connection, safety and predictability, and sometimes a lack of boundaries and self-control. The differences in the typical background of these two client groups are summarized in Table 1.2. There is often also a difference in temperament, with anger being more present and visible in cluster B clients than in cluster C clients (who sometimes deny ever becoming angry).

Table 1.2: Differences between clients with cluster C and cluster B personality disorders

Cluster C	Cluster B
Too much protection	Insufficient protection
Emotional abuse	Sexual, physical and emotional abuse
Too many rules	Too few rules
Deficits in parents 'more subtle'	Deficits in parents 'clearer'
Parents strict and guilt-inducing	Parents very abrasive
Greater loyalty to parents	Loyalty to parents less strong
Client cooperative	Client uncooperative
Virtually no anger	Too much anger

1.2.1 Explanation of Table 1.2

Clients with a cluster C personality disorder have often been too sheltered in their upbringing. Rather than lacking basic safety, they have been given insufficient room for self-expression, autonomy, spontaneity and play. There has usually been no physical or sexual abuse, but emotional abuse usually has occurred. For example, the client's parents might have been strict or inhibitive, but not in a very abrasive way. They may have shown disappointment or disapproval, but in a much more subtle way than the parents of clients with a cluster B personality disorder. Another possibility is that one or both parents leaned too much on the client for support, for help or to realize their own dreams, causing the client to feel responsible for the other person's well-being far too early in their lives. This may have caused the client to try much too hard, and to pay insufficient attention to their own needs.

The more subtle, indirect way in which their basic needs have remained unmet often makes it difficult for cluster C clients to recognize their parents' role in the development of their personality disorder. These clients experienced their parents as caring and loving in many ways, so they remain loyal to them. Loyalty and guilt are thus prevalent themes in the treatment of these clients. Combined with a less temperamental nature, this means that these clients are not quick to anger, even if treated badly. An 'advantage' of this is that cluster C clients tend initially to be very cooperative in treatment. However, when the time comes to really make changes, they shy away. The coping styles of Avoidance and Inversion continue to be so effective in the short term that this personality issue is remarkably persistent.

To summarize, the main characteristic differences between cluster C disorders and cluster B disorders are:

- Different basic needs are relevant in cluster C disorders. It is not so much about safety or connection; more about self-expression, autonomy, spontaneity and play.
- Coping modes are at the heart of the issues in clients with a cluster C disorder. There is a reason these are called Dependent, Avoidant and Obsessive-Compulsive Personality Disorders – the names typify the dominant persistent coping modes. This makes it difficult to achieve the main goals of schema therapy treatment by fulfilling the basic needs of the Vulnerable Child and strengthening the Healthy Adult.

Next, we will look more closely at the specific characteristics of each cluster C disorder. Although we assume that this diagnostic knowledge is already available to the reader, this description is necessary to define the framework for the rest of the book.

1.3 Dependent Personality Disorder

A person with a Dependent Personality Disorder has difficulty making decisions independently. That inability affects important matters as well as mundane ones. They subordinate their own needs to those of others. This means that they frequently ask others for advice, and that they cannot or dare not make their own decisions. The result is usually that they do what others advise them to do, without checking whether this is really what they want themselves. This can have far-reaching consequences for their choices in education or work, and also in terms of social contacts. They dare not stand up for their own opinions for fear that others will no longer like them or want to help them. They are even willing to take on unpleasant tasks or do things that could be harmful to them, just to avoid losing the other person's support.

They do not undertake things independently, because they are afraid that they won't be able do it and/or that others will disapprove. Because they think they won't be able to take care of themselves, they prefer to be in the company of others and go out of their way to avoid being alone. Some go so far as to prevent their partner or another important person from going away for an extended time. Or, for example, they might stay with their parents when their partner has to travel for work for a few days. In the case of a breakup or the death of a partner, they immediately look for another person to take care of them. They worry a lot about being left alone, even when that threat is not actually there.

Characteristics of Dependent Personality Disorder
- Has difficulty making everyday decisions.
- Leaves important decisions to others.
- Does not dare to disagree with others, even if they are wrong.
- Does not take initiative independently for fear of not being able to do something or of doing it wrong.
- Subjects themselves to the needs of the others.
- Does unpleasant things if necessary to get support and care from others.
- Cannot be alone because they think they cannot take care of themselves.
- Looks for another immediately after losing a partner.
- Has unrealistic worries about being left alone.

If someone answers affirmatively to at least five of the characteristics described here, and there is a sustained pattern of this over much of their life, they have Dependent Personality Disorder.

1.4 Avoidant Personality Disorder

The DSM-5 describes Avoidant Personality Disorder as a pervasive pattern of social inhibition, combined with feelings of inadequacy and a hypersensitivity to negative judgement by others. Clients with Avoidant Personality Disorder tend to avoid work or occupational tasks for fear of the social contacts involved. This avoidance can go so far that it causes them to miss out on promotion or development opportunities. They also avoid contact with other people in other areas of life, especially if they are not yet certain that others appreciate them. For instance, people with Avoidant Personality Disorder will almost never take the first step in making contact with someone they don't know.

Avoidance also plays a big role in these clients' relationships with people they do know well. In intimate relationships, for example, they avoid sharing anything about their deep feelings, thoughts, fantasies and desires for fear that they will be thought strange or ridiculed. This concern about the negative judgement of others occupies these clients so strongly that they worry about it long before or after a social situation. During encounters with people they don't yet know, or don't know well, they will often fall silent and wait to see the tenor of the conversation for fear of not being good enough. They often don't feel as worthy, intelligent or attractive as other people. Finally, the fear of making mistakes and then being judged negatively can be so great that it causes them to avoid new activities.

Avoidant Personality Disorder has significant overlap with generalized Social Anxiety Disorder. This too involves a persistent pattern of fear of negative judgement by others, which leads to avoidance of social interactions in various areas of life. Just as with personality problems, this avoidance out of fear of negative judgement by others in Social Anxiety Disorder also often occurs from early adulthood. In practice, this often makes it difficult to differentiate between the two disorders. Of course, it is possible that they overlap and partly describe the same phenomena, and it is also possible for a client to suffer from both. Some differential diagnostic considerations are described below.

Avoidant Personality Disorder involves personality traits that clients consider to be 'their own'. Avoidance is such a normal aspect of their existence that they often no longer perceive the underlying fear of negative judgement by others so acutely. They avoid social interactions because they 'don't feel like it' or they 'don't feel comfortable'. By contrast, clients with Social Anxiety Disorder do often still experience a phobic fear of negative judgement by others. They are more likely to feel genuinely anxious, and not just 'uncomfortable'. Clients with Social Anxiety Disorder also consciously avoid social situations because they are afraid, not because they find it uncomfortable or don't feel like it. There is also evidence that avoidance in Avoidant Personality Disorder also involves activities and experiences other than social interactions (Taylor *et al*, 2004).

Characteristics of Avoidant Personality Disorder
- Avoids tasks or positions at work out of fear of criticism or rejection.
- Avoids strangers unless they are certain that the other person likes them.
- Closed in intimate relationships for fear of being ridiculed or criticized when they share feelings or needs.
- Worries excessively about social situations and possible negative judgement by others.
- Withdrawn in new social situations for fear of not being good enough.

- Self-image is coloured by the feeling of not being good, intelligent or attractive enough.
- Avoids new activities for fear of making a fool of themselves in the process.

If someone answers affirmatively to at least four of the characteristics described here, and there is a sustained pattern of this over much of their life, they have Avoidant Personality Disorder.

1.5 Obsessive-Compulsive Personality Disorder

Obsessive-Compulsive Personality Disorder is described in the DSM-5 as a persistent pattern of compulsive perceptions and behaviours in various areas of life. Clients with this disorder often pay excessive attention to details, order and organization, and get so absorbed in them that they lose sight of the bigger picture or goal. They have a strong tendency towards perfectionism, as a result of which they require more time to complete tasks than other people. They often fail to meet deadlines because they are so occupied with work being absolutely right, and they are very focused on productivity and efficiency.

All this means that clients with Obsessive-Compulsive Personality Disorder work hard and long, and non-work activities often have to take second place. They also have high standards for what is right and wrong in other areas of life, and they can be annoyed by people who do not live up to those standards and rules. For instance, traffic can be a major source of irritation for them, because other people don't always adhere to the rules of the road. These high standards about 'how things should be' can make it difficult for these clients to delegate tasks, simply because they cannot be sure that the other person will do it 'properly'. This also gives them a tendency to check other people's work. As a result, others often see them as stubborn or rigid. A specific form of difficulty with letting go is a tendency in some clients towards stinginess, which can make it difficult for them to spend money on others and/or themselves.

Characteristics of Obsessive-Compulsive Personality Disorder
- Gets lost in detail, order and organization, and loses sight of the big picture.
- Perfectionistic, resulting in deadlines not being met or tasks taking more time.
- Workaholism that does not leave room for other activities or people.
- Overly strict standards and frequent irritation when others do not adhere to them.

- Pattern of stinginess and therefore not spending money on themselves or others.
- Difficulty delegating tasks if unsure that a person will adhere to strict standards.
- Often very sure that they are right, and perceived by others as stubborn and rigid.

If someone answers affirmatively to at least four of the characteristics described here, and there is a sustained pattern of this over much of their life, they have Obsessive-Compulsive Personality Disorder.

Obsessive-Compulsive Personality Disorder can be very similar in its clinical presentation to Autism Spectrum Disorder (ASD). Even so, there are clear differences in the underlying mechanisms (Spek *et al*, n.d.). Most of the overlap has to do with keeping to routines and rituals. In contrast to autism, however, the difficulty that clients with Obsessive-Compulsive Personality Disorder have in letting go of rituals and routines often arises somewhat later in their development, and is not as rigid in childhood. Furthermore, clients with Obsessive-Compulsive Personality Disorder often stick to routines and rituals out of a need for efficiency; in autistic people, the motivation is more often that 'it simply has to be right' and to keep things predictable in their lives.

Another overlapping feature between the two clinical presentations is that clients with Obsessive-Compulsive Personality Disorder, like those with autism, can lose themselves in activities and interests. In this aspect, Obsessive-Compulsive clients strive more for perfection, while for those with autism it is more about completeness. In clients with Obsessive-Compulsive Personality Disorder, the need for appreciation or approval from others also plays a role in this perfectionism, unlike in autistic people.

A characteristic of autism is limited social-emotional reciprocity. This is not found in clients with Obsessive-Compulsive Personality Disorder, who are able to sense and comfort other people. Also, unlike those with autism, clients with Obsessive-Compulsive Personality Disorder do not have impairments in non-verbal communication. They can make adequate eye contact, and they can generally also read non-verbal cues in other people correctly. While they are sometimes demanding, they are essentially able to build reciprocal friendships. This is less possible for autistic people. Autism is further characterized by stereotypical motor functions, language and behaviour, which are not characteristic of clients with Obsessive-Compulsive Personality Disorder.

Finally, the latter group does not have sensory hyposensitivity to hunger, thirst, heat and cold – although they can sometimes become so preoccupied with the high demands that they place on themselves that they are less aware of those bodily signals.

1.6 Chapter summary

To our knowledge, this is the first book about individual treatment with schema therapy for patients with a cluster C personality disorder. In this first chapter, key differences between cluster B and C personality disorders were described. Some considerations regarding differential diagnosis have also been touched upon, for example the differentiation between Obsessive Compulsive Personality Disorder versus autism.

1.7 A word on terminology

In general, throughout this book we use the 'formal' language found in most articles and manuals about schema therapy. For example, we discuss 'modes' such as Coping Modes and Critical Modes. In the chapters dealing with practical implementation, however, we have included client dialogues – and in these dialogues we substitute the word 'side' for 'mode'. For example, we use 'Critical Side' instead of 'Critical Mode'. We have done this in an effort to use terms that are recognizable to most therapists when working in clinical practice.

Chapter 2: Developments in schema therapy – concepts and definitions

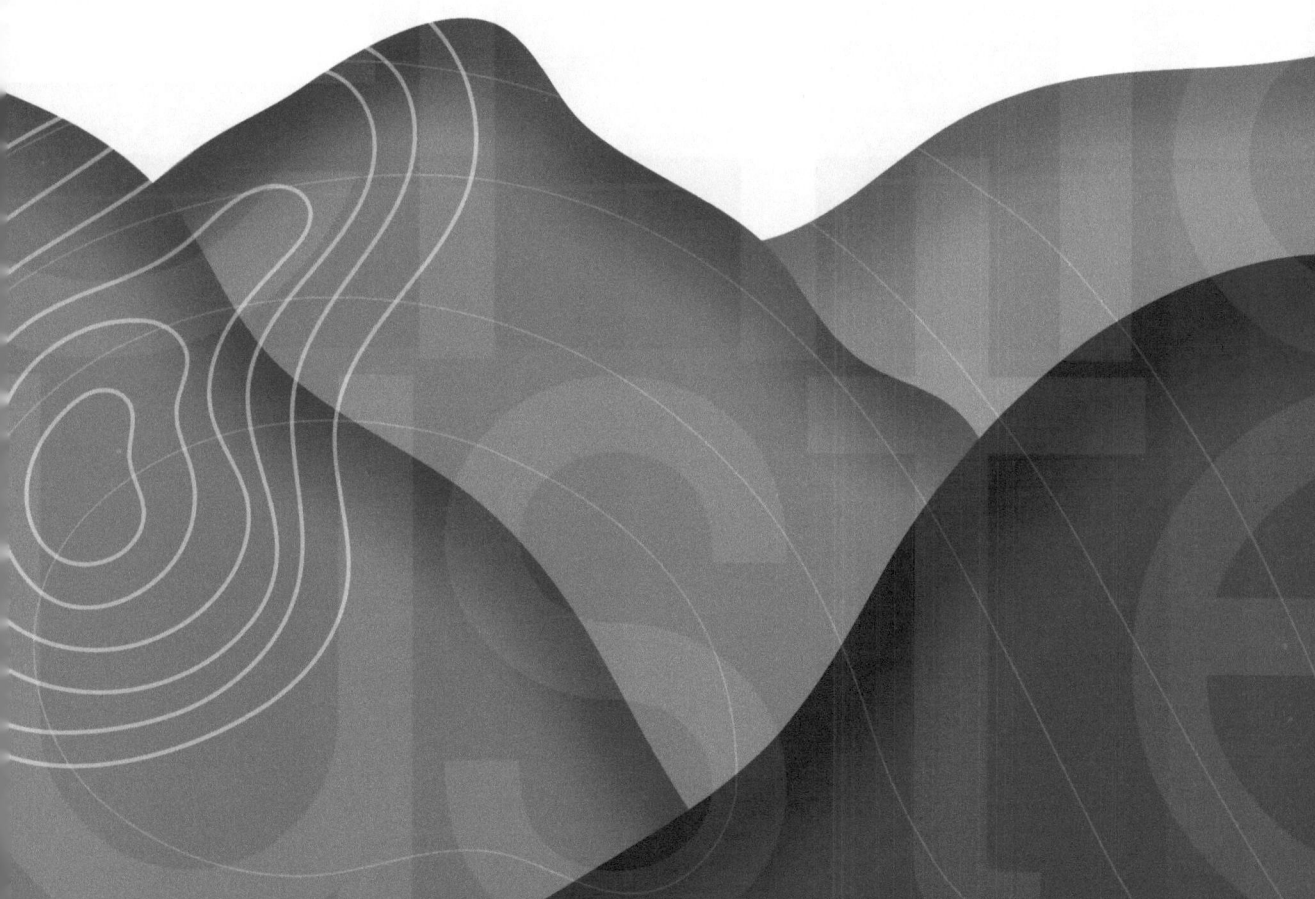

Chapter 2: Developments in schema therapy – concepts and definitions

Arnoud Arntz*, Hannie van Genderen and Remco van der Wijngaart

* Arnoud Arntz is Professor Emeritus of Clinical Psychology at the University of Amsterdam. He is also active as a clinical psychologist at the Academic Center for Trauma and Personality (ACTP). He contributed (and still contributes) to the development of schema therapy and its empirical validation.

Chapter map	
2.1	Introduction
2.2	The emergence of schema therapy for cluster C personality disorders
2.3	Research findings
2.4	Concepts and definitions
2.5	The therapeutic relationship
2.6	Methods and techniques
2.7	Phases and objectives
2.8	Chapter summary

2.1 Introduction

This chapter sets out the theoretical principles for this book, drawing on the new theoretical insights described in the article 'Towards a reformulated theory underlying schema therapy' (Arntz et al, 2021). This article proposed three new schemas and changed the formulation of coping styles and coping modes. Based on the new understanding of the relationship between schemas, coping styles and modes, a larger number of more differentiated modes were described.

After describing the concepts that are used (2.3), a brief overview of the methods and techniques used is given in the second part of this chapter (2.4).

2.2 The emergence of schema therapy for cluster C personality disorders

Traditionally, cluster C problems often went unrecognized, and clients were instead treated for syndromic issues such as depression, anxiety disorders or addiction. Of course, approaches such as psychodynamic psychotherapy and client-centred therapy did go some way to address underlying personality issues. When personality disorders gained more attention as an official diagnosis, these person-centred treatments were often the first choice for clients with a cluster C disorder. Furthermore, it was also often assumed that personality disorders were simply not treatable, and the result of this was that this diagnosis led only to low-frequency supportive contact.

Cognitive Behavioural Therapy (CBT) treatments for personality disorders were developed in the 1980s and 1990s, especially for Avoidant Personality Disorder – perhaps because exposure and assertiveness training seemed to be obvious treatments. However, early applications of CBT also found that effects were lacking in the domain of intimacy (Alden, 1989). An overview of early studies on the treatment of cluster C personality disorders is given in Simon (2009). With the validation of schema therapy for Borderline Personality Disorder (Giesen-Bloo *et al*, 2006), the research question arose as to whether schema therapy might also offer an effective treatment for cluster C problems. To this end, special schema mode models for cluster C disorders were developed and validated (Bamelis *et al*, 2011). By conceptualizing cluster C problems in terms of schema modes, a form of schema therapy adapted to these problems could be proposed and tested (Arntz, 2012). The studies on this are discussed in the section below.

2.3 Research findings

Only a few studies have so far been conducted on the effectiveness of schema therapy for cluster C personality problems. To the authors' knowledge, the first randomized clinical trial (RCT) was conducted by Bamelis *et al* (2012; 2014). In this study, individual schema therapy was compared with a modified form of client-centred therapy (CCT) called Clarification-Oriented Psychotherapy (COP; Sachse, 2001), and with the optimal form of treatment as usual (TAU) for the individual client. This multi-centre study was conducted in twelve mental health institutions in the Netherlands, and it involved three hundred and twenty clients with either a cluster C or paranoid, histrionic or narcissistic personality disorder as a primary diagnosis. The vast majority of participants (90%) had a cluster C personality disorder as their primary diagnosis, with 51% having Avoidant, 11% Dependent and 28% Obsessive-Compulsive Personality Disorder. Because cluster C personality disorders dominated, and because the primary diagnosis has no effect on outcomes, we can consider the results of this study as being valid for cluster C disorders.

If a participant was randomized to TAU, the intake staff determined what the optimal treatment would be for this specific participant. Afterwards, it was found that in 74% of cases this was a form of psychodynamic psychotherapy; CBT was provided in 19% of cases, and 5% received no treatment (initially). The schema therapy protocol consisted of forty individual sessions in the first year, followed by a maximum of ten individual booster sessions in year two. Three years after the start (i.e. one year after the last booster session in the case of schema therapy), independent evaluators who were unfamiliar with the treatment condition administered Structured Clinical Interviews for DSM (SCID) again to establish diagnoses.

The results showed that one year after treatment ended, 82% of those who had received schema therapy no longer had a personality disorder diagnosis. This was significantly better than the 55% achieved with TAU and the 61% achieved with COP. The improvement in the Global Assessment of Functioning (GAF) and Social and Occupational Functioning Assessment Scale (SOFAS) scores was also significantly higher with schema therapy than with TAU or COP. Comorbid depression, present in 45% of the sample at baseline, disappeared significantly more often following schema therapy than following TAU (13.5% vs 25.2% with a depressive disorder at three years). However, it was striking that, unlike the interview-based results, the self-reports did not show any variation between treatments. The authors postulate the possible explanation that there may be more improvement with objective indicators than in the client's perception. In line with this, the drop-out rate from schema therapy was found to be much lower than from TAU (15.4% vs 40.5%) – in other words, schema therapy was more acceptable and tolerable for participants than TAU. There was no significant difference with COP (20.8% drop-out).

An unexpected finding was that the method of schema therapy training had a substantial effect on the outcomes. While the first cohort of therapists was primarily trained through verbal instruction and watching videos, the second cohort was trained with a focus on practicing specific schema therapy techniques. It is estimated that in the first cohort, 25% of training time was spent practicing, compared to 75% in the second cohort. From independent assessments of recordings of sessions, the second cohort of schema therapists was found to use more schema therapy techniques than the first cohort, especially in the middle phase. The superior effects of schema therapy were primarily achieved by the second cohort, which had a much lower drop-out rate and much better clinical outcomes than the first cohort. This study (Bamelis et al, 2014) was therefore one of the few to examine the relationship between the method of training and patient-level effects, and furthermore to find a clinically relevant effect.

The same study also included economic data on the cost-effectiveness of the treatments. It found that schema therapy was more cost-effective than TAU or COP: there were better outcomes and lower costs with schema therapy over the entire three-year study period than with the other treatments (Bamelis et al, 2015). The higher drop-out rate with TAU did not lead to lower healthcare costs, because participants then received other treatments. Overall, the costs of schema therapy and TAU were similar, and the cost of COP was significantly higher – related to the fact that this was an open-ended treatment. The lower total cost of schema therapy was primarily related to more and earlier returns to the workforce. In summary, while fifty sessions of schema therapy might seem expensive, in practice this treatment is no more expensive than TAU in terms of healthcare costs, and it provides more societal benefits.

Qualitative studies have examined the experiences of patients and therapists (De Klerk et al, 2017; Ten Napel-Schutz et al, 2011; 2017). The De Klerk study found among other things that the schema therapy model and techniques were very appealing to therapists and met a need, but that therapists were often critical of the limited duration of treatment (a maximum of fifty sessions) and about the training – there was a greater need to practice techniques themselves and to safely discuss experiences and any resistance to techniques that they experienced. This feedback has (or should have) influenced the way in which today's therapists are trained in schema therapy. Therapists further indicated that peer supervision was essential, and that they would have wanted frequent supervision by an expert.

Feedback from clients in the same study indicated that the mode model was seen as very useful, the therapeutic relationship was appreciated, and experiential techniques were seen as emotionally taxing but ultimately very important. There was, however, a need for more explanation about experiential techniques. Clients also indicated that they had difficulty with the limited duration of therapy. Because of the very good results of the fifty-session protocol, instead of recommending open-ended therapy, the researchers decided to incorporate a proper explanation of the fifty-session approach into the protocol to reassure clients. It was actually found that many participants improved further even after treatment ended, and that they were better able to handle life without help (sometimes by using schema therapy techniques themselves). We now explain to clients how valuable it is to try a year without therapy, as this provides an opportunity to grow in self-confidence and helps to free them from the self-stigma of the chronic patient who is dependent on care for their whole life (many participants in the study had experienced many treatments and/or been in care for a long time).

2.3.1 Special populations

2.3.1.1 Autism

A common idea among clinicians is that autism is a contraindication for schema therapy. Needless to say, autism cannot be 'treated' (though psychoeducation and skills training can be given), but the combination of autism and personality disorders is common, and cluster C disorders are strongly represented (Vuijk *et al*, 2018). Note that the current understanding is not that there is either an autism (ASD) diagnosis or a personality disorder diagnosis, but that these disorders can be comorbid. Vuijk *et al* (2023) conducted a multiple-case-series study to test whether schema therapy is effective with these kinds of comorbid conditions, and whether CBT techniques differed from experiential techniques in their (short-term) outcomes. Among the twelve participants, several personality disorders were usually diagnosed based on SCID-II, with Obsessive-Compulsive (10) and Avoidant (8) being the most common. Most participants had positive outcomes with schema therapy, but in about a third of participants there was no effect. We do not know exactly what the characteristics of this subgroup of non-responders were, so we certainly cannot say that autism is a contraindication for schema therapy. It was further noteworthy that the experiential techniques certainly did not do worse than CBT techniques, again disproving a widely held idea.

2.3.1.2 Older people

A second clinical idea that is gradually disappearing is that schema therapy cannot be used to treat older people. Videler *et al* (2018) used a multiple-baseline case-series design to test the effects of schema therapy in a sample of elderly people with a mean age of sixty-nine, all with a cluster C personality disorder. While no changes in idiosyncratic core beliefs occurred during baseline, the changes during schema therapy were significant – and these effects were maintained during a follow-up period after therapy. Seven of the eight participants no longer had a diagnosis of a personality disorder after treatment. This study therefore indicates that a higher age is not a contraindication for schema therapy.

2.3.2 Group schema therapy

Interest in group schema therapy (GST) as developed by Farrell *et al* (2016) has also led to the development of forms of GST for cluster C disorders. An early pilot study by Skewes *et al* (2015) found major effects of a twenty-session GST protocol supplemented by five individual sessions. The group initially included two people with Borderline Personality Disorder, but they withdrew because they felt their stronger emotional expressions were too stressful for the other participants (all cluster C). This indicates that it is better to offer GST for cluster C separately from that for Borderline Personality Disorder. Group treatment calls strongly for a semi-closed format, because the moments of participant exit and entry facilitate clinical implementation. Also, it avoids large numbers of clients waiting (possibly for a long time) to start treatment, and any drop-outs can be replaced fairly quickly.

To this end, Tjoa (see Tjoa & Muste, 2021) developed a protocol, which was compared with group CBT in an RCT on the treatment of dual diagnoses of Social Anxiety Disorder and Avoidant Personality Disorder (Baljé *et al*, 2016). The GST protocol consisted of thirty sessions of group therapy and up to three hours of individual schema therapy; the group CBT protocol followed Heimberg *et al* (1990) and primarily focused on cognitively challenging dysfunctional thoughts and exposure in vivo. The study found no significant differences in clinical effectiveness, although group CBT did produce stronger effects on some measures and the study noted that, in cases of strong avoidant behaviour, the use of exposure should be considered. However, treatment drop-out was much lower with GST than with group CBT (35% vs 62%), indicating that schema therapy is an acceptable and tolerable treatment for more participants.

This protocol by Tjoa was tested further in a slightly modified form (see Tjoa & Muste, 2021) in a large multi-centre open trial as a treatment for cluster C (Wibbelink et al, 2023). Of the one hundred and thirty-seven participants, 78% had Avoidant, 8% had Dependent and 14% had Obsessive-Compulsive Personality Disorder as their primary diagnosis. Major effects were found, with the improvement again continuing in the year after therapy. Indeed, in the case of Dependent Personality Disorder, this post-therapy effect was so strong that the improvement only occurred after therapy had ended (suggesting that time-limited treatment does have a therapeutic effect). Participants with Obsessive-Compulsive Personality Disorder seemed to benefit less than the other participants, but they also had fewer severe problems at baseline so there was less room for improvement. It is also possible that GST is less indicated for obsessive-compulsive issues.

Drop-out during the thirty GST sessions was low (12%), again indicating high acceptability of the treatment. Based on feedback from participating therapists, it was decided to increase the duration of individual therapy to five hours and to reduce the number of booster sessions to four. This modified protocol is currently being tested in a large multi-centre study in which GST is being compared with individual schema therapy and TAU (Groot et al, 2022). An important question is whether the client has certain characteristics – such as autistic traits, introversion or a history of childhood trauma – that predict whether individual or group schema therapy is more indicated. These findings can help in future needs assessment.

2.4 Concepts and definitions

The concepts of basic needs, schemas, coping styles and modes are well-known in the schema therapy literature. Therefore, we will not spend time explaining them here; readers seeking more background information are referred to the available literature (Arntz & Jacob, 2012; Brockman et al, 2023; Van Genderen & Arntz, 2021; Young et al, 2005).

There has been discussion about the use of these terms for some time in the international community of schema therapists. Early in the development of schema therapy, the emphasis during treatment was on the use of early maladaptive *schemas*, but gradually this shifted over to *modes*. The two concepts were used side-by-side, leading to potential confusion because the relationship between schemas, coping styles and modes was not elaborated.

The very similar terms 'coping styles' and 'coping modes' often compounded these difficulties. In short, there was a need for more clarity about the links and differences between the different concepts.

The first study on the relationship between schemas, coping styles and modes (Rijkeboer & Lobbestael, 2012) clarified the relationship between the concepts of schemas, coping styles and modes. An international working group, led by Arnoud Arntz and Marleen Rijkeboer, then sought to gain a better understanding of the theoretical foundations of schema therapy and the concepts it uses. They came up with a number of new theoretical insights into the connection between basic needs, schemas, coping styles and modes (Arntz et al, 2021). Although this research, involving more than sixty researchers from thirty-two countries, is still ongoing, we think these new insights are already relevant enough to us to use in this book – and we offer a brief explanation of them below.

2.4.1 The relationship between basic needs, schemas, coping styles and modes

Schema therapy assumes that personality disorders arise because a number of basic needs were not met during the client's childhood. Jeffrey Young (1990) formulated five (universal) basic needs that must be met for a child to develop into a Healthy Adult. Later, partly based on research by Dweck (2017), two more basic needs were added: fairness and self-coherence. The definitions of these two further needs and their corresponding schemas, as taken from the article by the international working group (Arntz et al, 2021) and personal communication with Arnoud Arntz (2023), are given below.

Fairness is the need to be treated justly and fairly. If it is insufficiently met, it can lead to the schema of *Unfairness*. A person with the *Unfairness* schema experiences the world as unfair and unjust. They perceive a lack of fairness in society and feel like a victim of this unfairness. This schema leads to strong feelings of outrage, anger and powerlessness.

Self-coherence: a clear self-image and view of the world relates to the need to feel psychologically intact and rooted, both over time and in different contexts. It is the need to experience the self as integrated (a sense of identity) and the environment as an understandable and predictable place (a meaningful world). It is therefore the need to answer the questions 'Who am I?' and 'How does/should the world work in ways that matter to me?' This basic need is of a higher order, as it were, and is fulfilled by the successful integration of the six other basic needs. If the need for a clear self-image and picture of the world is not met, this can lead to two schemas:

- *Lack of a Coherent Identity:* The person experiences themselves as diffuse, dissociated or consisting of disconnected parts. This leads to confusion, alienation and existential angst.
- *Lack of a Meaningful World:* The person experiences the world as meaningless or unpredictable and feels disconnected from the processes going on around them. This leads to feelings of being lost and no longer having a grip on anything.

Table 2.1 shows how inadequate fulfilment of all seven basic needs can lead to various schemas, and briefly describes what each schema entails.

Table 2.1: The relationship between (insufficient fulfilment of) basic needs and schemas *Based on Van Genderen (2023).*

Unfulfilled basic needs	Can result in schema	Concepts
Acceptance, connection, security and predictability	1. Mistrust / Abuse	No one can be trusted. Others will take advantage of me, cheat, manipulate or humiliate me.
	2. Abandonment / Instability	Everyone lets me down sooner or later. I can't assume that others will really support me or be there for me when I need them.
	3. Social Isolation / Alienation	I don't belong. I am very different from other people. In groups, I'm always an outsider.
	4. Emotional Deprivation	No one loves or understands me. I won't get attention, warmth or good advice from others. They don't listen to me, and I can't share my feelings with them. I am on my own.
	5. Defectiveness / Shame	I'm intrinsically bad, inferior and worthless. I am unattractive. If others really get to know me, they'll discover this and reject me. I am ashamed of myself.

Self-expression (expressing your own opinions and feelings)	10. Subjugation	I must always obey or I will be punished. I must suppress my needs and feelings, otherwise conflicts and negative reactions will follow.
	11. Self-sacrifice	I must always take care of others and subjugate my own needs. Others are weaker than I am, so I gladly sacrifice myself for them. If I don't do this, I feel guilty.
	12. Approval-seeking / Recognition-seeking	I can't manage without attention and recognition. I value status and good looks to gain social appreciation. I consider that to be more important than my other needs or personal development.
Realistic limits and self-control (overconfidence)	13. Entitlement / Grandiosity	I'm better than others. I'm superior to most people. I don't have to follow the rules that apply to them. I can do whatever I want without considering others. I like to have power and control over others.
	14. Insufficient Self-control / Self-discipline	I want to get my way, and I tend to do everything impulsively. I can't handle frustrations. I don't like obligations. I can't stand discomforts such as pain or arguments. If I have to make an effort or do a boring task, I have the urge to give up.
Spontaneity and play (overcontrol)	15. Negativity / Pessimism	Everything always goes wrong anyway. I always have bad luck. I only see the negative side of things and dismiss the positive. The future is hopeless and dark.
	16. Emotional Inhibition	I always hold back all my emotions and impulses because I'm afraid that this could harm others or that they will leave me. If I don't restrain my emotions, I could lose self-esteem and feel ashamed of myself. I prefer to approach everything rationally. →

Spontaneity and play (overcontrol) (continued)	17. Unrelenting Standards	I must do everything perfectly and I can't make any mistakes. I can never do well enough, because there is always room for improvement. I'm critical of myself and also of others. I want everything to be well organized, and done efficiently and on time. Fun, relaxation or socializing always come second for me.
	18. Punitiveness	People should be punished harshly for their mistakes. I'm impatient, intolerant and rarely forgive mistakes.
Fairness	19. Unfairness	I can't stand dishonesty or unfairness. I'm always aggrieved and can't do anything about it.
Coherent self-image and clear picture of the world	20. Lack of a Coherent Identity	I'm confused. I don't perceive myself as unified. I've lost my grip on myself. I don't know who I am, and I feel lost.
	21. Lack of a Meaningful World	Not only have I lost my grip on myself, I also have no grip on the world around me. I don't understand how it works. Everything seems to keep changing, and I feel alienated from the things happening in my environment. I'm afraid of existence because I don't understand what's happening and what it means.

2.4.2 Coping styles and Coping Modes

Jeffrey Young (1990) proposed that there are three broad coping styles, or ways to deal with schema activation:

- **Surrender:** You feel, think and behave as if the schema is true.
- **Avoidance:** You try to avoid activating the schema and experiencing the feelings evoked by it.
- **Overcompensation:** You feel, think and behave as if the exact opposite of the schema is true.

Young related these terms to the survival strategies of animals: freeze (surrender), flee (avoidance) and fight (overcompensation). However, Arntz *et al* (2021) point out that these innate animal defence mechanisms have evolved to deal with external threats. They argue that schemas are more about reactions to 'internal' threats, and specifically to negative feelings and thoughts evoked by activated schemas. The international research group therefore defined these concepts differently.

2.4.2.1 Surrender
Surrender in the new model means the same as it did previously, which is that you completely believe that the schema is true.

2.4.2.2 Avoidance
The avoidance coping style is still used for the tendency to avoid schemas being activated. This term can therefore be used among other things to switch off your feelings or avoid situations, but also to become submissive or seek distraction.

2.4.2.3 Inversion
The term 'overcompensation' has been changed to 'inversion' in the new model. In this context, this word is more accurate. After all, this is about dealing with schemas through the tendency to think, feel and do the *opposite* of what the schema dictates. The word 'overcompensation' suggests that this always involves externalizing forms of behaviour, such as being tough, bragging or attacking. But the opposite of *Unrelenting Standards* is actually quite passive – lazinesss – just as the opposite of *Punitiveness* is excessive leniency and forgiveness.

Now that we have explored the new definitions of the three coping styles, we will turn our attention to modes.

2.4.3 Modes

Schema activation combined with one of the three coping styles leads to a state of mind, or a 'mode'. In other words, a mode is a combination of an activated schema (strong feelings and negative thoughts) and a coping style (behaviour to believe, avoid or invert that schema) and it determines what a person feels, thinks and does in that moment (see Figure 2.1).

There are three types of modes that lead to symptoms and problems: Child Modes, Critical Modes (Parent Modes) and Coping Modes. There are also two healthy modes: the Healthy Adult Mode and the Happy Child Mode. In the literature, the latter mode is also sometimes called the Free or Contented Child.

The term 'Parent Mode' is given a different name in the new model, the 'Critical Mode'. Previously, Critical Modes were usually called Parent Modes because it was often the client's parents who were a negative influence. But Critical Modes are not always primarily caused by parents. Other support figures (teachers, coaches, etc.) or peers (bullies or siblings) might also have given critical messages that clients have internalized. That is why we propose using the term 'Critical Mode' from now on, divided into a Demanding Mode, a Punitive Mode and a Blaming Mode.

Surrendering to most schemas means going into a Child Mode. Surrender to *Unrelenting Standards* and *Emotional Inhibition* leads to a Demanding Mode, and surrender to *Punitiveness* leads to a Punitive Mode. Arntz *et al* do not mention a Blaming Mode, but we will add this variant of the Critical Mode because we often see clients suffering from these kinds of blaming messages in clinical practice. Processing the Blaming Mode also often requires a different approach than processing the other two Critical Modes. We see the Blaming Mode as surrendering to the *Punitiveness* and *Subjugation* schemas.

The other two coping styles (Avoidance and Inversion) lead to Coping Modes. This is also shown in Figure 2.1.

Figure 2.1: The relationship between schemas, coping styles and modes
Based on van Genderen (2023) and Arntz et al (2021)

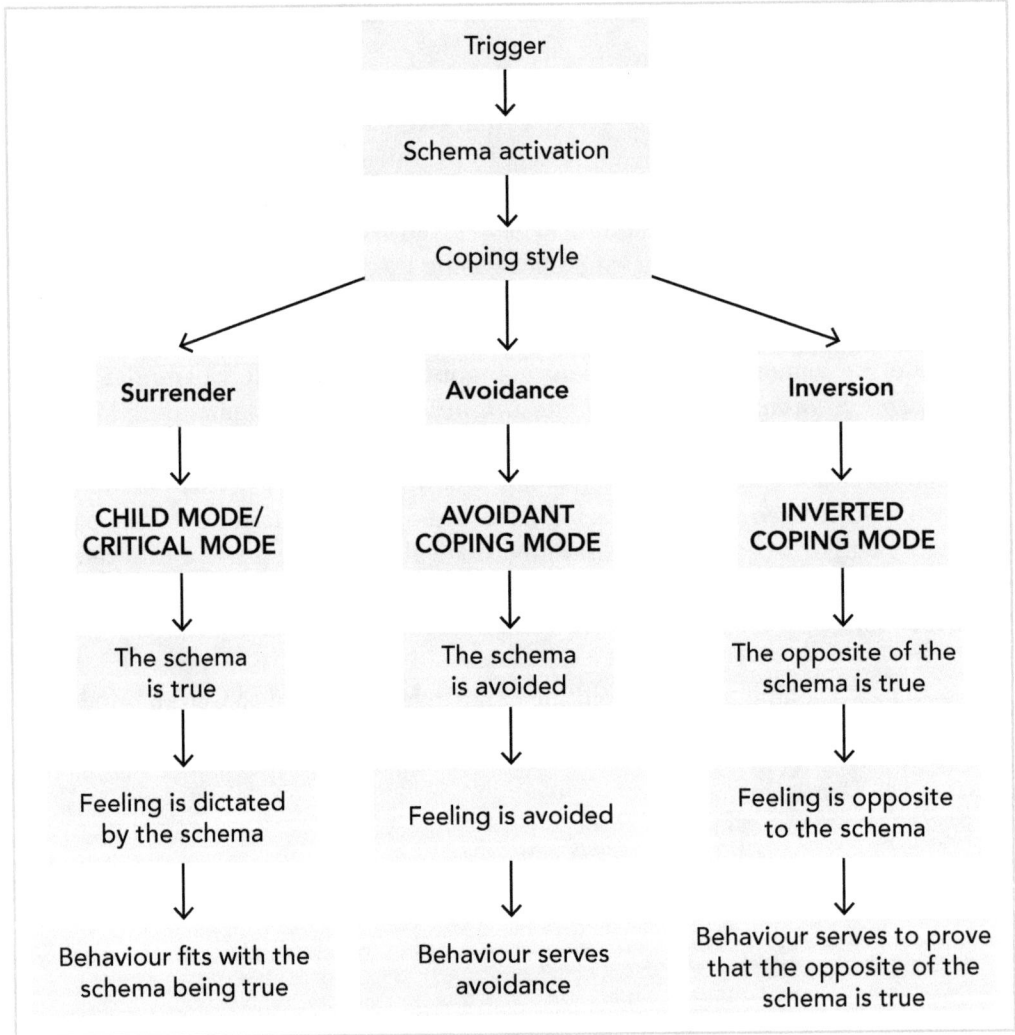

The schemas that are relevant for a specific client's modes are determined in the case conceptualization phase. This is explained further in the sections on the three individual cluster C personality disorders.

2.4.3.1 Child Modes

Surrender to almost any schema can lead to Vulnerable, Angry or Impulsive Child Modes.

If one or more of your basic needs are not adequately met, the primary emotional response may be fear or sadness, or indeed it could lead to very angry or impulsive behaviour. Such strong emotional reactions are typical of Child Modes. These Child Modes are explained in more detail below. In practice, you usually use the client's first name with these modes – for example 'Little Claire', 'Angry John' or 'Impulsive Marian'.

Vulnerable Child Mode
Depending on which basic needs are not met, the Vulnerable Child Mode, or the Vulnerable Child Part, may have a different cause and therefore a different theme in which other schemas are involved. A review by Panagiotopoulos *et al* (2023) investigated which schemas were most common among the different cluster C personality disorders. We adopt those schemas and add *Emotional Deprivation* and *Vulnerability to Harm or Illness* because we also frequently encounter these in clinical practice. Each of these schemas will lead to a different variant of the Vulnerable Child Mode (Arntz *et al*, 2021). For example, among clients with Dependent Personality Disorder, one of the most common schemas is *Dependence/Incompetence*. With this schema, there is a Dependent, Failing Child. In Avoidant Personality Disorder, *Defectiveness/Shame* is one of the most common schemas (Panagiotopoulos *et al*, 2023). And within this schema, there is a Defective/Ashamed Child (Arntz *et al*, 2021).

Angry Child Mode
Irritation or anger because your basic needs are not being met (again) can lead to an Angry Child Mode. In clients with a cluster C personality disorder, the Angry Child Mode (or a variant of it) is not often apparent. Anger is more likely to express itself in a sulking or rebellious form. Table 2.2 shows possible variants of the Angry Child Mode depending on which basic need is not met in your client.

Impulsive, Undisciplined or Spoiled Child Mode
These modes relate to an impulsive, undisciplined or spoiled reaction to failure to fulfil one or more basic needs. As far as we can determine, these modes never occur in clients with a cluster C personality disorder. Accordingly, we do not give further explanation here.

Table 2.2 describes the most common schemas in cluster C personality disorders with their corresponding Child Modes as described by Arntz *et al*. The last column lists the experience in those modes.

It should be noted that, with Obsessive-Compulsive Personality Disorder, the *Unrelenting Standards* schema is the most common. Other schemas are reported, but the results of a meta-analysis are not as clear for them. Arntz *et al* write that the *Unrelenting Standards* schema does not seem to lead to Vulnerable Child Modes, but it does lead to a Demanding Mode. They postulate two possible associated Child Modes – 'The Disappointing and Underperforming Child' and 'The Over-diligent Child', but research on this is still in progress.

Table 2.2: Vulnerable and Angry Child Modes in cluster C personality disorders with associated schemas and experiences *(Based on Van Genderen (2023) and Arntz et al (2021))*

Schema	Vulnerable Child / Angry, Sulking, Rebellious child	Form of expression
Acceptance, connection, security and predictability		
Emotional Deprivation	Lonely and Unloved Child	You feel like no one really understands you or realizes how you feel or cares about you.
	Angry Child	Can also be the belief that your feelings are too much for others.
Abandonment / Instability	Abandoned Child	You get angry at others when they don't consider your feelings, even if you haven't expressed them.
	Angry Child	You feel intense despair because you think you won't get love, security or acceptance. You easily feel let down. Because of this, you cling to people.
Social Isolation / Alienation	Alienated and Misunderstood Child	You react angrily to the (perceived) threat of abandonment or actual abandonment. Sometimes you angrily break up a relationship so that the other person cannot leave you.
	Angry Child	You feel like you are very different from other people. You feel like you don't fit in or belong to a group. You react angrily to the (perceived) threat that you don't belong, or when someone does not understand what is going on within you.

Defectiveness / Shame	Inferior and Ashamed Child	You feel inadequate and bad. This can be accompanied by feelings of shame.
	Angry Child	You are angry at others who give you the impression that you are inferior and that they think you should be ashamed of yourself
Competence and autonomy		
Dependence / Incompetence	Dependent and Incompetent Child	You feel anxious and unable to handle everyday responsibilities. You can't do anything without help from others.
	Angry Child	You get angry at the impression that too much responsibility is placed on your shoulders.
Failure	Failing Child	You believe you will fail at your tasks. You believe that your own skills, knowledge and ideas are inferior to those of others.
	Angry Child	You get angry when others criticize your behaviour or when others do better, and also when others put you in a situation where you fail.
Vulnerability to Harm or Illness	Anxious Child	You feel anxious and unsafe. You feel overwhelmed by perceived dangers. You are constantly worried that you are not safe and seek reassurance from others.
	Angry Child	You get angry when others don't take your fears and concerns seriously.
Enmeshment / Undeveloped Self	Non-individualized Child	You think that one or several significant others cannot survive if you separate from them. You feel a duty to stay connected to these others and feel guilty if you try to do something independently of them.
	Angry Child	You get angry when others put pressure on you to individualize more.
	Sulking Child	You passively aggressively resist the duty of always having to be connected to others.
	Rebellious Child	You rebel against the suffocating atmosphere of enmeshment by acting defiantly.

Self-expression; expressing your needs, opinions and feelings		
Subjugation	Intimidated Child (Subordinate Child)	You feel intimidated by others and believe that expressing your own needs will have negative consequences. You feel small and powerless.
	Angry Child	You get angry at the feeling of not getting a chance to express your own wants and needs, or when you think others do not take them seriously.
	Rebellious Child	You act defiantly and do forbidden things in protest. You refuse to follow the rules and do not consider the consequences.
Self-sacrifice	Parentified Child	You firmly believe that you need to care for others, ignoring whether this is needed or refused.
	Angry Child	You have outbursts of angry accusations because you have to constantly sacrifice yourself and others do not recognize your concern.
	Victimized Child	You perceive the imbalance between giving and receiving care as unfair. You feel you have been wronged and that you are being treated unfairly.
Spontaneity and play (excessive vigilance and control)		
Negativity / Pessimism	Pessimistic Child	You tend to interpret situations in a negative, pessimistic way. You expect that things will go wrong. The future is dark and disasters are likely. You usually feel hopeless and dejected. You don't let others cheer you up.
	Angry Child	You get very angry when others are optimistic, or even realistic, because you really believe in your pessimistic and gloomy expectations.
Emotional Inhibition	Inhibited Child	You don't dare to express emotional needs. You are sub-assertive, feel easily embarrassed and lack spontaneity and playfulness. This is perceived by others as cold, rigid and overly formal. →

Emotional Inhibition (continued)	Frightened and Panicking Child	You are afraid of losing control over negative feelings, including anger, sadness and fear.
Unrelenting Standards	Disappointing and Underperforming Child	You are disappointed in yourself with regard to your own performance and standards.
	Over-diligent Child	You work hard, are obedient and behave well and nicely.
	Angry Child	You get angry because of unrealistic or unreasonable demands. You are often angry at others or organizations and you don't realize that you are actually angry at your own Unrelenting Standards. You feel angry because you feel that others demand too much of you.
	Rebellious Child	You are not overtly angry, but you deliberately do things badly in protest against the high demands.
	Sulking Child	You protest in a passive, indirect, non-verbal way against excessive demands and expectations.
Punitiveness	Bad Child	You feel bad and guilty, and think you deserve punishment.
	Angry variant: Protesting Child	You protest emotionally against the punishment you are experiencing. Usually, you direct your anger at others, who are perceived as critical.
	Sulking Child	You protest passive aggressively, indirectly, and non-verbally against excessive punishments, accusations and restrictions.

2.4.3.2 Critical Modes

The Critical Modes (formerly called Parent Modes) are the result of surrender to a specific set of schemas resulting from unmet basic needs in the areas of spontaneity, play and relaxation (excessive control). These are primarily schemas that dictate how you should behave and what the consequences are if you don't, namely *Emotional Inhibition, Unrelenting Standards*, and *Punitiveness*. All the Critical Modes can occur in people with a cluster C personality disorder (see Table 2.3). In any case, the Demanding Mode occurs in clients with Obsessive-Compulsive Personality Disorder and the Punitive Mode often occurs in Avoidant and/or Dependent Personality Disorder.

As noted above, in this book we deviate from the model of Arntz *et al* by adding a Blaming Mode to the Punitive Mode. This mode emphasizes the sense of guilt that many cluster C clients feel when they don't do exactly what significant others (for example, parents) dictate to them. In such cases, the significant others were not overtly negative or dismissive of the child. However, they indirectly showed that the child had fallen short of their expectations when, at far too young an age, they were made responsible for the care and well-being of others (such as a sick parent or sibling). Given that the child cannot handle this indirectly communicated responsibility, it can also lead to feelings of failure, inferiority or guilt.

Table 2.3: Critical Modes
(Based on van Genderen (2023) and Arntz et al (2021))

Critical Modes

Critical Mode	Schema	Expression
Demanding Mode	■ Emotional Inhibition ■ Unrelenting Standards	You have to keep going until things are finished and perfect. It can always be better. You can only relax once everything is finished.
Punitive Mode	■ Punitiveness	You are bad, stupid and ugly. If something goes wrong, it is your own fault and you shouldn't complain.
Blaming Mode	■ Punitiveness ■ Subjugation	You should always be there for others. You are a burden to others when you think of yourself. It is your fault if family or friends are unhappy.

2.4.3.3 Coping Modes

If a schema is activated and someone reacts to it with the coping styles of avoidance or inversion, then a Coping Mode becomes active. The function of these Coping Modes is to avoid having to feel the unpleasant feelings and thoughts that threaten to arise due to the activation of schemas. In the client's childhood, not feeling or denying negative feelings were probably more or less functional survival strategies. But in their present life, precisely those strategies can get in the way of fulfilling basic needs. For example, if all kinds of social situations are avoided, it becomes impossible to discover that there are people who do respond with understanding or assistance. Inversion often activates a Coping Mode that involves displaying behaviour that repels other people, for example by being much too perfectionistic (Obsessive-Compulsive Personality Disorder) or by behaving extremely independently, as if they don't need anyone (Dependent Personality Disorder). Inversion can also take the form of overly optimistic or forgiving behaviour (Avoidant Personality Disorder). This fails to meet the person's basic needs. The different types of Avoidant and Inversion Coping Modes are explained in more detail below.

Avoidant Coping Modes

Avoidance is probably one of the most strongly developed coping styles of many clients with a cluster C disorder. The tendency to deal with (impending) schema activation with avoidance can lead to different Coping Modes. In this chapter, we will discuss all possible Avoidant Coping Modes according to Arntz *et al.* From Chapter 3 onwards, we will look a little more closely at the Avoidant Coping Modes for each Cluster C personality disorder.

Table 2.4 shows the types of Coping Modes. The first column lists the name of the Avoidant Coping Mode as it is called in the current literature and questionnaires (along with a name you could use for clients in brackets). The second column gives the schema that is avoided by this Coping Mode, and the third column describes the behaviour(s) by which that mode can be recognized.

Table 2.4: Avoidant Coping Modes
(Based on van Genderen (2023) and Arntz et al (2021))

Avoidant Coping Modes

Avoidant Coping Mode	Schema	Expression
The Detached Protector (The Feeling Blocker)	All schemas, except: ■ Entitlement / Grandiosity ■ Insufficient Self-control / Self-discipline	*Shutting off feelings:* You ignore your feelings, do not react, dissociate or abuse numbing drugs.
The Joker	■ Mistrust / Abuse ■ Abandonment / Instability ■ Social Isolation / Alienation ■ Emotional Deprivation ■ Defectiveness / Shame ■ Dependence / Incompetence ■ Failure ■ Vulnerability to Harm or Illness ■ Enmeshment / Undeveloped Self ■ Subjugation	*Making jokes:* When something unpleasant happens, you make jokes about it.
The Angry Protector (The Angry Cynic)	■ Mistrust / Abuse ■ Social Isolation / Alienation ■ Defectiveness / Shame ■ Emotional Inhibition	*Getting cynical or angry:* When someone does something annoying or is critical, you react angrily or cynically.
The Avoidant Protector	All schemas	*Avoiding situations:* You literally avoid situations, awkward contacts or difficult tasks.

The Detached Self-Soother (The Stupefier)	All schemas except: ■ Subjugation	*Seeking distraction:* You avoid lingering on your feelings by constantly engaging in activities that distract you from your feelings.
The Compliant Surrenderer (The Subordinate)	■ Abandonment / Instability ■ Emotional Deprivation ■ Dependence / Incompetence ■ Enmeshment / Undeveloped Self ■ Subjugation	*Making yourself subordinate:* You always do what others want and deny your own needs or allow yourself to be abused.
The Reassurance Seeker	■ Abandonment / Instability ■ Dependence / Incompetence ■ Failure ■ Vulnerability to Harm or Illness	*Seeking reassurance:* You constantly seek advice and reassurance with big and small concerns so you don't have to feel or endure your fears and insecurities.
The Suspicious Overcontroller (The Suspicious Person)	■ Mistrust / Abuse ■ Abandonment / Instability	*Paranoid need for control:* You are constantly alert and watch others to prevent them from taking advantage of you or letting you down.

Inverted Coping Modes

Inverted Coping Modes are more common in cluster B personality disorders than in cluster C personality disorders. However, there are various Inverted Coping Modes that can also occur in people with a cluster C disorder. Dependent Personality Disorder can involve inversion, where the client pretends to be super independent (the Independent). In Avoidant Personality Disorders, when the *Vulnerability to Harm or Illness* schema is activated, you sometimes actually see inversion of the schema manifested in high-risk behaviour (the Daredevil). And with Obsessive-Compulsive Personality

Disorder, the Perfectionistic Overcontroller (inverting *Failure*) might be relevant or, at the other extreme, the Slacker (inverting *Unrelenting Standards*). These are only a few examples. Starting in Chapter 3, we will go into the relevant Inverted Coping Modes for each personality disorder in a bit more depth.

We give all the possible Inverted Coping Modes according to Arntz *et al* in Table 2.5, which shows the types of modes that can occur and how they are related to schemas. As before, the first column lists the name of the Inverted Coping Mode as it is called in the current literature and questionnaires (along with a name you could use for clients in brackets). The second column gives the schema that is inverted by this Coping Mode, and the third column describes the behaviour(s) by which that mode can be recognized.

Table 2.5: Inverted Coping Modes
(Based on van Genderen (2023) and Arntz et al (2021))

Inverted Coping Modes		
Inverted Coping Mode	**Schema**	**Expression**
The Independent	■ Abandonment / Instability ■ Dependence / Incompetence ■ Enmeshment / Undeveloped Self ■ Subjugation ■ Self-sacrifice ■ Approval-seeking / Recognition-seeking	*Extreme independent behaviour:* You act like you don't need anyone. But you're really afraid of being abandoned or forced into something you don't want.
The Clown	■ Mistrust / Abuse ■ Abandonment / Instability ■ Emotional Deprivation ■ Social Isolation / Alienation ■ Defectiveness / Shame	*Ridiculing needs:* You deny your needs by calling them ridiculous, petty or excessive. You pretend that your experiences or shortfalls are no big deal to avoid feeling pain about them. →

The Clown (continued)	■ Dependence / Incompetence ■ Failure ■ Vulnerability to Harm or Illness ■ Enmeshment / Undeveloped Self ■ Subjugation ■ Self-sacrifice ■ Negativity / Pessimism ■ Emotional Inhibition	*Ridiculing needs:* You deny your needs by calling them ridiculous, petty or excessive. You pretend that your experiences or shortfalls are no big deal to avoid feeling pain about them.
The Attention and Approval Seeker (The Attention-Grabber)	■ Emotional Deprivation ■ Defectiveness / Shame ■ Social Isolation / Alienation ■ Emotional Inhibition	*Drawing attention to yourself:* You can invert your insecurity and sense of not belonging by attracting attention to what you can do or have experienced.
The Daredevil	■ Vulnerability to Harm or Illness	*Seeking danger:* While you are actually afraid, you suppress that feeling precisely by seeking out danger.
The Perfectionistic Overcontroller (The Perfectionist)	■ Emotional Deprivation ■ Failure ■ Insufficient Self-control / Self-discipline	*Continuing until it is perfect:* To avoid the feeling of failure or sloppiness, you try extremely hard.
The Slacker	■ Unrelenting Standards	*Deliberately being lazy and inactive:* You do little or nothing, you cut corners, you don't try at all.
The Over-Optimist	■ Negativity / Pessimism ■ Unfairness	*Being excessively optimistic:* You close your eyes to unfairness or abuse by pretending that everyone always has good intentions.

The Merciful	■ Punitiveness ■ Entitlement / Grandiosity	*Acting overly humble and forgiving:* You do feel superior, but out of fear that people will think you are arrogant, you act very humble.
The Self-Aggrandizer (The Braggart)	■ Defectiveness / Shame ■ Social Isolation / Alienation ■ Subjugation ■ Self-sacrifice ■ Approval-seeking / Recognition-seeking	*Bragging:* You pretend to be very special and brag about who you are and what you do.
The Bully and Attack Mode (The Attacker)	■ Mistrust / Abuse ■ Abandonment / Instability ■ Subjugation ■ Unfairness	*Attacking and intimidating:* You think that offence is the best defence to avoid being deceived, abused or suppressed.
The Conning and Manipulation Mode (The Pretender)	■ Abandonment / Instability ■ Unfairness	*Lying and cheating:* You manipulate others to avoid being cheated or abandoned.
The Predator	■ Unfairness	*Threat:* You take out potential threats, rivals or enemies in a cold, calculated way.

Now that all the terms have been explained, we can describe how to change the dysfunctional modes and strengthen the Healthy Adult and the Happy Child.

2.5 The therapeutic relationship

2.5.1 Handling the therapeutic relationship

The central concept within the therapeutic relationship in schema therapy is 'limited reparenting'. This means that, as a therapist, you take on the role of the 'good parent' that the client should have had in their past – ensuring that those basic needs that were not sufficiently met in childhood are fully met now. Limited reparenting is achieved by offering the client corrective emotional experiences.

For clients with a cluster C personality disorder, building a good therapeutic relationship will not typically be as difficult as for those with a cluster B personality disorder. Clients with a cluster B disorder have deficits in the realm of safety and connection; for cluster C clients, basic needs such as competence and autonomy, self-expression, and spontaneity, play and relaxation are more central. As a result, the therapist will have to fill the role of a 'good parent' differently for cluster C clients than for cluster B clients.

A client with Dependent Personality Disorder will appeal to the therapist to provide good advice and help. The therapist can seize on this behaviour to explain that they need to learn to develop more autonomy, and so he will not give them any advice in this instance.

A client with Obsessive-Compulsive Personality Disorder will attend sessions reliably, but they will often want to give such detailed explanations that the case conceptualization phase takes much too long. Limited reparenting for this client therefore involves communicating that explaining everything in so much detail is related to the need for control, for fear that something might go wrong. Consequently, therapy is precisely aimed at letting go more and learning to develop spontaneity and play.

By contrast, a client with Avoidant Personality Disorder may attend therapy less reliably because they want to avoid activating unpleasant feelings as much as possible, and those feelings will inevitably be evoked during sessions. With this client, the therapist will therefore encourage self-expression, but also offer reassurance that the therapy will proceed step-by-step and that they can ask the therapist not to go too fast. Specific components of limited reparenting are discussed in more detail below.

2.5.1.1 Schema activation

A corrective emotional experience, needless to say, must first be an emotional experience. Some schema activation is therefore necessary for these healing experiences. Without some emotional arousal, no new information is processed. However, too much emotional arousal can also prevent new information from being processed.

In the initial phase of the treatment, there is often a lot of schema activation in clients with a cluster C personality disorder. For example, your client may be emotional when they come to the session because of something that occurred outside or during therapy. If that spontaneous schema activation has not yet occurred, there are various methods and techniques to generate it using chairwork, imagery rescripting or an empathic confrontation. These therapeutic methods and techniques are described below.

2.5.1.2 Good care and giving direction

The corrective emotional experience you offer in schema therapy is actually the validation of basic needs. It is therefore important to know which basic needs have not been met, or have been insufficiently met, in your specific client. The Coping Modes are often the first obstacle to connecting with the Vulnerable Child, because despite being problematic in the long term, they generally do bring clients many short-term benefits in their everyday lives. For example, if the client always does their best (the Perfectionist), their employer thinks this is a very good trait and compliments them for it. If the client adopts a dependent attitude (the Subordinate), this is often seen as accommodating and friendly. If the client avoids everything (the Avoidant Protector), they have few intense emotions and no conflict at all, and they would rather avoid therapy than change.

Whatever the basic need is, as a therapist you must have explicit compassion for what your client is lacking. This means being very understanding of the client's behaviour on the one hand, but also very insistent on change on the other. Showing understanding is essential for a client to feel seen and recognized, but warmth and understanding alone generally leads to stagnation rather than change in cluster C clients. You must also work on a cognitive restructuring of the assumptions that ensue from the activated schemas.

For this group, giving advice is more about encouraging the client to try things they are afraid of than literally giving direct guidance. If a dependent client asks how they should approach something, suggest that they think of a few ways to approach it themselves and let them try them all to find out what works best for them. This is comparable to how you teach a child to become independent. Advise an avoidant client to try something they have avoided, and to predict what outcomes they expect. Perfectionist Obsessive-Compulsive clients should not be given advice on how to do something even better; instead, they can be advised to start making mistakes on purpose to see what the consequences are. You will also often have to advise obsessive-compulsive clients on how to relax more and develop playful activities.

Unlike clients with a cluster B personality disorder, good care and giving direction in patients with a cluster C disorder consists of several components, all of which are aimed at fulfilling basic needs such as autonomy, competence, self-expression and spontaneity. This is different for each personality disorder and for each client. The specific possibilities for each personality disorder are explained in Chapters 5 to 7.

2.5.1.3 Empathic confrontation and boundary setting

In clients with a cluster C disorder, empathic confrontation is primarily necessary if the client, usually under the influence of their Coping Modes, seems persistently uncooperative (avoidant behaviour) or overly cooperative (dependent or obsessive-compulsive behaviour) in therapy. This involves all the Coping Modes that get in the way of making contact with the Child Mode and prevent the client from fulfilling their basic needs. The therapist would then typically try other methods such as imagery rescripting, chairwork or cognitive techniques. Only if these approaches are insufficiently effective can an empathic confrontation be useful. In such situations, you can explain to the client that you notice the usual approach does not seem to be working adequately because a Coping Mode is getting in the way. There are several ways to set up an empathetic confrontation. Although this intervention is familiar, the step-by-step plan in the box below can help to guide you in this important intervention. Each step is explained further below the box.

Empathic confrontation step-by-step
Step 1 – Preparation: what behaviour is interfering with therapy? Can you understand this behaviour from the case conceptualization?
Step 2 – Indicate to the client that you want to spend some time thinking and talking about communication (meta-communication).

Step 3 – Deliver the empathic confrontation.
 	
    Confrontation: Ask if your client recognizes the behaviour described. Explain in a friendly and personal way how your client's behaviour is affecting you.
 	
    Empathy: name the behaviour as a side of your client, not as the whole person.

Step 4 – Reflection (consolidation): How is this conversation perceived by your client, what did they learn from it, and how can that insight be remembered?

Step 1: Empathic confrontation focuses on client modes that interfere with communication. Because these are modes that can be understood from the case conceptualization, you can prepare for the empathic confrontation in advance. What behaviour is interfering with the therapy? What are your primary emotional and behavioural responses when confronted with this behaviour? How can you reformulate them for a helpful empathic confrontation?

Step 2: The second step is a clear explanation that you want to discuss what is happening in the communication taking place between you and your client.

Step 3a: Confrontation: You explain in a friendly and personal way how your client's behaviour is affecting you. When doing this, be specific and check first whether the client recognizes the behaviour. In your choice of words, be careful not to put the client off, as they are likely to be very sensitive to criticism under the influence of messages from their Critical Mode. Even with careful formulation, the client might still be alarmed. Keep their Window of Tolerance in mind. A confrontation, even if it is empathic, usually leads to schema activation. Give your client some time to receive the message.

Step 3b: Empathy: You show understanding for your client's behaviour. Discuss the learning history in which your client's basic needs were insufficiently met. Indicate that survival is only one side of your client, and they have other sides too. Use the mode language for this as much as possible. Also mention your appreciation for your client. In this way, the intervention also becomes a corrective emotional experience.

Step 4: You acknowledge the fact that your client is able to listen, even though it is hard for them. As a final step, discuss how the client experienced this confrontation, and pay attention to the positive or corrective aspects of this discussion. This could, for example, be that you discussed something difficult in a constructive way, and your client was still able to bear it. Or that they have had the experience of taking negative feedback without feeling completely rejected as a person. In this review, also provide psychoeducation on possible alternative (healthier) behaviours to meet the relevant basic need(s).

If the client is already very tense and shuts down or becomes very emotional, sometimes it is better to start with empathy rather than confrontation. In such cases, start by expressing your appreciation for your client's qualities and show understanding that this is how the client has had to learn to survive in difficult circumstances in their past. Begin by making the connection between this behaviour and their schemas, modes and childhood experiences. Only then say what this behaviour evokes in you.

Boundary setting
Setting boundaries is generally not often required in clients with cluster C disorders, but the behavioural change can be so difficult in these clients that sometimes you do end up having to set boundaries. If this is necessary, do it incrementally, giving the client enough space to correct their own behaviour (see e.g. Van Genderen & Arntz, 2021).

2.5.1.4 Consolidation of the corrective emotional experience

The forms of care mentioned above are new, corrective emotional experiences for many clients. They will therefore need to be consolidated to form the basis for a Healthy Adult.

A first form of consolidation is to pay explicit attention to the experience during the session. Take time to reflect on the different modalities of this new experience. What is the pleasant feeling? Where do you feel that in your body? Questions like 'What colour or temperature is this feeling?' can help your client to reflect on the experience and become aware of all aspects of it.

Consolidation also means keeping this experience 'alive' using homework. Ask your client to take notes about the experience and what it means. For example, record an audio flashcard so your client can hear the messages you gave during the session again.

With this strategy, your client can learn to internalize healthy experiences that will serve as the basis for the Healthy Adult during the course of treatment.

2.6 Methods and techniques

The techniques used to treat clients with a cluster C personality disorder are also used for other personality disorders (Van Genderen & Arntz, 2021; Van der Wijngaart, 2020; 2022; Young et al, 2005). However, recommendations to adapt the techniques to better suit particular issues are made in the specific chapters on the three separate cluster C personality disorders. This is because the basic needs that are lacking in this target group are different from those with other personality disorders. The experiential techniques used will mainly focus on competence and autonomy, self-expression, and spontaneity and play. The cognitive techniques will therefore also involve correcting other thoughts.

Changing behaviour is perhaps the most difficult aspect of therapy with this target group because, as mentioned above, their adaptive, avoidant or perfectionist coping behaviours also bring them many apparent short-term benefits.

2.6.1 Experiential techniques

2.6.1.1 Imagery rescripting

Clients with a cluster C personality disorder will usually have more difficulty finding unpleasant memories from the past than clients with a cluster B disorder. This is partly because their Coping Modes are very highly developed, and partly because this target group has greater loyalty to their parents. They typically describe their childhood as good, and they do not want to speak ill of their parents. This makes it more difficult to use the affect bridge from present to past to recall memories of similar situations.

It helps if you acknowledge that their parents had a good side, and that what they did 'wrong' was often done with good intentions. Furthermore, it is important to explain early on that the messages we receive from our parents are communicated in different ways, not only verbally but also – and often more importantly – non-verbally through the behaviours they model. Another possibility when doing imagery rescripting with cluster C clients is to go directly to difficult situations from the past in which the basic needs were not met, rather than using an affect bridge.

In the rescripting, the therapist will also have to adjust their refutation in such a way that it does not scare the client or make them want to defend their parent.

2.6.1.2 Chairwork

The recommendations above on the best tone for the therapist to use when addressing the Critical Modes apply equally to chairwork. The client will seem to cooperate easily and sit in the other chair without complaint (for example from their Compliant Surrenderer Mode), but the question is whether they can actually connect with the Vulnerable Child.

One way to facilitate this is for the therapist to sit in the chair of the Vulnerable Child and articulate what they believe the child's needs are at that moment. The basic needs of autonomy and competence, self-expression, and spontaneity and play are often so strongly suppressed that the client no longer knows what they need, what they would really like, or what their opinion is. The therapist can initiate feeling and thinking about these needs by naming them from the child's perspective.

Furthermore, the beliefs of the Demanding and/or Blaming Critical Mode can sometimes seem difficult to negate, unlike the assumptions of the Punitive Mode. As a result, another adaptation of chairwork for cluster C disorders is that, as a therapist, you will have to prepare more cognitive argumentation when you want to combat those modes.

2.6.1.3 Historical roleplay

To do a historical roleplay, the client will need to actively think of examples of restrictive, guilt-inducing or failure experiences from their past. There is a high chance that this will not come easily to clients with a cluster C disorder, just as with the other experiential techniques. Once the therapist has made a comprehensive summary of relevant events from the client's past, he can suggest a situation himself and propose re-enacting it.

In the second roleplay, in which the roles are reversed, the client can gain more insight into the motives and shortcomings of one of their parents. This gives a better understanding that this parent had problems of their own which hindered the client's development. As a therapist, you will have to guide this process of cognitive restructuring more explicitly than with cluster B clients. With that help, a client might, for example, discover that their mother was depressed and relied on them too much as a result, or that their father used to have learning difficulties himself, which is why he now values achievement too highly.

The third roleplay gives the client a chance to stand up for their needs. Here too, you will need to provide more active guidance because avoidant and dependent clients have more difficulty standing up for their own opinions and needs than cluster B clients.

2.6.2 Cognitive techniques

The self-inquiry circle can be used quite early on to explore situations in which one or more modes were activated. Because treatment of cluster C disorders takes less time than cluster B treatments, and you do not want to deviate from the predetermined number of sessions, it is particularly important to manage the available time efficiently with these clients. More than in cluster B treatments, you deploy and actively use this self-inquiry circle early on, so your client learns to use this tool independently in good time.

In the first phase of therapy, the client may have difficulty recognizing the modes, but later on this is a good way to recognize modes in everyday life and to learn to describe the client's unmet needs. A cognitive diary is particularly useful in the second half of therapy to strengthen the Healthy Adult at the cognitive level.

A common problem in applying cognitive techniques in clients with a cluster C personality disorder is that they will have great difficulty coming up with arguments against their dysfunctional thoughts, or thinking about what they actually need or would want to do. After all, they are used to thinking that their parents do everything out of good intentions, and as a result they tend to accept their opinions and standards.

2.6.3 Behavioural techniques

In clients with a cluster C personality disorder, behavioural change is one of the most difficult components. Unlike borderline clients, dependent or avoidant clients finds it particularly difficult to 'take action'. And although an obsessive-compulsive client may find taking action somewhat easier, they have their own difficulties with doing this in a different way than they are used to. Even if a client knows where their avoidant, dependent and/or perfectionist behaviour comes from, and what its disadvantages are, they will be hesitant to really change their behaviour. And to some extent they are right about that, because the behaviour has helped them, and their environment largely perpetuates it.

For these reasons, it takes some courage and tolerance of frustration for them to make their own decisions, give their own opinions, make their own choices, or perform a task anything other than perfectly. It may create conflicts, and sometimes the client's attempt to take action will fail. The therapist's role in these moments is to encourage the client as much as possible to change their behaviour anyway. Clients must learn to handle setbacks in order to discover the benefits of new behaviours – such as being more relaxed, getting what they need, and feeling more 'seen'.

There will be some skills that cluster C clients have never adequately learned. Unlike for cluster B clients, experiencing and expressing anger can be particularly problematic. Self-expression, flexibility, spontaneity and play may also require explicit practice, because there was not enough attention paid to these during the client's childhood.

2.6.4 Strengthening the Healthy Adult

Aside from combating the dysfunctional modes, strengthening the Healthy Adult is a key focus of schema therapy. Clients with a cluster C disorder were not stimulated sufficiently to develop their Healthy Adult mode during their development. In particular, dependent and avoidant clients are likely to have experimented far too little with developing their own will, opinions, tastes and skills. As a result, they must develop them during therapy. For obsessive-compulsive clients, the emphasis is more on learning to be less perfectionistic, being allowed to make mistakes and finding relaxation.

Because the therapy time is limited, you cannot start too early with introducing the Healthy Adult. Indeed, for some therapists, the timing may seem rather too early because the cluster C client still has so much difficulty recognizing and processing the different modes. Nevertheless, given the limited number of sessions (see also section 2.6), the therapist must bring in the Healthy Adult and increasingly address it. Therapists may feel supported in this by the results of research showing that cluster C clients improve significantly in this treatment with a limited duration, even if therapists themselves sometimes have doubts (De Klerk *et al*, 2017; Ten Napel-Schutz *et al*, 2011; 2017).

Because strengthening the Healthy Adult is such an important part of the therapy, Chapter 8 of this book is devoted to the topic.

2.6.5 Stimulating the Happy Child and learning to express anger

Clients with a cluster C personality disorder were never really allowed to be children. They had to adapt much too early, and were busy fulfilling others' needs, feeling responsible and doing everything well. As such, playing and relaxing were badly neglected. Expressing anger was also often out of the question, which is why these clients are poor at doing that. Many claim never to feel anger, and while obsessive-compulsive clients may get annoyed more often than avoidant and dependent clients, it is usually in the wrong way and about the wrong issues. Specifically, cluster C clients do not express themselves about their basic needs not being met. For this reason, each of the chapters on the three specific cluster C personality disorders devotes a lot of attention to expressing anger and encouraging relaxation and play.

2.7 Phases and objectives

Schema therapy for cluster C personality disorders is divided into four phases. The therapy starts with the analysis phase, in which the case conceptualization takes place. This is followed by the beginning, middle and end phases of treatment, within which the process of change takes place. Table 2.6 illustrates this phasing, along with an appropriate number of sessions per phase. This example represents the study protocol in the cluster C study (Bamelis *et al*, 2014), in which a time-limited treatment protocol was deliberately chosen because clients with a cluster C personality disorder tend to procrastinate about actual change. Therefore, it is good practice to remind the client regularly of how many sessions of therapy are left in their treatment. In clinical practice, the total number of sessions per treatment will vary somewhat, as will the distribution of the available sessions throughout the treatment.

Table 2.6: Phases of therapy with cluster C personality disorders	
Phase 1: Sessions 1–6	Introduction, case conceptualization and discussion of treatment plan.
Phase 2: Sessions 7–25	The initial phase of treatment.
Phase 3: Sessions 26–40	The middle phase of treatment.
Phase 4: Sessions 41–50	The final phase of treatment.

2.7.1 Introduction and case conceptualization

We assume that the choice of schema therapy has been preceded by an indication phase. If this is not the case, it is important to clearly address the choice of personality disorder treatment right from the first interview. The client must understand that this is an intensive process, and that they will need to take an active role in it. This evokes some tension or anxiety in all clients with a cluster C personality disorder. The dependent client is afraid of having to solve everything themselves and never getting help again. The avoidant client is afraid of having to do all sorts of scary things and failing. And the obsessive-compulsive client is afraid of no longer being in control or that things will become chaotic if they do less than their best. It is a good idea to put those fears into perspective, and to revisit why the client sought help in the first place.

Together with the client, the therapist creates a case conceptualization and mode model (see Chapter 3) and draws up a treatment plan (see Chapter 4). The therapist makes it clear that there are a limited number of sessions. There are a total of forty sessions in the first year and ten sessions in the second year, so in total the treatment will take about two years. Unlike clients with cluster B personality disorders, clients with cluster C disorders should be aware that reduction of Coping Modes will also be part of their therapy. In short, they will have to learn to become less avoidant, dependent or obsessive-compulsive. To motivate these clients, it is important to explain that you will teach them about other, healthier coping strategies by reinforcing the Healthy Adult and that this will equip them to fulfil their basic needs better going forward.

2.7.2 Treatment in three phases

In the first phase of treatment, about twenty weekly sessions, the client continues to receive a lot of support and instruction. During the middle phase of about fifteen weekly sessions, they are increasingly given the role of working on their changes independently, and behavioural change is initiated. The final phase consists of ten monthly sessions in which the client mostly tries to break their patterns and practice behavioural change themselves. At the end of each phase, there is a moment for evaluation to discuss which goals have already been achieved and the goals that are yet to be worked on.

Chapter 4 explains these phases of treatment in detail.

2.8 Chapter summary

This chapter has set out the theoretical principles for the case conceptualization and treatment of cluster C personality disorders with schema therapy. We have drawn on the latest insights in the field of schema therapy to outline the techniques used, and to explain the goals, duration and phasing of therapy. These concepts and techniques are explained in more detail, and are adapted for the treatment of each of the three specific cluster C personality disorders, in the chapters that follow.

Chapter 3: Case conceptualization for cluster C disorders

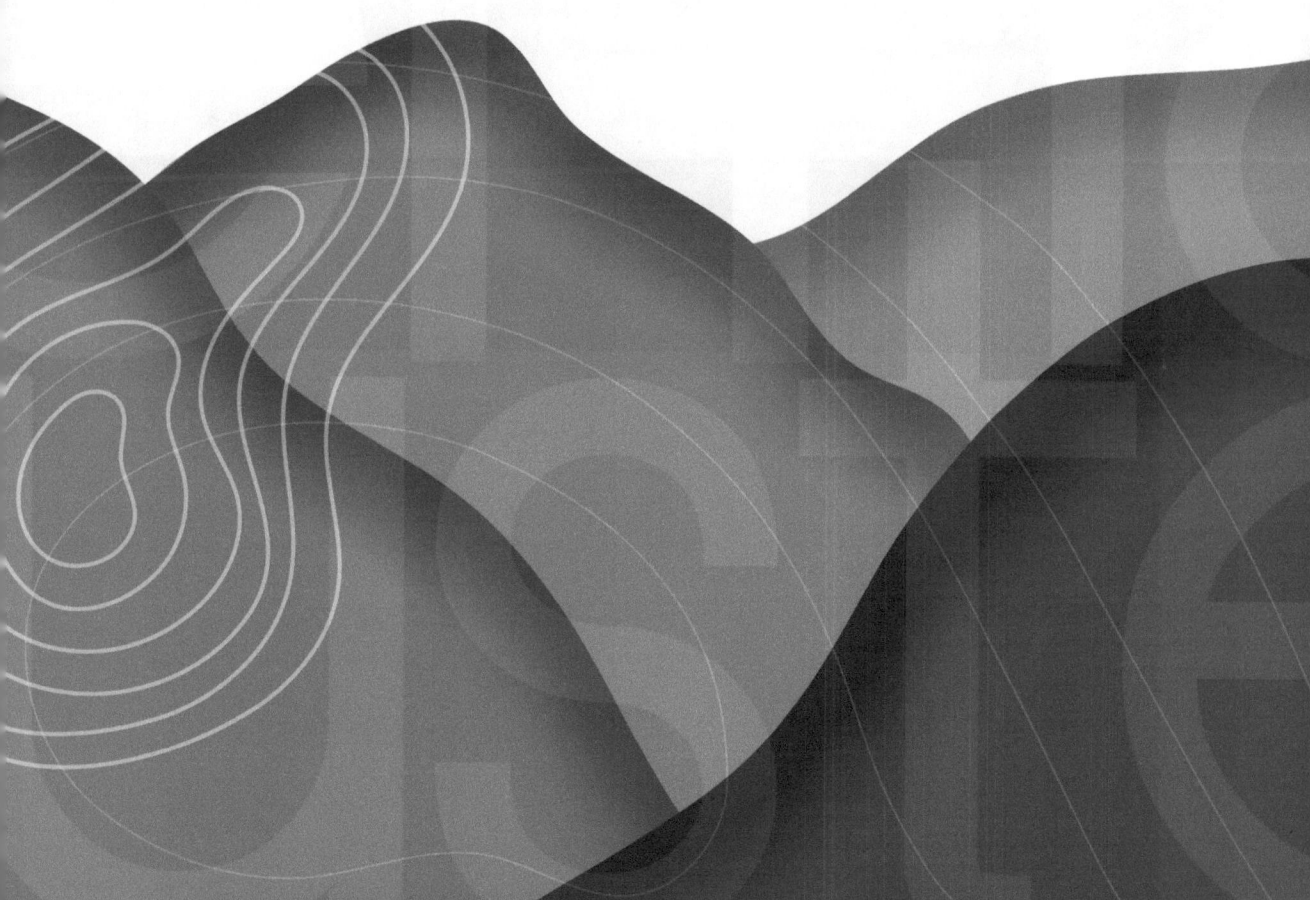

Chapter 3: Case conceptualization for cluster C disorders

Chapter map	
3.1	Introduction
3.2	The structure and process of case conceptualization
3.3	Dependent Personality Disorder
3.4	Avoidant Personality Disorder
3.5	Obsessive-Compulsive Personality Disorder
3.6	Mode models for anxiety and mood disorders
3.7	Chapter summary

3.1 Introduction

In the case conceptualization phase, you work with the client, using the concepts and language from schema therapy, to try to understand their patterns and problems. The symptom patterns are related to unmet basic needs in youth and the client's schemas, coping styles and modes have formed from them. A second goal in this phase is to introduce your client to some methods and techniques that will be frequently used in therapy. Diagnostic imagery exercises and chairwork are therefore an essential part of the case conceptualization phase. This gives your client the important message that, in addition to talking, experiential exercises will also form part of their treatment.

3.2 The structure and process of case conceptualization

The five to six sessions of the case conceptualization can become quite jam-packed with various objectives, methods and techniques. It is therefore best to structure these sessions in advance, and to put the various components on the agenda. The sample format of sessions shown in Table 3.1 does not necessarily have to be strictly followed, but we recommend using all the methods and techniques we describe in this phase.

Table 3.1: Division of sessions during case conceptualization	
Session	Method/technique
1	Explain the procedure and features of schema therapy. Explore symptoms, for example using downward arrow technique. Introduce the concept of modes as 'sides of the person'.
Preparation for session 2	Fill in case conceptualization form with the information available. Draw up a provisional mode model.
2	Hand out schema questionnaire and schema mode questionnaire. Ask the client to bring childhood photos.
Preparation for session 3	Further fill in case conceptualization form. Supplement/modify mode model. Look at the outcomes of completed questionnaires.
3	Start discussing questionnaires and making links to causal factors. Look at childhood photos and diagnostic imagery.
Preparation for session 4	Further fill in case conceptualization form. Supplement/modify mode model. Formulate a provisional treatment proposal.
4	Chairwork for diagnostics and put provisional mode model on board. The client takes photo of mode model. →

Multidisciplinary intake meeting with discussion of proposed treatment	
5	Go through the report and proposed treatment.
	Give report to the client, including the case conceptualization form (except the section on interaction with their own schemas) as well as the mode model.
6	Discuss any questions and changes.
	Submit treatment plan.
	Recommend the book *Breaking Negative Thinking Patterns*.

3.2.1 Exploring patterns and introducing modes

During the case conceptualization phase, on the one hand you zoom in on specific moments when symptomatic patterns manifest themselves, and on the other you zoom out and discuss more general patterns with your client. Look at contrasts in your client's state of mind to identify modes. For example, your avoidant client talks about avoiding situations in which they feel uncomfortable or insecure. With this, they are describing two sides to their experience, or two aspects of themselves. There is the experience in which they are preoccupied with anxiety and uncertainty, and then there is the experience where they are preoccupied with avoiding situations and people. These two sides of their experience can be illustrative of two different modes: a Dependent/Incompetent Child Mode, which is anxious and afraid of failure, and an Avoidant Coping Mode. Support the naming of those two modes ('sides', to the client) with gestures. Gesture to a place in the room when talking about the Child Mode. Then gesture to another place in the room when talking about the Avoidant Coping Mode. In this way, you bring the modes almost 'to life', like two different people in the room. This allows them to become more than just theoretical constructs.

Section 3.2.7 explains more ways to help a client discover their modes.

3.2.2 The downward arrow technique

Symptoms can be explored in different ways. The most common way is to examine the different aspects of a client's experience in a given situation: How did you feel in that moment? What were you afraid of? What went through your mind? What did you think about yourself and others? What did you do when you felt so anxious? How did it go after that?

However, with the downward arrow technique, the therapist goes on asking more questions about the meaning of the fears experienced by the client (Bögels & Van Oppen, 2019; Van Genderen & Arntz, 2021; Brockman *et al*, 2023). After using the above questions to form a picture of the situation, continue this technique with the following:

- What were you afraid of in that moment?
- What if that was true; what would that mean for you?
- What would it say about you as a person if that was true?

These deeper questions are why this is called the *downward* arrow technique. It is a way to identify underlying schemas, which are revealed when deep-seated emotional 'wounds' become visible and stronger emotional responses are provoked.

> ### Example of the downward arrow technique
>
> **>>Client:** "Then they laughed, and I just left..."
>
> **>>Therapist:** "Why did they laugh then, do you think?"
>
> **>>Client:** "Well, it was clear they were laughing at me..."
>
> **>>Therapist:** "Okay, well that doesn't sound very nice... But suppose it was true and they were laughing at you, what would that mean for you?"
>
> **>>Client:** "Uh, well, just that they thought I was different; weird, maybe."
>
> **>>Therapist:** "And if that was true, what would that mean for you?"
>
> **>>Client:** "I don't know... people thinking I'm weird again, something like that..."
>
> **>>Therapist:** "Okay, I can imagine all kinds of reasons why that's an unpleasant thought. But what would bother you about it personally if they really did think you were weird?"
>
> **>>Client:** "I don't know... that I just don't belong, that's how it feels..." *[tears]*
>
> **>>Therapist:** *[soft voice]* "Okay, then I understand why this was such an awful moment for you. For you, it wasn't just a situation where people laughed at something you said, for you it was more evidence that people think you're weird and you don't belong..."
>
> *(Client nods)* →

>>**Therapist:** "And I think that's a familiar feeling for you, isn't it?"

(Client nods again)

>>**Therapist:** "So the situation when they laughed was an unpleasant moment for you. But it's really about that underlying feeling, the feeling that people think you're weird and you don't belong. It's as if you're on an island and everyone else lives on a continent that you'll never really connect with. Does that feel accurate?"

(Client nods again)

>>**Therapist:** "That old wound, that wound of feeling socially isolated, of not belonging, is called the schema of *Social Isolation*. This is an old emotional wound, a sensitive spot, that you carry with you and bump up against in moments like the one we just discussed. In a moment like that, it's not just a difficult situation – it's also an overwhelming pain from the past causing you so much trouble."

3.2.3 Discussing the questionnaires

During the case conceptualization, always administer both the schema questionnaire (YSQ) and the Schema Mode Inventory (SMI). This measures the severity of the problem at the start of treatment. You can also use these questionnaires in subsequent phases as a source of information during evaluation moments in the course of treatment, in the interim, and when concluding. Several versions of these assessments are in circulation.

Broadly, the outcomes of the YSQ and SMI can be discussed during the session in two different ways. One is simply to present a summary of outcomes to your client. The advantage of this is that you can see and discuss all the outcomes and all the relevant schemas and modes in one place. The downside of this approach is that the volume of information can be a bit overwhelming for your client. This can sometimes lead to the discussion about it remaining rather cognitive, and not being felt vividly.

Another approach is to playfully weave the YSQ and SMI outcomes into conversation during sessions. When your client talks about a feeling or theme that also scored high in the questionnaires, you can link to the questionnaire. The advantage is that this can make discussions more vivid, and therefore more meaningful. However, a drawback of this approach is that it takes more time to discuss the schemas, so you may run out of time in the limited number of sessions allocated to the case conceptualization.

If more than five or six schemas seem to be relevant (an average score of 2.5 or higher), we recommend selecting five schemas. These can be the ones with the highest average scores, or those you consider most important in your client's treatment. An example of a schema you might choose to include despite it not scoring high could be *Emotional Deprivation*. Clients often give this schema a low score at the start of therapy. However, it may turn out to be a very important theme in their life history. Because this schema involves a deficiency, it is quite possible that your client does not yet recognize it when therapy has just begun. In such circumstances, you can still include it in the 'top five'.

> ### Example of questionnaire discussion
>
> **>>Client:** "And then I had a terrible feeling, like I was alone or something…"
>
> **>>Therapist:** "And was that the feeling that you don't really belong, that you're different from others?"
>
> **>>Client:** "Yes, exactly, as if I'm a bit of an outsider."
>
> **>>Therapist:** "That reminds me of what you said in the questionnaire. There, too, you identified this theme of being different from others. For example, there was that question 'I sometimes feel as if I'm a complete outsider', which you gave a high score. Is that a feeling you've experienced frequently in your life?"
>
> **>>Client:** "Yes – always, actually."

The current schema and mode questionnaires do not include all the schemas and modes that we have mentioned in this book, because research on them is still ongoing. This doesn't mean that you can't include one of the new schemas or modes in your case conceptualization. The same applies to schemas or modes that your client does not score highly, but that you think are still relevant based on other information. After all, questionnaires are based on self-reporting, and sometimes they do not adequately reflect whether a schema or mode is relevant.

For example, if the downward arrow technique or diagnostic imagery reveals a theme that is better explained by one of the new or low-scoring schemas, then you should include this one in your list of relevant schemas and modes.

3.2.4 Using the client's childhood photos

The use of childhood photos is a valuable tool during case conceptualization. Ask your client to bring some photos from their childhood to the next session. Sometimes a dependent or obsessive-compulsive client will ask how many photos to bring, and what are the 'right' photos to bring. Your first answer could be that any photo will be fine. If your client still needs or wants to make a choice, they can bring photos that are illustrative of the atmosphere in their original family or frequent childhood feelings.

You will look at the photos in the next session. There is no protocol for how this discussion should go. In practice, you reflect on the images from your client's past together, discussing the atmosphere those images exude and the feelings you think you detect on your client's face as a child. Link these discussions to previously discussed topics and themes. In this way, the images from the photos can become part of your mode model. These photos put a face to the Vulnerable Child, both for you and for the client.

Ask your client if you can keep a copy of one or two photos in the file. Choose images that are a good reminder for you of the feelings your client experienced as a child, or that are illustrative of the family in which your client grew up. These photos can help you and the client to stay aware of the Vulnerable Child's feelings and needs throughout the treatment.

3.2.5 Diagnostic imagery

Diagnostic imagery is an experiential technique that extends the more standard cognitive verbal exploration of patterns. The client's current problems are examples of recurrent schema activation. Explain that you understand that the situation sometimes feels very difficult and painful for the client, but that this event might be triggering pain from the past. This exercise helps both of you to understand that pain better.

The following schema-activating event can be used during the exercise as a starting point to identify the underlying meaningful events in the past. First, ask your client to put themselves into that recent symptom situation. Then ask them to concentrate on the emotional experience in that recent situation, and whether this is a familiar feeling. If it does seem like a familiar feeling, ask them to let images and memories from their childhood come up. Explore these early images and memories. In the review, you can discuss the unmet basic needs, the schemas formed, and the coping reactions that emerged in your client.

The box below gives steps that can serve as a guideline to conduct diagnostic imagery.

Diagnostic imagery step-by-step
Step 1: Introduction.
Step 2: Good place.
Step 3: Unpleasant situation in the present.
Step 4: Affect bridge to the past.
Step 5: Exploring meaningful experiences in the past.
Step 6: Back to the Good place.
Step 7: Review.

This step-by-step plan is intended only as a guide and does not need to be followed strictly. Ultimately, the essence of the exercise is that current symptom situations are linked to schema-forming experiences in the past. Because of this, other step-by-step plans are possible for this exercise. For instance, the exercise can be initiated with a past memory, after which the affect bridge is used to make the link to current symptom situations. Alternatively, the strong emotional feelings that the client is talking about can be used as an affect bridge directly, without visualizing the recent situation first.

The later sections of this chapter on the different cluster C personality disorders describe examples of diagnostic imagery and possible variations of this technique.

3.2.6 Chairwork in the diagnostic phase

With chairwork, chairs are used to represent meaningful aspects of clients' symptoms or problems. Using this technique, chairs can, for example, represent a deceased significant other, an internal or interpersonal conflict, feelings, thoughts, or a substance such as alcohol. In schema therapy, chairs are used as representations of the person's different modes. By sitting in a different chair and speaking from a specific mode, this chair is 'charged' with the experience of that mode. You can then ask the client to stand up and look back at that experience with you from a distance. This distance is not only physical, but also emotional, and this makes chairwork a powerful tool in the process of becoming aware of modes and breaking free from them.

The box below explains how to explore a mode using chairwork step-by-step.

Step-by-step plan for chairwork in the diagnostic phase
Step 1: Choosing chairwork.
Step 2: Naming the mode (or 'side', to the client).
Step 3: Explaining the rationale of the technique.
Step 4: Having the client sit on another chair.
Step 5: Interviewing the mode.
Step 6: Adding an extra chair or chairs for any other modes.
Step 7: Back to the original chair for reflection. This reflection can also be done in a standing position.
Step 8: Review.

As with diagnostic imagery, these step-by-step instructions for chairwork in the diagnostic phase are not intended as a rigid directive, but more as an aid. Therefore, they do not need to be followed strictly.

In this way, chairwork can contribute to a better understanding of the perceptions and thoughts associated with a given mode. However, chairs can also be used to visualize the mode model being worked on. Put a separate chair in the room for each mode and indicate where each mode is sitting. You can also put a sheet of paper or a mode card on each chair to make it clearer which mode the chair represents. Like a mode model on a whiteboard or flip chart, the mode model represented in the form of chairs provides an overview and insight into your client's internal dynamics. This is strengthened by standing up and discussing the arranged chairs from that position of oversight.

3.2.7 The Healthy Adult in the case conceptualization phase

In the case conceptualization phase, you are actually already working on strengthening your client's Healthy Adult. Although the Healthy Adult is not the main focus of the conversations in this phase, you are already making interventions that contribute to shaping and strengthening that Healthy aspect of the client. The way in which the Healthy Adult is already part of the case conceptualization is described below.

3.2.7.1 Becoming aware of modes

An important goal of case conceptualization is to translate symptom patterns in terms of the client's modes. Instead of being overwhelmed by intense experiences, your client must learn to put those experiences into words. Looking at and talking about those experiences is already a substantial change relative to being overwhelmed by them. For many clients, this distancing, looking at themselves in terms of modes, or sides of themselves, is not easy. Their assumptions about themselves, others and the world around them are their reality: for them, they are true. Merely saying that this is a 'side', a mode, might make sense to you as a therapist, but it is too big a step for many clients.

> **Example of becoming aware of modes (see 3.4)**
>
> *In the session, John complains about colleagues not following rules and procedures. The therapist thinks he recognizes John's Perfectionistic Overcontroller. The aim of their initial conversations is for them to gain insight into the patterns in John's life together. The therapist therefore decides to call this the Perfectionistic Overcontroller.*
>
> **>>Therapist:** "As you talk about your colleagues, it sounds a lot like your controlling side. Could it be the controlling side that I'm hearing now?"
>
> **>>John:** "No, that's what I really think! I think it's ridiculous that they can just get away with it like that. It's not a side within me, it's the reality. They're just careless people!"
>
> **>>Therapist:** "Well, I really do think that your controlling side is also at play here. The side that wants to do everything by the rules. Could that be the case?"
>
> **>>John:** "No, that's really what I think!"

Going directly to naming experiences as a 'side' at this early stage of therapy doesn't fit well with John's experience up to this point. After all, he doesn't have a well-developed Healthy Adult yet, so he isn't able to acknowledge or recognize that it is an aspect of him. A first intermediate step in learning to name modes is to concretely mirror the states of mind that you notice. Naming the contrasts in your client's presentation is an accessible way to teach them to think in terms of sides, and to develop a Healthy Adult perspective.

Example of becoming aware of modes – continued

>>Therapist: "As you sit there today, I notice that you're very concerned with how unfair it is that others don't play by the rules. (*As the therapist describes this, he calmly gestures to a spot next to John, as if describing a third person in the room.*)

>>John: "Yes, but it is odd isn't it, that they think they can just get away with it!?"

>>Therapist: "Exactly, that's what I notice: you're completely in that experience. (*Calmly gestures again to the same place.*) You're completely immersed in it, and to you it feels like you're just talking about reality."

>>John: "But that's what it is!"

>>Therapist: "Exactly, you're so worried about it that there's nothing else on your mind. And I do understand that when I talk about 'that side of you', it feels like it doesn't fit at all, it's almost weird. Is that right?"

>>John: (*slightly calmer*) "Yes, exactly…"

>>Therapist: "Perhaps it's worth emphasizing first that I'm not trying to say anything about your colleagues at all. That's not my point. My point is more that, as you sit there today, so full of how unfair those colleagues are, it's different from what else I've seen from you. To put it simply, you've been different at other times. For example, when you talked about your concerns that your wife wants to leave you, you sounded very different. (*Here, the therapist gestures to where the client is sitting now.*) You sounded more concerned – a bit uncertain. Do you see what I'm saying?"

>>John: "But… but that's natural! That's about something completely different! The issue with my wife bothers me, yes, but I get so angry about those…"

>>Therapist: (*interrupting John*) "Exactly! Exactly that! You say it well: that when you talk about those colleagues, you have a very different perspective than when you talk about your wife. And that's part of you – sometimes you're completely frustrated that others don't keep to the rules (*points again to the spot next to John*) and other times you have a different perspective, for example when you're talking about your wife (*gestures to where John is sitting now.*) Apparently, there are different sides to your experience, different sides of you. At least, I can't say that you feel exactly the same way when you talk about your colleagues as when you talk about your wife, right?"

(*John nods hesitantly.*)

>>Therapist: "And what would you call that perspective, when you get so worked up about your colleagues, that side of you?"

>>John: "I don't know… my strong side?"

>>**Therapist:** "Well, it certainly is strong. But then it sounds as if that's the only characteristic. What strikes me is that when you're in that state (*points again to spot next to John*) you're wrapped up in the rules and you also try your very best to make sure everything goes well. Is that true?"

>>**John:** "Yes…"

>>**Therapist:** "And Couldn't we include that when we're looking for a name for him?"

3.2.7.2 Identifying sources of strength

When clients sign up for therapy, naturally a lot of the attention is on their symptoms and problems. After all, that is why they sought help. However, even within the case conceptualization phase, you should already be looking for early signs of the Healthy Adult. Given that your client may be struggling with a number of problems and symptoms, such signs are easy to miss. But they are definitely there. For example, the fact that your client is going to therapy at all is very healthy. The Angry, Happy and Vulnerable Child Modes are also healthy aspects of your client. And as we said, naming those modes is the first therapeutic intervention for some cluster C clients.

Furthermore, in the case conceptualization phase, you can also take an inventory of activities that give your client strength and self-confidence, such as hobbies. These can then be used during treatment to keep the difficult change process going.

3.2.8 Case conceptualization form and mode model

During this phase, you will continue to fill in the case conceptualization form after each session. Do not use the form as a sort of questionnaire during sessions. The conversations are not only meant to obtain factual information, but also to build the therapeutic relationship. By using the form as a questionnaire, you run the risk of making the conversation more like ticking off a checklist. Do take some notes for yourself during sessions, and use these notes after the session to further fill in the form. And do prepare for each session with a brief agenda, for example, 'diagnostic imagery'.

3.2.9 Discussion of report and treatment proposal

To conclude the case conceptualization phase, you report the insights gained back to your client. This 'story' becomes the basis or blueprint for further treatment. In it, the current symptoms and problems are related to unfulfilled basic needs in the past and the schemas and modes/sides that emerged as a result. The story can be shaped in different ways, and you may have already developed your own style in this. The box below gives a sample structure for the concluding summary of the report with useful wording. With this version of the form, we assume that a firm decision to use schema therapy has not yet been made. That is why the form includes a detailed explanation of the choice of therapeutic approach (*in italics*). If the choice is already made, you can skip this part.

> **Summary and conclusion**
>
> **Symptoms**
> The client reports the following symptoms ...
>
> These symptoms occur in different areas of life. There are recurrent patterns, both in the client's current life and in their past, and they are linked to an encumbered past history.
>
> The symptoms have been present since ...
>
> **Current situation**
> (description of living and working situation, marital status, other relevant details)
> In the current situation ...
>
> **Background**
> (description of relevant life events)
> The person concerned is the ... child from a family of ...
> Father is described as a ... ... man, mother as a ... ... woman.
> The client's disposition seems to be ...
>
> **Basic needs and schemas**
> The client grew up in an atmosphere of ...
> All this seems to show a lack of (basic needs) ...
> The consequence of this lack has been that persistent patterns (schemas) have formed. The client has the schemas ...   →

Modes

The client experienced this feeling as a child, but in their current adult life, the client often still experiences this as an overwhelming feeling of ... In those moments, the client slips into a state of mind in which they feel the same pain as the child they literally used to be: Little (Client's name).

The client has internalized the negative messages from the past into a Critical Mode. In various situations, the client enters a state of mind in which their own feelings, behaviour and thinking are regarded in a negative way, matching the disapproval, parentification, and high demands that the client experienced as a child.

As a survival strategy, the client developed a pattern of (examples of Avoidant Coping Mode and/or Inverted Coping Mode). In their current life, the client regularly slips back into that survival strategy.

With these modes, the client managed to maintain a certain functional balance as a child. However, in their current life, the client is increasingly troubled by these patterns.

Request for help

The impetus to seek help now was ...

The request for help aims to ...

Diagnosis according to the DSM-5

Treatment proposal

The client's request for help focuses on patterns in personality and interpersonal functioning.

Given the request for help with regard to changing these long-standing issues and patterns, psychotherapy aimed at giving insight and making these changes can be considered. Forms of psychotherapy that may be appropriate include psychodynamic psychotherapy, client-centred therapy or schema therapy.

Based on the available research, schema therapy appears to be an appropriate form of therapy (Giesen-Bloo et al, 2006; Nadort et al, 2009; Bamelis et al, 2014). Given that the client's early childhood development was coloured by a deficit in (state the relevant basic needs), schema therapy seems to be the most appropriate, because this form of psychotherapy focuses on active validation of these basic needs.

Schema therapy is an integrative form of psychotherapy that uses experiential, cognitive and behaviour-altering methods and techniques.

The aim of schema therapy is to gain more insight into recurring patterns in a client's interpersonal functioning. To do this, it is necessary to fight the client's internalized Critical Mode and to reduce the influence of old Avoidant and Inverted Modes. At the same time, the client will learn to make contact with underlying unmet basic needs. The client learns to validate those needs in order to understand and support the Vulnerable Child Mode. This triggers emotional growth, and enables the client to develop a stronger Healthy Adult Mode.

Duration of treatment

Based on research, a change-oriented (for this personality disorder or other persistent problems) and time-limited schema therapy of about fifty sessions is indicated.

The therapy will have a beginning, middle and end phase. The beginning and middle phases each consist of twenty sessions and the end phase of ten sessions.

The goal of the initial phase is, on the one hand, to build awareness of the different sides of oneself, and on the other hand to gain new corrective emotional experiences.

The middle phase aims to strengthen the Healthy Adult Mode so that the client becomes able to recognize and validate their needs themselves, in combination with learning to handle their Critical and Coping Modes in a healthy way.

The end phase primarily focuses on actual behavioural change and breaking unhelpful patterns of thinking and behaviour.

Each phase will be followed by a moment for evaluation.

In the sections below, the case conceptualization phase is described for each of the three cluster C personality disorders. Typical basic needs, schemas and modes are associated with the characteristic patterns of each disorder. A case study is then developed for each disorder, and the mode model of that specific case is described as an example from clinical practice.

3.3 Dependent Personality Disorder

Case study: Claire

Claire has been referred to a psychotherapist by her doctor, who thinks that her fatigue and panic symptoms are caused by her mental health issues. She regularly asks him for advice, but he cannot find a somatic explanation for her symptoms. Claire has already received some cognitive behavioural therapy for her panic symptoms, but it had limited results.

Claire lives with her boyfriend, Jonas. He is usually very supportive, but he can also trigger her fear of being abandoned because sometimes he doesn't keep appointments or doesn't have the patience to give her advice. They do not have children.

Claire currently does not have a job. She has not learned a profession because she was told by her parents that she could not manage that much, and that it would be best to become a housewife. She did spend some time as a domestic helper with elderly and disabled people. She worries a lot and constantly feels tired. Because of this, she feels unable to work.

Claire was an only child. Her father was an alcoholic and could unexpectedly become angry or even aggressive. Her mother was an anxious woman who could not stand up to her father. She shared her worries and fears with Claire, which made Claire feel responsible for her mother's well-being. Consequently, she did not manage to discover her own needs. She lived at home until the age of twenty-four out of concern about the situation at home. Then she moved in with her first boyfriend.

Her parents divorced a few years ago. Since then, her mother has leaned on Claire even more than before. Conversely, Claire also often calls her mother to ask for advice or reassurance when she is not feeling well.

How can you tell if someone has Dependent Personality Disorder?

When dealing with someone with Dependent Personality Disorder, you will notice that they ask you for advice much more often than other people you know. At times, you might feel that they are clinging to you and cannot stand being alone. This can sometimes cause irritation because they demand too much of you. They always consider your wishes, so you won't find it easy to express that irritation with them. That means you will not easily have a difference of opinion with them, unless you want to do something independently of them.

Of course, determining whether someone meets the official criteria for Dependent Personality Disorder requires testing against the DSM-5 (see Chapter 1).

3.3.1 Basic needs and schemas

In people with Dependent Personality Disorder, almost all basic needs in the areas of competence, autonomy and self-expression are unfulfilled (see Table 2.2). This can lead to various schemas, or pitfalls, that result in a person not being able to manage independently in adulthood. A review by Panagiotopoulos *et al* (2023) found that the most common schemas in people with Dependent Personality Disorder are *Dependence/Incompetence, Subjugation, Abandonment/Instability* and *Enmeshment/Undeveloped Self*. In clinical practice, we often also see *Failure* and *Vulnerability to Harm or Illness*.

While the schemas that are present can vary from person to person, there is a high chance that at least five of these seven schemas are relevant. For clients with Dependent Personality Disorder, it is important to during treatment spend a lot of time on the unmet basic needs, because typically they are barely aware of these deficits. For example, Claire will be convinced that she is clumsy and that is why she is dependent on others. She doesn't know what she lacks, and she has not learned that it is normal to make mistakes and to learn to make her own choices or have her own opinions through trial and error. However, now that she feels despondent and anxious more frequently, she is still seeking help and wants to cooperate to find out what is wrong with her.

3.3.2 Modes in Dependent Personality Disorder

In this section, we take a closer look at the possible modes of a client with Dependent Personality Disorder (see Table 3.2). The modes ensue from the schemas above that are relevant to this personality disorder, and the associated modes as described by Arntz *et al* in the appendix to their article (Arntz *et al*, 2021). Table 2.2 and Appendix 1 explain the substance of all the modes in more detail.

As explained in Chapter 2, surrender to the schemas involves Child Modes or Critical Modes. When there is avoidance or inversion of the schemas, this involves Coping Modes.

Table 3.2 describes the relevant modes for a client with Dependent Personality Disorder. Where appropriate, we give another name for the mode in parentheses that can be used with clients (see also Van Genderen, 2023). We summarize all the possible modes here, but this does not mean that a client will have developed all these modes. For instance, with Claire, we will see that she does not have all these modes.

Table 3.2: Possible modes in Dependent Personality Disorder	
Child Modes (with related schemas)	
Dependent/Incompetent Child (Dependence/Incompetence)	You feel anxious and unable to handle everyday responsibilities.
Angry Child	You get angry when you feel that too much responsibility is placed on your shoulders.
Intimidated Child (Subjugation)	You feel intimidated by others and believe that expressing your own needs will have negative consequences. You feel small and powerless, allowing others to dominate you.
Angry Child	You get angry at the feeling that you don't get the chance to express your own wants and needs, or that others do not take them seriously.
Rebellious Child	You act defiantly and do forbidden things in protest. You refuse to follow rules and do not consider the consequences.
Abandoned Child (Abandonment/Instability)	You feel intense despair that you won't get love, security or acceptance. You feel easily let down.
Angry Child	You react with anger to the (perceived) threat of abandonment or actual abandonment.
Non-individualized Child (Enmeshment/Undeveloped Self)	You believe that one or several significant others cannot survive if you separate from them. You feel a duty to stay connected to these others.
Angry Child	You get angry when others put pressure on you to individualize more.
Sulking Child	You resist passive-aggressively: while you have given in, there is also resistance against the obligation.
Rebellious Child	You rebel against the suffocating atmosphere of enmeshment by acting defiantly.
Anxious Child (Vulnerability to Harm or Illness)	You feel anxious and unsafe, feeling overwhelmed by the dangers and constantly worried that you are not safe.
Angry Child	You get angry when others don't take your fears and concerns seriously.

	Critical Modes
Punitive Mode	You reject yourself and feel ashamed of yourself. 'I am bad, worthless, stupid and unattractive.'
	Avoidant Coping Modes
Detached Protector (Feeling Blocker)	You switch off your feelings.
Compliant Surrenderer (The Subordinate)	You subordinate yourself. You do what others say.
Detached Self-Soother (The Stupefier)	You seek distraction compulsively.
Avoidant Protector	You avoid situations.
Reassurance Seeker	You ask for reassurance much too often.
Funny Protector	You make jokes about unpleasant situations as if nothing is the matter.
	Inverted Coping Modes
The Independent	'I don't need anyone.'
Daredevil	You seek out danger.
Clown	You light-heartedly ridicule your need for autonomy or self-expression.
Perfectionist	You excessively try your best.

The way Claire's case conceptualization was designed is described below.

3.3.3 Gathering information for the case conceptualization

3.3.3.1 Listing the current problems

Claire initially seeks help for her panic symptoms, bouts of gloominess and fatigue. These symptoms prevent her from working. Claire has already received some CBT, but it had limited results. An investigation was therefore carried out into the causes of her panic symptoms, which revealed that she mostly panics when she has to function independently and when she fears she will be abandoned. She lives with her boyfriend, Jonas, who does usually support her, but not always. He has problems of his own, which gives her the feeling that he will abandon her. She also says that her mother often relies on her. She finds this a bit difficult, but at the same time she is very understanding of it. Claire was diagnosed with Dependent Personality Disorder. Schema therapy has now been selected to investigate and treat the underlying patterns.

3.3.3.2 Description of life history

The factors that can lead to Dependent Personality Disorder come from a combination of temperament and upbringing. With Claire, we see that most of the ingredients for Dependent Personality Disorder to develop are present. The factors in the upbringing that may have influenced the development of relevant schemas are described below.

> **Case study: Claire – continued**
>
> An only child, Claire was a sweet and shy girl.
>
> She was often criticized by her father, which made her insecure about almost everything in her life. He was very strict, and everything had to be done his way. This taught her that she is stupid, clumsy and gets everything wrong (*Failure*), and that she is not allowed to express her own opinion (*Subjugation* and *Dependence/Incompetence*).
>
> Claire's mother was a sweet but anxious woman who did not stand up to Claire's father and had difficulty making decisions for herself (*Dependence/Incompetence*). She warned Claire about all kinds of dangers, both health-related and external (*Vulnerability to Harm or Illness*). She involved Claire in her own problems far too much and was emotionally dependent on her. This gave Claire little room to develop her own identity (*Enmeshment/Undeveloped Self*). Claire tried to help and support her mother as much as she could, and her mother was very grateful for that. In this way, Claire learned that always being there for others could make you feel good (*Self-Sacrifice* and *Approval Seeking/Recognition Seeking*).
>
> In this way, neither parent taught Claire how to solve problems herself or how to deal with setbacks. She did not receive emotional support from either of her parents, and she was constantly called in as a mediator between them. This, of course, was an impossible task, which made her feel even more like a failure.
>
> The schemas above are hypotheses that you will test later by collecting information in other ways.

3.3.3.3 Questionnaires

Claire completes the YSQ-S3 and scores high on all the schemas described in Table 3.3. She also completes the SMI, and the modes that are relevant also score high there (see Table 3.4).

Table 3.3: Claire's YSQ scores	
Dependence/Incompetence	5
Failure	4.5
Enmeshment/Undeveloped Self	4.5
Vulnerability to Harm or Illness	3
Subjugation	4.5
Self-sacrifice	4
Approval-Seeking/Recognition-Seeking	3.5
Punitiveness	3

Table 3.4: Claire's SMI scores	
Vulnerable Child	4
Angry Child	1.2
Compliant Surrenderer (referred to as the Subordinate for clients)	5
Punitive Mode	4.5
Healthy Adult	4.3
Happy Child	1.4

N.B. *The SMI has not yet been updated to reflect the new terms and concepts described in the article by Arntz and others (2021).*

When Claire hands in the questionnaires, she asks you if she has filled them in properly. She is worried that she has filled in some questions incorrectly, and she wants reassurance from you. Looking at the results, you have no reason to believe that Claire has filled in anything wrongly, and you realize that the high scores on *Dependence/Incompetence* and *Failure* probably explain why she feels so insecure about it. You explain this to her when discussing the questionnaire.

Even though Claire scores relatively low on *Punitiveness*, she is often hard on herself during the conversations. You look at the items related to that with her, and you find that she scores somewhat lower on some items because she did not perceive her father's negative reactions as punishments. Rather, she felt that he was right – and this is why she scores those items lower than expected.

The scores on all the other schemas are discussed during the course of conversations when Claire talks about something from her life history or a current situation in which one of those schemas is clearly in play.

Looking at the results of the completed SMI, it is notable that Claire scores very low on the Angry Child. When this is discussed, she says she is never angry. You explain that anger is a universal, and therefore a normal, primary emotional response. Claire evidently finds it difficult to recognize anger in herself, but the angry, irritated reactions will certainly be there. In therapy, Claire will have to learn to recognize and acknowledge that anger. This is important because that anger can serve as a source of strength, which is needed to break the patterns in her life. Anger is also a way of regulating tension. The Angry Child is therefore included in Claire's mode model, but drawn very small to acknowledge that Claire has difficulty recognizing that anger.

Claire also has an inverted mode that is not yet included in the current version of the SMI: 'The Clown'. In cases like this, you can name this mode and include it in the case conceptualization.

3.3.3.4 Childhood photos

Claire brings in a few photos from her childhood. In most of them, you see a nice girl who looks well cared for. It is striking that she is with her mother in all these photos. She sits on her lap or holds her mother's hand. In one of the pictures, she is wearing the same dress as her mother. You notice that she always seems to be doing something together with her mother. In the only photo showing her with both her parents, her father does not seem particularly happy. When asked about the meaning of this, Claire explains that he usually didn't want his picture taken and would get irritated.

3.3.3.5 The downward arrow technique

Claire regularly asks you for help or advice about everyday situations. You decide to apply the downward arrow technique to find out which schemas are being activated, because you prefer not to give advice to a client with Dependent Personality Disorder.

Example of applying the downward arrow technique

>>Claire: "I have to go to the dentist at that time because I have a toothache. I don't know how to cancel this arrangement with my friend without getting into an argument with her. What's the best way to do it?"

>>Therapist: "I notice that you often ask for my advice about things like that. I wonder why you have difficulty doing it yourself?"

>>Claire: "I'm not sure I'm doing it right."

>>Therapist: "What are you afraid of?"

>>Claire: "That she won't want to reschedule the arrangement and will be annoyed."

>>Therapist: "Suppose that were true, what would that mean?"

>>Claire: "That she won't want to make a new arrangement with me, and she'll think I'm difficult."

>>Therapist: "And if it is difficult for her, what does that say about you?"

>>Claire: (*tense*) "That I'm doing something she doesn't like."

>>Therapist: "And what's so bad about that?"

>>Claire: (*sad*) "Then she won't like me and might not want to hang out with me anymore."

>>Therapist: "That certainly wouldn't be nice, so now I understand better why you're afraid to reschedule the arrangement. You always try to make others feel good, and you'd rather adapt than ask for something for yourself. Even in this case, when there is no alternative to rescheduling the arrangement because you have to go to the dentist. You usually subordinate yourself to others, is that right?"

3.3.3.6 Diagnostic imagery

Claire finds it very difficult to make the links between her problems, her schemas and her past. On the one hand, she wants to believe what you tell her about this (*Dependence/Incompetence* and *Subjugation*), but on the other hand, she is very afraid to say anything bad about her parents (*Enmeshment/Undeveloped Self*). In particular, she sees her mother as a caring woman who could not help being anxious and insecure. She has always helped her mother, and she still does (*Self-Sacrifice*).

To address this feeling that she always has to consider the other person, an imagery exercise will be done to explore where it comes from.

Example of an imagery exercise within the case conceptualization

Claire says that she arranged to go to the movies with a friend. Her friend suggested a film that Claire would rather not go to because it was too scary for her. She agreed to it anyway, and as expected she had a horrible experience.

\>\>**Therapist:** "Let's take a closer look at the moment when you agreed to your friend's idea, even though you didn't want to. We're going to do an imagination exercise. (*You should explain the exercise first; see 3.2.5*)

\>\>**Claire:** "Sure."

\>\>**Therapist:** "Just close your eyes and try to imagine a pleasant situation where you feel at ease."

\>\>**Claire:** "I'm sitting in the garden in the sun."

\>\>**Therapist:** "Do you feel the sun?"

\>\>**Claire:** "Yes, I feel the warmth on my skin."

\>\>**Therapist:** "Do you hear sounds too, like birds?"

\>\>**Claire:** "I hear the birds singing."

\>\>**Therapist:** "How do you feel?"

\>\>**Claire:** "I feel relaxed."

\>\>**Therapist:** "Keep your eyes closed, and let go of that pleasant situation, that good place. Let it fade away. Now think of the moment when your friend proposed that scary movie. Really put yourself back into that moment. Where are you?"

\>\>**Claire:** "We're at her house."

\>\>**Therapist:** "Do you see her?"

\>\>**Claire:** "She looks very happy because she loves this kind of film."

\>\>**Therapist:** "How do you feel now?"

\>\>**Claire:** "I feel insecure and anxious, but I don't think I can say I don't want to see that film, because she'd be disappointed."

\>\>**Therapist:** "Where do you feel that in your body?"

\>\>**Claire:** "Heart palpitations and abdominal pain."

\>\>**Therapist:** "Focus on that anxious feeling, the fear that you can't say what you think. You're afraid you'll disappoint the other person if you do. Let the image of that situation fade away, but hold on to that feeling, and see if you've ever felt this way in your childhood. You don't have to 'invent' a situation – just wait and see if a memory comes up."

>>**Claire:** "I'm reminded of my mother… She asks if I'll go with her to the doctor because she's not comfortable going alone."

>>**Therapist:** "Where are you?"

>>**Claire:** "We're in the room."

>>**Therapist:** "Roughly how old are you?"

>>**Claire:** "I don't know… I think I'm eight years old."

>>**Therapist:** "How do you feel? What do you say to your mother?"

>>**Claire:** "I feel tense and anxious because I think there's something seriously wrong with my mother. I'd rather not go because I've arranged to meet a friend. But when I say that, my mother sighs and looks very unhappy. So I say I'll cancel my friend."

>>**Therapist:** "Is there anyone who can help you? Or who can go with your mother?"

>>**Claire:** "No, I'm the only one she asks for help."

>>**Therapist:** "Okay, then we'll stop the exercise now by going back to the good place you imagined. Go back to the garden in the sun, with the birds singing around you."

After Claire has returned to the good place, the exercise is calmly concluded and reviewed. Through the exercise and review, Claire discovers that she learned very early on to give more consideration to others than herself, and that she did not dare oppose her father and mother. That is why she still habitually adapts to others to this day.

3.3.3.7 Using chairwork to get to know modes

At this stage, another way to explore which schemas and modes are relevant, and to find out what these modes look like specifically with your client, is chairwork (see 3.2.6). Below we see how chairwork goes for Claire when her Avoidant Mode, the Pleaser, is in the foreground. Of course, the same technique can also be used for other modes.

Chairwork with one of Claire's Coping Modes

Claire pays very close attention to your reactions and regularly asks if what she is saying is what you want to hear. You will explore this submissive side of her using chairwork.

>>Therapist: "I've noticed that you always pay close attention to how I react and check if what you say is right. When I ask you a question, you often ask what I want to hear. Does that sound right?"

(Claire nods and looks at you expectantly.)

>>Therapist: "Today, we could do an exercise to find out why this is the case."

>>Claire: "Sure."

>>Therapist: (*takes an extra chair and places it diagonally across from Claire's chair*) "I'd like to ask you to sit in that chair, and when you're there get into that feeling of 'wanting to do it right for the other person, wanting to say the right thing'. I think it shouldn't be hard for you, because you were already kind of in that feeling."

>>Claire: "Okay, so you want me to sit there?" (*Immediately gets up and sits there.*)

>>Therapist: "Thank you. So, in this chair, I want you to get totally into that feeling where you check if you're doing things right. I'm going to address you now as the sidet of Claire that wants to get it right and say the right thing. Tell me, why do you think it's important that you do everything right from the other person's point of view?"

>>Claire: "Because then I know for sure what I should do."

>>Therapist: "What could go wrong otherwise?"

>>Claire: "I might make a mistake."

>>Therapist: "What would happen if you did make a mistake?"

>>Claire: "You'd think that was annoying or maybe get angry with me."

>>Therapist: "So, by paying such close attention, you're not only trying to avoid mistakes but also trying to avoid me getting irritated? So, in a sense, you're trying to prevent me from getting irritated with Claire (*gesturing to the original empty chair*) if you (*gesturing to the chair Claire is now sitting on*) don't do what I ask or need?"

>>Claire: "Yes, that's true…

>>Therapist: "That's clear. Now I understand why you're there so often, trying to protect her (*gestures to empty chair*). Now you can come back and sit in the chair next to me, but leave that perspective behind in the chair where you're sitting now."

(Claire sits down on the original chair.)

>>**Therapist:** (*looks at the empty chair*) "That side of you is always checking whether you're doing everything right and not irritating others. She is actually trying to help you. As you sit here now, how do you feel?"

>>**Claire:** "Yeah, that feels good."

>>**Therapist:** "I understand that it helps you, but I can also see that you're afraid of doing anything wrong. I think you've been afraid of doing anything wrong since you were a little girl. Your father could get angry at unexpected moments and say you were stupid. As a result, you became insecure and started paying closer attention to make sure you weren't doing anything wrong, to prevent him from getting angry. Does that sound right?"

>>**Claire:** "Yes, that was the best I could do."

>>**Therapist:** "And your mother probably also said it was best not to contradict your father, even if he was wrong. So that's how you tried to help keep the atmosphere in the house calm."

>>**Claire:** "Yes, she used to say: 'Quiet, he's had too much to drink, so you'd better leave him alone'."

>>**Therapist:** "Adapting and submitting to your father's will was probably the best way to deal with the situation back then. So that's what she does (*gestures to empty chair*), but she isn't actually helping you that much anymore, in your present life. You still don't dare to do what you really want, and you let others decide for you. You're afraid that everyone will react like your father, so you often remain silent and adapt. So, from being a side of you that was helpful then, now she's become an unhelpful side of you. Perhaps we might call her 'the Pleaser'.

3.3.4 Claire's schemas and modes

Claire has a number of schemas that are common in clients with Dependent Personality Disorder, and she yields to the associated feelings and beliefs much of the time. In her Dependent/Incompetent Child Mode, she feels insecure and dependent on others. She then believes that she can't do it herself anyway (surrender to *Failure*) and so she had better adapt to others and do what they say (surrender to *Subjugation*). This not only makes her anxious and gloomy, but also makes her very tired.

At the same time, surrender to *Punitiveness* leads to a Punitive Mode, which says that she really does do and say the wrong things all the time.

To deal with this, Claire developed Avoidant and Inverted Coping Modes in her childhood. She usually uses avoidance, but sometimes also inversion. She adapts to the needs and wishes of others as much as possible, and frequently asks for their reassurance and advice (avoidance of *Dependence / Incompetence* and *Failure*). We call this mode the Pleaser. In her case, inverting *Dependence / Incompetence* and *Approval-Seeking / Recognition-Seeking* consists of ridiculing her own needs (the Clown).

See also Table 3.5.

Table 3.5: Claire's modes	
\multicolumn{2}{c}{Child Modes}	
Subordinate Claire (Dependent/ Incompetent Child)	Does not express opinions and feelings. Gets anxious when she can't do something or doesn't know how to make the other person feel good.
Angry, sulking Claire (Angry Child)	Gets angry (sometimes) when people put too much pressure on her to do something herself. Then she does things reluctantly or deliberately does not do what is expected of her.
Critical Modes	
The Strict One (Punitive Modet)	Rejects herself because she thinks she can't do anything and is worthless. Believes that she deserves punishment for everything that goes wrong.
Avoidant Coping Modes	
The Pleaser (Compliant Surrenderer) (Reassurance seeker)	Does what others expect of her. Doesn't dare to set boundaries. Frequently seeks reassurance about health, relationships or other things she is uncertain about.
Inverted Coping Modes	
The Clown (Attention and Approval Seeker)	Ridicules Claire's need for independence and desire to be allowed to express her own opinions.

> ### Example of Claire's Punitive Mode
>
> Claire had to cancel a plan to help her father clean up the shed because she had the flu and a sore throat. She is in bed with a 39-degree fever. The whole time she is lying there, she is worried about how to solve this because she is very afraid that her father will get angry. She has already asked her boyfriend, Jonas, if he could go help her father instead of her, but he refused. He thinks it would be best to postpone the job for a couple of weeks, but Claire is afraid that her father will be angry with her. She asks Jonas to call her father to ask when it would be convenient for her father to reschedule. Jonas says it would be better for her to wait until she feels a bit better before making another appointment. Now Claire feels even worse, because if she does what Jonas says, her father will definitely get angry, and if she pressures Jonas to call her father, she will have a conflict with Jonas instead. So she calls her father to make a new appointment herself, even though she can barely speak because of her sore throat.

In this example, we see that the Punitive Mode is so strong that Claire wants to do everything she can to relieve the sense of fear that it generates. Her Dependent Child Mode does not know how to solve this, so she asks her boyfriend for help. She asks him to take over her obligation (*Approval-Seeking/Recognition-Seeking*). If that fails, she will call her father herself to make another appointment, despite the fact that she can barely speak due to her sore throat (*Subjugation*).

Here, we see that Claire suffers from both her Dependent/Incompetent Child Mode (Subordinate Claire) and her Avoidant Coping Mode (the Pleaser). It is sometimes difficult to keep these two modes separate from each other. The difference is that when the Dependent/Incompetent Child Mode is activated, the client is in a panic and does not know what to do. She feels she has failed in her duties and is afraid of being rejected. You notice that she is really desperate and scared. Her voice sounds like a frightened child. You also notice in yourself that you can sympathize with her and want to fix everything for her.

The Avoidant Coping Mode (the Pleaser) becomes active shortly afterwards to salvage the situation by doing everything possible to avoid the other person being disappointed or angry with her. If necessary, Claire even comes up with things that are harmful to herself to accommodate the other person. In the example, she makes a phone call despite barely being able to speak. In that call, she might even promise to help her father in a few days anyway, even though she hasn't fully recovered from the flu. As the therapist, you notice that now you feel more distance – and you might even get slightly irritated because

Claire wants to do things that are not good for her. You also notice the Pleaser in the way she speaks. Less panicked, more rational and focused on resolving her discomfort.

> **Example of Claire's Avoidant Coping Mode**
>
> Claire calls her father while she can hardly speak due to a sore throat. She tells him she is very sorry that she cannot come. Then, when her father also begins to complain about the cat being sick, she continues to listen patiently and encourages him. She says she'll come to help as soon as possible and promises that she'll be there in a few days, even though she knows from experience that she'll need much longer to recover. Afterwards, she also apologizes to Jonas for bothering him with her concerns.

Once all of Claire's modes have been mapped sufficiently using the techniques above, a mode model is created.

3.3.5 Claire's mode model

In the phase where Claire's problems, schemas and modes are surveyed, the links between the different components are described at the end of each session. In this way, an increasingly complete picture of how the issues fit together is formed. The mode model is different for each client and tailored to your client's specific problems. It will become a guide and blueprint for further treatment, both for you and for your client.

Each mode (or side) is given its own name. In each mode, both the schemas and some thoughts are given to indicate the client's experience in that mode.

Chapter 3: Case conceptualization for cluster C disorders

Figure 3.1: Claire's mode model

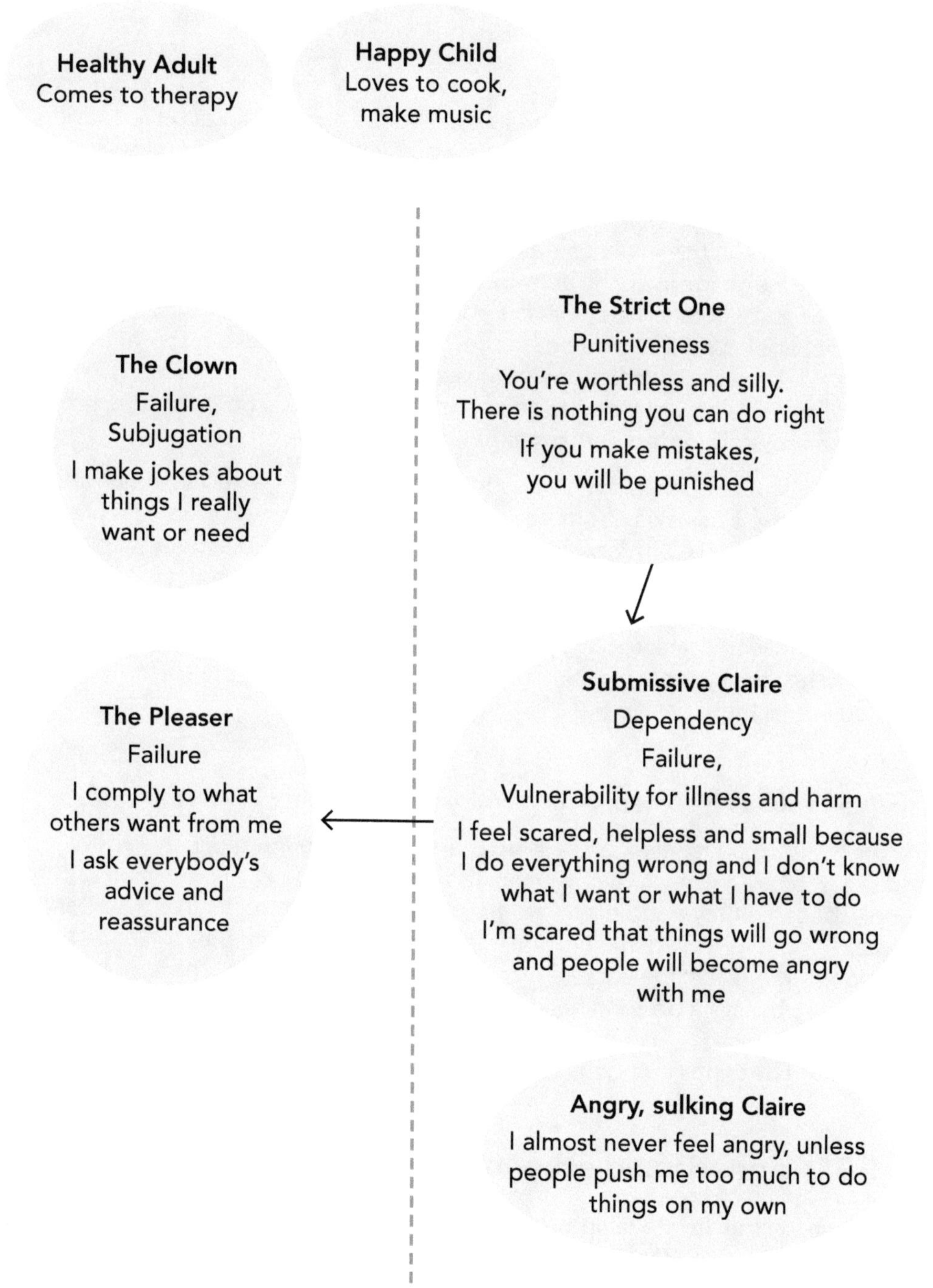

Healthy Adult
Comes to therapy

Happy Child
Loves to cook, make music

The Strict One
Punitiveness
You're worthless and silly. There is nothing you can do right
If you make mistakes, you will be punished

The Clown
Failure, Subjugation
I make jokes about things I really want or need

Submissive Claire
Dependency
Failure,
Vulnerability for illness and harm
I feel scared, helpless and small because I do everything wrong and I don't know what I want or what I have to do
I'm scared that things will go wrong and people will become angry with me

The Pleaser
Failure
I comply to what others want from me
I ask everybody's advice and reassurance

Angry, sulking Claire
I almost never feel angry, unless people push me too much to do things on my own

3.3 Avoidant Personality Disorder

Case study: Jenny

Jenny is a shy, introverted woman, who often looks away during conversations and speaks in a soft voice, which sometimes makes her difficult to understand. She has recurrent bouts of depression, without knowing quite what makes her despondent. She does experience a distinct fear of critical judgement from others. Further, she has many somatic pain symptoms, which often make her feel unable to engage in social activities. She does part-time administrative work for the local library. This work is a source of stress for her, but it has been manageable because she is one of the few employees to have her own office, and rarely needs to face colleagues. However, this situation has recently changed, and she now shares her office with a colleague. The increased stress and gloominess prompted her to see her doctor, who referred her.

Jenny is not in a relationship, and although she often fantasizes about having a boyfriend, she shies away from actually making contact with men. She has a limited social network with one friend, Linda. In her spare time, Jenny drank a lot of alcohol for a long time, which felt like a 'warm blanket' over all her worries. She stopped doing this when one of her colleagues made a negative comment about people who drank too much. Her depressive feelings have increased since then, and her doctor noticed this during one of her visits for pain symptoms and referred her to therapy.

How can you tell if someone has Avoidant Personality Disorder?

People with Avoidant Personality Disorder are rarely encountered in everyday life and seem to be very much on their own. It is not easy to build a connection with such people, because they avoid making arrangements. Arrangements that have been made often get cancelled. If there finally is a firm appointment, they will often be late, won't say much in the conversation, and will look away a lot. This avoidance can be so strong that it's a bit irritating; it seems like they don't like talking to you. When the conversation gets a bit more personal, they often seem very uncomfortable and embarrassed by things that don't seem odd or strange to you at all.

3.4.1 Basic needs and schemas

There is no 'recipe' for developing a personality disorder, including Avoidant Personality Disorder. However, there are certain factors that often seem to occur in the development of this personality disorder. For instance, avoidant clients seem predisposed to shyness and inhibition. As children, they may have preferred to wait and see and were reluctant to approach new, unfamiliar situations or people.

The upbringing of these avoidant clients was usually not characterized by abuse or other forms of an obvious lack of safety, but rather by a lack of emotional support or care, which often left them feeling somewhat alone and vulnerable. They may also have been confronted with critical messages from attachment figures, which were conveyed either in an indirect, blaming way, or in a demanding way. In these clients, who were already somewhat sensitive by disposition, these critical messages might have had a major impact on how they formed their self-image and images of others.

In their perceived lack of appreciation and validation, these clients tend to see themselves as deficient and failing. In contrast, they see others as critical and judgemental. Their predisposition gives them a tendency to withdraw, and avoidance has become the way to survive the tensions they experience. This can take different forms, ranging from literally staying away from situations that can trigger feelings of inadequacy, to substance dependence or developing psychosomatic symptoms that seem to continuously hinder them in their social activities.

In terms of basic needs, clients with Avoidant Personality Disorder are often deficient in self-expression and esteem. These clients have not felt the safety or freedom to speak out about their thoughts and feelings. To the extent that they did do this, they often felt they were not good enough. The schemas that emerge from these deficits are often *Social Isolation/Alienation, Negativity/Pessimism, Emotional Inhibition, Subjugation, Defectiveness/Shame*, and *Failure* (Panagiotopoulos *et al*, 2023). We also often see the *Emotional Deprivation* schema as relevant in clinical practice.

3.4.2 Modes in Avoidant Personality Disorder

This section describes the modes that can occur in clients with Avoidant Personality Disorder. These modes are based on the most common schemas and the modes that are linked to them by Arntz and others (2021). A case conceptualization will need to be made for each individual client in which the modes are identified. This can mean that Table 3.6 omits modes that are relevant to your specific client. It is also possible that not all the modes mentioned seem relevant to your particular client (see mode model for Jenny).

The description in Table 3.6 is therefore more of a starting point, an overview of the modes that are most likely to be present in a client with Avoidant Personality Disorder.

Table 3.6: Possible modes in Avoidant Personality Disorder	
Child Modes (with related schemas)	
Lonely, Unloved Child (Emotional Deprivation)	You feel like no one really cares about you or understands how you feel. You might also feel that your feelings are too much for others.
Angry Child	You get angry at others when they don't consider your feelings, even if you haven't expressed them.
Inferior/Ashamed Child (Defectiveness/Shame)	You feel inadequate, bad. This can be accompanied by feelings of shame.
Angry Child	You are angry at others who give you the impression that you are inferior and that they think you should be ashamed of yourself.
Pessimistic Child (Negativity/Pessimism)	You tend to interpret situations in a negative, pessimistic way. You expect that things will go wrong. The future is dark, and disasters are likely. Hopelessness and dejection are the prominent feelings.
Angry Child	You get very angry when others are optimistic or even just realistic, because you really believe your pessimistic, gloomy expectations.
Inhibited Child (Emotional Inhibition)	You don't dare to express emotional needs. You are sub-assertive, feel easily embarrassed and lack spontaneity and playfulness. This is perceived by others as cold, stiff and overly formal.
Frightened/Panicking Child (Emotional Inhibition)	You are afraid of losing control over negative feelings, including anger, sadness and fear.
Alienated/Misunderstood Child (Social Isolation/Alienation)	You feel like you are different from other people. You feel like you don't fit in or belong to a group.

Angry Child	You react angrily to the (perceived) threat that you don't belong, or when someone does not understand what is going on within you.
Failing Child (Failure)	You believe you will fail at all your tasks. You believe that your own skills, knowledge and ideas are inferior to those of others.
Angry Child	You get angry when others criticize your behaviour or do better than you, or when others put you in a situation where you fail.
Intimidated Child (Subjugation)	You feel intimidated by others and believe that expressing your own needs will have negative consequences.
Angry Child	You get angry at the feeling of not getting a chance to express your own wants and needs, or that others do not take them seriously.
Rebellious Child	You act defiantly and do forbidden things in protest. You refuse to follow rules and do not consider the consequences.
Critical Modes	
Blaming Mode	You feel that giving attention to your own needs or desires is a burden to others, and that the suffering of others is your fault.
Avoidant Coping Modes	
Avoidant Protector	You avoid situations and people to avoid confronting feelings of inferiority.
Detached Self-Soother (e.g.: 'The Stupefier')	You subdue insecurity and anxiety with alcohol, binge-watching, marijuana, etc.
Detached Protector (e.g.: 'The Feeling Blocker')	You suppress or ignore your feelings and needs. In this state, you feel flat, neutral.
Inverted Coping Modes	
Perfectionistic Overcontroller (e.g: The Perfectionist)	To avoid the feeling of failure or sloppiness, you try extremely hard.
Overly humble side (e.g.: 'The Saint')	You do feel superior to others, but out of fear that people will think you are arrogant, you act very humbly.

3.4.3 A closer look at some Avoidant Personality Disorder modes

A few of the most common modes are described in more detail below.

3.4.3.1 Avoidant Coping Modes

In this state, interpersonal contact and the possible criticism of others are avoided. This mode prevents others from seeing the client's shortcomings and criticizing or ridiculing them. From this mode, your client avoids eye contact, speaks quietly and talks about their feelings or needs as little as possible. Avoidance may lead them to cancel arrangements or arrive late to sessions. Homework is not completed, because they would have to present their thoughts and experiences in the diaries. In sessions, when in this mode, they will be more inclined to talk about physical symptoms than emotional experiences.

Avoiding situations can lead to attention being directed to other things to minimize lingering on emotions and insecurities. For example, this mode leads your client to watch a lot of TV, spend time on the Internet, drink alcohol, take medication, use substances or do any other activity that helps to distract from their feelings and needs.

Avoidance is also the active coping style of the Detached Self-Soother and the Detached Protector. How does avoidant coping (literally avoiding situations) differ from the avoidance seen in these two modes? Some differential diagnostic considerations are given below that can help distinguish how the Detached Self-Soother and the Detached Protector avoid situations.

The Detached Protector is a state in which your client can still look at the therapist and factually recount the events of the past week. Avoidance in this state is a detachment from the fears that are felt internally, a disconnection from them. In the Avoidant Protector, that disconnection is not there, and your client still feels the fears. However, they try to keep those vulnerabilities from you, the therapist, by looking away and not speaking much, or by speaking quietly. With the Avoidant Protector, you feel the underlying fear as the therapist, but you cannot make contact with it properly. In the Detached Protector, the feeling of fear seems to be missing completely.

The Detached Self-Soother (described to clients as, for example. 'the Stupefier') is an escape away from fear into a pleasant, soothing feeling, laid over pain like a warm blanket. In this way, for a client with a Detached Self-Soother, watching

TV, gaming or drinking can be experienced as a pleasant high – an oasis of calm after all the anxiety and stress. A client with an Avoidant Protector experiences these activities more as a fog in which the stress and turmoil of all their uncertainties fade somewhat, but do not vanish completely.

3.2.3.2 Blaming Mode

Guilt is familiar to most of us. For example, perhaps you said something that another person didn't seem to like much, and afterwards you keep worrying about it with thoughts like: 'If only I hadn't said anything. Now I've made them feel bad, when they're always so supportive of me.' In this sense, guilt is a normal emotional experience and familiar to almost everyone. However, an avoidant client might feel excessive guilt, inadequacy and shame for what they have done or said, even when there is no objective basis for this.

In their youth, these blaming messages were not usually communicated directly, but implicitly. For example, avoidant clients might have had parents who were struggling themselves, or who were depressed or anxious. Even if this was not expressed explicitly, clients inferred a message of blame from the suffering of these attachment figures. In seeing the suffering of the parent, for example, the child understood the message 'you are a burden to me'. When the parent did not respond to expressed feelings or needs, the child read the subtext 'You are not important to me'. When the parent cried or talked about their own suffering, it gave the child the clear message 'You must be considerate of me, and if you want something for yourself, I'll feel even worse'. In other words, you are punished for having your own needs and not always considering (the suffering of) the other.

With these kinds of internalized messages, avoidant clients regularly slip into this Blaming Mode in their current lives. In this state, they dwell on the suffering and problems that their actions, or lack of actions, have caused for others. Their thoughts are mostly about how badly the other person is feeling because of something they said or did. With a Punitive Mode, the focus seems to be mostly on the self, but with a Blaming Mode, the focus is mostly on someone else's suffering. In seeing and thinking about that suffering, there is again that implicit message: 'The other person is suffering because of me…'.

> **Example of Jenny's Blaming Mode**
>
> Jenny has cancelled an arrangement with a friend because she was so tense that she slept badly and has a headache. Although cancelling the arrangement eased the tension somewhat, she now feels bad. In her mind, she is still worried about that friend. She keeps thinking back to the phone call and the silence she heard when she said she would not come. In that silence, she sees her friend in front of her with a disappointed look on her face. Following that image, Jenny feels a cramping pain in her chest, shame and a bad feeling about herself. In that disappointment, she sees what she did to that friend. Maybe she needed a chat very badly, but now she can't because of Jenny…

3.2.3.3 Child Modes

For many avoidant clients, the biggest problem is speaking out spontaneously and expressing their emotions or opinions. As a result of the Blaming Mode, such spontaneity and self-expression is immediately associated with feeling like a burden to others – and as a result, it quickly activates the Vulnerable Child Mode. In this state, avoidant clients feel anxious, insecure, lonely, inadequate or guilty. Depending on the schemas present, other feelings may also be evoked in the Child Modes.

As with dependent clients, the Angry Child is not very visible. Avoidant clients can sometimes feel primary feelings of anger more easily in the safety of their avoidance. Expressing or acknowledging that anger can be a strong trigger for the Blaming Mode and activate feelings of worthlessness and inferiority. Again, you still put the Angry Child in the mode model. As with dependent clients, you explain that anger is a primary, universal emotional response, and a source of strength that is needed to break stubborn patterns.

3.4.4 Gathering information for the case conceptualization

3.4.4.1 Listing the current problems

Jenny has suffered from recurrent episodes of depression for many years. In her past she had a period of alcohol dependence, although she has a strong tendency to downplay this. She drank as a way to relax, especially after days involving lots of social contact. Socializing makes her very tense, and, when Jenny engages in this kind of contact, she worries a great deal about what others think of her.

Because of this tension, Jenny tends to avoid socializing. When this isn't possible, she prefers to stay in the background and say as little as possible.

Although she has felt uncomfortable around others all her life, the trigger to seek help now was a change in her work situation. After years of having had her own office in the company, she has recently been told that she will have to share this workspace with a colleague. The announcement upset the unstable equilibrium that she had managed to maintain for years. Now she is suffering from anxious thoughts, physical tension symptoms and insecurity. She was referred to specialist help by her doctor.

3.4.4.2 Description of life history

Jenny was naturally sensitive and shy as a child. Her mother often had physical symptoms that demanded a lot of attention and care, and which caused her to feel tense and stressed (Blaming Mode). Her mother did not cope well with normal childlike behaviour such as running, being lively or making noise. Jenny often heard remarks that made her feel guilty when her spontaneity and playfulness made her too lively and noisy for her mother (*Defectiveness/Shame, Failure*). Her father was a somewhat closed man who was often depressed (*Emotional Inhibition*). During those depressive episodes, he often felt guilty about his depression and frequently asked Jenny for forgiveness for being such a bad father to her (Blaming Mode). Jenny mostly learned to withdraw in such circumstances, and not to 'bother' her parents in any way.

3.4.4.3 Questionnaires

You have sent questionnaires, and discussing their outcomes is on your agenda for the next session. However, the day before the appointment, you realize that you have not yet received the completed questionnaires. You send Jenny a friendly reminder to send them as soon as possible, so that you can prepare for the discussion. The next day, she replies that she will send them immediately. However, it takes until just before the appointment for one of the two questionnaires to be sent. When you open the document, you see it is only half-filled in. You therefore plan to discuss Jenny's experience of filling in the forms. However, Jenny comes to the appointment fifteen minutes late, and when you discuss filling in the questionnaires you find that she is terribly embarrassed by her answers. Even before knowing the average scores from the questionnaires, you can already see that the schema *Defectiveness/Shame* seems to be relevant.

In the following session, all the results are known, and you can discuss the most relevant schemas and modes with Jenny (see Table 3.7 and Table 3.8). Although *Emotional Deprivation* scores low, you still include it in the list of relevant schemas. This is because Jenny had insufficient emotional care in her childhood.

In both questionnaires, you notice that the scores are somewhat lower than you would have expected based on the severity of Jenny's problems. It does not immediately become clear in the conversation why those scores are that much lower. Your hypothesis is that the same shame that made Jenny avoid filling in the questionnaires in the first place also made her somewhat restrained in her answers.

Table 3.7: Jenny's scores on the YSQ	
Emotional Deprivation	2.1
Defectiveness/Shame	3.5
Unrelenting Standards	3.1
Social Isolation/Alienation	4.8
Emotional Inhibition	2.7
Punitiveness	3.2

Table 3.8: Jenny's scores on the SMI	
Vulnerable Child	3.3
Happy Child	2.3
Angry Child	1.9
Detached Protector	2.6
Detached Self-Soother	3.1
Punitive Mode	3.5
Healthy Adult	2.5

When discussing the SMI, it is notable that Jenny does not recognize her own anger clearly. She acknowledges being angry at times, but mostly calls it irritation. You explain that anger is a universal, natural reaction. You also explain that anger can help to break persistent patterns. You decide to include it in the mode model as 'Grumpy Jenny'.

3.4.4.4 Childhood photos

In her childhood photos, Jenny is often alone. In the earlier photos, she comes across as a cheerful, active child, although she does also seem a bit on guard.

Her parents are rarely, if ever, smiling in the pictures. Her mother looks tense and anxious. Her father looks unhappy. It is striking that Jenny seems to find this quite normal. When you remark that her parents are never smiling in the photos that Jenny brought, she doesn't quite understand why you seem to think this is important. In the later childhood photos, Jenny's cheerfulness seems to have disappeared and she comes across as more timid and shy.

3.4.4.5 The downward arrow technique

Jenny talks about cancelling a recent arrangement with Linda, a good friend of hers. She describes the strong feeling of guilt that doing this has left her with. You decide to use the downward arrow technique to gain more insight into the underlying schemas that could explain this guilt.

> **Example of the downward arrow technique**
>
> **>>Therapist:** "And what did you feel so guilty about?"
>
> **>>Jenny:** "Well, that I disappointed her by cancelling our arrangement."
>
> **>>Therapist:** "Okay, but suppose that's true, that she's disappointed… What would that mean, do you think?"
>
> **>>Jenny:** "I'm not sure, maybe that she'd be fed up…"
>
> **>>Therapist:** "And suppose that were true, that she really was fed up, what are you afraid that would that mean?"
>
> **>>Jenny:** "That she'd no longer be my friend…"
>
> **>>Therapist:** "That doesn't sound very nice, and I can imagine how awful that would feel. But what exactly would be so bad for you if she was no longer your friend?"
>
> **>>Jenny:** "That I'd have no one left… but mostly that she'll be fed up with me… that she'd think I'm difficult… annoying…"
>
> **>>Therapist:** "And what would it mean for you if Linda found you annoying or difficult?"
>
> **>>Jenny:** "That it's really how I am… if she thinks so too, then I really am annoying…"
>
> **>>Therapist:** "Is that a familiar feeling? That feeling of being annoying? As if there's something wrong with you that makes others leave?"
>
> **>>Jenny:** "Yes…" (*There is sadness in her voice, she looks down.*)
>
> **>>Therapist:** "Hey… it feels a bit like this is what's making you so sad, doesn't it? That idea that there really is something wrong with you…"
>
> (*Jenny nods.*)

> **>>Therapist:** "Now I understand better why you were so upset about the idea that Linda didn't like your arrangement being cancelled. For you, it wasn't just about that arrangement; it might be proof that Linda, like others, found something wrong with you. That you're so annoying that people don't want to spend time with you, not even Linda."
>
> **>>Jenny:** "..."
>
> **>>Therapist:** "I think that pain has been there all along, and it comes up at moments like that. It's old pain, perhaps the pain, the fear that you felt as a child?"
>
> *(Jenny nods.)*
>
> **>>Therapist:** "That feeling that something is wrong with you – that sense of inferiority, of shame."

3.4.4.6 Diagnostic imagery

When you suggest doing diagnostic imagery, you notice Jenny becoming more tense. When you ask why she is tense, she hesitantly says that she doesn't like closing her eyes. You explain that this isn't necessary; she could focus on a point on the floor in front of her instead. However, you notice that the tension remains, and even seems to increase a little. The explanation of the exercise method and procedure don't seem to alleviate the anxiety either. Apparently, closing her eyes is not the (only) problem.

At this point, the easiest way to avoid resistance would be to tell Jenny that she doesn't have to do the exercise. However, you realize that other imagination exercises will need to be done in the course of Jenny's therapy. By avoiding diagnostic imagery now, you run the risk that this valuable technique will be more difficult to use in the future. You therefore decide to put aside the question of whether diagnostic imagery will be used, and first explore Jenny's anxiety further using the downward arrow technique.

> #### Example of lead-up to diagnostic imagery
>
> **>>Therapist:** "We can come back to the exercise in a moment. But for now, I'd like to get a better understanding of what is making you so tense. You don't have to justify yourself, you know, I don't mean it that way. But I can see that you feel uncomfortable. Can you let me in to what's making you tense, just a little bit?"
>
> **>>Jenny:** *(softly and looking away)* "Yeah, I don't know… with me sitting like that and you sitting there… I just don't like being looked at like that…"

>>**Therapist:** "And what would bother you about me sitting here and observing?"

>>**Jenny:** "I don't know… what you'd be thinking, or something…"

>>**Therapist:** "So I guess you're making an assumption that my thoughts about you aren't positive or friendly? Because otherwise you wouldn't feel so tense, would you?"

>>**Jenny:** "No, no, it's not that, it's that you'd think what I'm saying is weird…"

>>**Therapist:** "That doesn't sound very nice… but now I understand your anxiety and tension a bit better. You think that if you do that kind of exercise, you'll run the risk of saying something that I'll think is weird…"

(*Jenny nods.*)

>>**Therapist:** "Well, I can promise that I won't think what you say is weird. I don't think your experiences are weird, they're actually very important! But just to make sure I understand you: suppose I did think something you said was weird, what would that mean to you to make you so tense?"

>>**Jenny:** (*barely audible*) "That you think I'm weird, that I'm…"

>>**Therapist:** "Weird?"

>>**Jenny:** "Yes…"

>>**Therapist:** "And that idea makes you feel anxious, tense…"

>>**Jenny:** "Yes…"

>>**Therapist:** "And where do you feel that in your body, that tension and fear?"

(*Jenny points to her chest and stomach area.*)

>>**Therapist:** "And is that a familiar feeling for you? A familiar anxiety and tension that you feel in your chest and in your stomach? A fear of being thought of as weird?"

>>**Jenny:** "Yes, very much so…"

In the exploration, Jenny's focus has shifted from the fear of what you might think as a therapist to memories of other situations. Exploring the experience has actually created an affect bridge to the past. You decide to suggest an imagination exercise again.

> ### Example of diagnostic imagery
>
> **>>Therapist:** "It sounds like you have all kinds of images and memories of situations where you felt tense and anxious like that, is that right?"
>
> **>>Jenny:** "Yes, very often really…"
>
> **>>Therapist:** "Yes, I get that impression. It's almost as if I see all kinds of thought balloons appearing above your head with images and memories. So that seems to have been your reality, that you've had this feeling and experience very often. I'd love to know what those experiences were so I can understand what it must be like for you to live with that anxiety… Could you tell me about one of those images or memories?"
>
> *(Jenny nods.)*
>
> **>>Therapist:** "Keep thinking about those memories, but with your eyes focused on the floor in front of you so that you can really concentrate. And then just tell me what you see with your mind's eye, as if you really were there again. Is that okay?"
>
> *(Jenny nods hesitantly.)*
>
> **>>Therapist:** "Just keep thinking of all the times that you felt as anxious as you do now, the fear that the other person might think you're weird… what images do you see?"
>
> **>>Jenny:** "I don't know… it's actually always been that way…"
>
> **>>Therapist:** "Okay, just pick one then. There isn't a right or wrong choice, it isn't about that here. Just pick an image and focus your attention on it… what do you see now?"

From then on, Jenny recounts a memory from when she was twelve. She had just started secondary school and, to get to know each other better, the teacher had asked everyone to say what hobby they had. When Jenny said that she played the violin, several children started laughing and mimicking how weird that looked. Jenny was already shy and anxious, but to her this experience was only confirmation that others think she is weird when she speaks up and shows who she is. In the review, you explain that this feeling can be seen as an old emotional wound that opens up every time she finds herself in similar situations. You also explain that there is a name for that wound, or schema: *Defectiveness/Shame*.

3.4.4.7 Using chairwork to get to know modes

It's the last session of the case conceptualization, and you realize that you haven't yet done any chairwork in this diagnostic phase. If you're honest, you've thought about it at times but avoided suggesting it. For instance, there was an opportunity when Jenny talked about her Avoidant Protector, the Silent One, but you didn't do it. That was because, with Jenny, you constantly feel her anxiety and tension, and you don't want to make it even harder for her than it already is. But now you realise that out of that sense of care, you have overlooked chairwork even though you plan to use it more often going forward. So you decide to use it in this last session to help build the mode model.

Example of chairwork with one of Jenny's coping modes

>>**Therapist:** "I was thinking about what we've discussed so far. We've talked about these different sides of you. And by that, I mean we've talked about how you have an Avoidant Side, the Silent One, with which you tend to avoid tense situations." (*At this, the therapist gestures to a spot next to Jenny, as if pointing at a person.*)

(*Jenny nods.*)

>>**Therapist:** "And we talked about other sides of you too, for example your Blaming Side, the Prosecutor. But I'd like to go through them step-by-step. To do that, I want to do an exercise where I bring in extra chairs."

(*Here, the therapist stands and pulls over an extra chair, which is put in the place where the Silent One was just indicated.*)

>>**Therapist:** "I'd like to ask you to sit on that chair and be the Silent One for a while. In that chair, you can get completely into the experience of being the Silent One. After that, I'll ask you to come and sit here next to me again, and then we can have a good look together from these chairs and talk about what the Silent One is actually thinking and doing, and why she does that."

(*Jenny looks very doubtful.*)

>>**Therapist:** "I see you're doubtful, like 'What's this now, and do we really have to do it?' And that's understandable. It's a new exercise – and why would you switch chairs, when you could just as easily talk about it from this chair."

>>**Jenny:** "Yes, exactly... I don't understand why yet..."

>>**Therapist:** "It's good that you say that. Well, experience and research have shown that this kind of exercise is very helpful. It helps to gain more insight into the patterns we're talking about here. But it also helps to start making changes in the patterns that you came here to deal with. Shall we just give it a try?"

>>**Jenny:** "I don't know..." (*She looks away and seems to withdraw further.*)

Arriving at this point, you realize that this is just what you feared: that Jenny would become even more uncomfortable and anxious. Your worry is that she will withdraw from therapy if she has so much anxiety during sessions.

However, you also realize that you aren't speaking to Jenny's Healthy Adult in these conversations so much as to her Avoidant Protector, the Silent One. You'll need to do a lot of negotiating with the Silent One in order to connect more with Lonely, Shy Jenny, and those negotiations have now begun.

Keeping the idea in the back of your mind that you're negotiating with Jenny's Avoidant Protector, and not her Healthy Adult, you give some more explanation about the procedure and benefits of the chairwork technique. You emphasize to Jenny that she can always stop if she really doesn't like it; she is always in control. You can also agree to do the exercise for only three minutes at first and then stop. Despite all your efforts, Jenny keeps avoiding. She does this rather subtly and indirectly, with sighs, silences and answers like 'I don't know...', but in fact it is still the Silent One speaking.

You could let the exercise go at this point, in order to avoid building more pressure. However, you decide to risk one more attempt to introduce chairwork 'under the radar'. With this approach, Jenny does not have to sit in the chairs herself. Instead, as the therapist, you articulate all the different modes while sitting in the different chairs. Jenny continues to observe from her own chair and in this way, almost without realising it, she can still get something of the experience and benefits of a chairwork exercise.

Example of 'under the radar' chairwork

>>**Therapist:** "Well, maybe I can show you what it looks like. You won't have to do anything except sit here and take it in. So, I'd just like to grab some extra chairs and show you what that exercise looks like. Sounds good?"

>>**Jenny:** "Uh... okay, and I can just stay sitting here?"

>>**Therapist:** "Yes, exactly. Okay, so now I've put a chair in the spot where I already mentioned the Silent One. If I just sit here for a moment..."

(*Therapist sits on the chair assigned to the Silent One.*)

>>**Therapist:** "And here, as the Silent One, I believe it's best to show as little of what I'm feeling and thinking as possible (*with this, the therapist gestures to a place behind him, as if that's where the feelings and thoughts are*), because if I say what I'm feeling or thinking, people will think it's weird..."

(*The therapist gets up from the chair and sits next to the client.*)

>>**Therapist:** "Does that make sense at all?"

(*Jenny nods hesitantly.*)

>>**Therapist:** "So the Silent One there (*points and looks at the empty chair*) actually protects against the fear that people will think that the thoughts and feelings that are being hidden behind that silence (*therapist points to the area behind the Silent One's chair*) are weird. Let me put a chair there too..."

(*The therapist stands, puts a chair behind the Silent One's empty chair and sits on it.*)

>>**Therapist:** "If I try to imagine what that must be like for Jenny, the idea that people think she's weird, then it's scary – actually terrifying. And I think Jenny also feels shame here, as if she isn't good enough. That hurts. And people don't even have to say it, that she's weird; in this chair, as Lonely, Shy Jenny, I think so myself."

(*Here, the therapist gets up from the chair and puts a third chair next to it, close to Lonely, Shy Jenny's chair, facing it. The therapist sits in that third chair.*)

>>**Therapist:** "When I put myself in your place, Jenny, and I think about what you told me, I think I could slip into this state very easily. This is the side that looks at Jenny, but not kindly. This is the side that mostly looks at how others might be bothered by Jenny or disappointed in her, and then I always get the message that 'It's because of you'. (*Here, the therapist looks at Lonely, Shy Jenny's empty chair. After a short silence, he gets up and comes back to sit next to Jenny. They look at the chairs in front of them together.*)

At this point, you and Jenny talk about the chairs and the dynamics between the different sides of her. In this conversation, an extra chair is added for Jenny's Self-Soothing Side. Jenny seems to be participating actively in the discussion, and there is not much of the earlier anxiety and tension regarding chairwork. You do make a point of saying that this method will be used more often in the rest of therapy. Now that it has been mentioned, it will be somewhat easier to use the full technique next time.

3.2.5 Jenny's schemas and modes

Jenny has a number of modes that are common in Avoidant Personality Disorder (see Table 3.9). Surrender to the schemas of *Punitiveness* and *Subjugation* has led to a Blaming Mode, which you have agreed with Jenny to call the Prosecutor. Surrender to the schemas of *Defectiveness/Shame, Social Isolation/Alienation* and *Emotional Deprivation* has led to two Child Modes – Lonely, Shy Jenny and Grumpy Jenny. Jenny mostly has Avoidant Coping Modes. The Silent One is the Avoidant Protector. In this mode, Jenny avoids the schemas of *Defectiveness/Shame* and *Social Isolation/Alienation*. Avoidance of *Emotional Deprivation* can lead Jenny to consume alcohol, and this is her Detached Self-Soother, called the Cocoon.

Table 3.9 Jenny's modes

\multicolumn{2}{c}{Child Modes}	
Lonely Shy Jenny (Lonely/Unloved Child, Inferior/Ashamed Child, Alienated/Misunderstood Child)	In this mode, Jenny feels sad and feels that no one cares about or is interested in her. She believes that this is because of who she is, and that when others really get to know her, they will lose interest in her.
Grumpy Jenny (Angry Child)	This is the feeling Jenny very occasionally has when she is alone, when she feels a bit irritated that others don't pay attention to her.
\multicolumn{2}{c}{Critical Modes}	
The Prosecutor (Blaming Mode)	In this mode, Jenny thinks a lot about how bad others must feel because of something she did or didn't do. Then she feels it is her fault the other person is suffering.
\multicolumn{2}{c}{Avoidant Coping Modes}	
The Silent One (Avoidant Protector)	This is the mode in which Jenny cancels arrangements. She also has a lot of headaches, and that is a common reason she gives for cancelling arrangements.
The Cocoon (Detached Self-Soother)	In this mode, Jenny stays up very late and drinks a bottle of wine while watching a TV series or surfing the Internet. The Cocoon feels safe and soft, and Jenny has a sense of participating in the world while remaining within the safe environment of her room.
\multicolumn{2}{c}{Inverted Coping Modes}	
	Not present
\multicolumn{2}{c}{Healthy Modes}	
Big Jenny (Healthy Adult)	This is the mode in which Jenny is slightly more confident, for example when she is working on her own. It is also the mode that led her to seek help.
Playful Jenny (Happy Child)	Jenny mainly knows this mode from the night-time hours when she's had a few glasses of wine. When she is in this mode, she gives in to impulses a bit more and can dance to music. She feels that, were she in a relationship, she might show this playful side of herself much more.

3.4.6 Jenny's mode model

Figure 3.2: Jenny's mode model

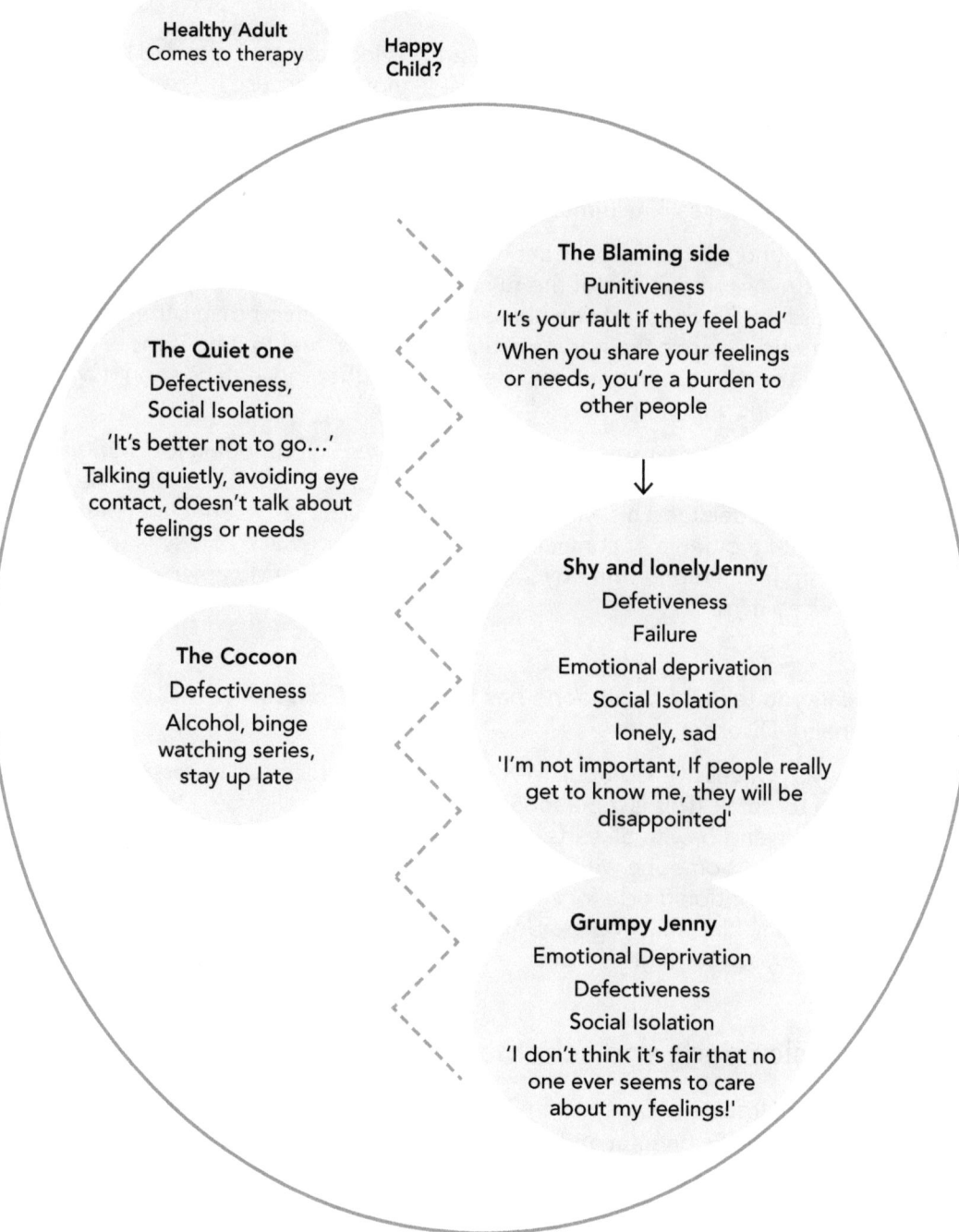

3.4 Obsessive-Compulsive Personality Disorder

Case study: John

John entered therapy because his wife, Laura, is increasingly bothered by the fact that he is constantly at work. She is also annoyed because he pays little or no attention to her anymore. As a result, they engage in fewer and fewer fun activities together. At the same time, work is often a source of frustration for John. While working, he is often confronted by people who do not follow the rules, and this irritates him immensely.

John can sound a bit self-important when he talks about how he is the only one who seems to be aware of the rules and regulations. Unlike in clients with narcissism, he does not see himself as a better person than others or as someone who is above the rules. He does, however, feel that he is more aware than others of how useful rules are. He also feels that those rules should apply to everyone, including him.

Laura has indicated that she is considering divorce if John does not change. The idea of a divorce is difficult and painful for John. At the same time, he struggles to understand his wife. He finds her feelings to be annoying, and talking about moments of conflict is laborious for him. Such conversations quickly turn into a monologue by John on why he cannot do anything other than work so hard.

How can you tell when someone has Obsessive-Compulsive Personality Disorder?

People with Obsessive-Compulsive-Personality Disorder pay excessive attention to detail. This is a person who, for example, tells you a story at tremendous length, with all sorts of information that doesn't necessarily seem relevant to you. Someone with this personality disorder is also always busy, either at work or doing odd jobs at home. You also notice that they look critically at anything that you are doing or have done, and that critical eye might make you feel slightly insecure or irritated.

3.5.1 Basic needs and schemas

Clients with Obsessive-Compulsive Personality Disorder have always been prone to perfectionism and were very sensitive to responsibilities and prohibitions as children. Many of them seem to have grown up in an environment with little explicit emotional care and warmth. Unlike individuals with Borderline Personality Disorder, many clients with Obsessive-Compulsive Personality Disorder grew up in stable, predictable and safe environments where they often lacked nothing in a material sense. However, the focus was typically more on work and performance than on the children's emotional needs.

Family rules could include sayings and proverbs such as 'If a job's worth doing, it's worth doing well' and 'There is always room for improvement'. Such rules may have been conveyed to the child both explicitly and implicitly. Perhaps the parents always told their child to have fun playing but, at the same time, they were constantly hard at work themselves. In their modelled behaviour, the importance of hard work was emphasized as a message that the children could read as a subtext. In addition, the fact that appreciation was expressed only for performance can be interpreted by children as a message that relaxation, play and spontaneity are not valued.

In such circumstances, the basic needs of spontaneity, play and unconditional appreciation are not fully met. The most common schema in this personality disorder is *Unrelenting Standards*; other schemas frequently reported include *Self-Sacrifice, Negativity/Pessimism* and *Punitiveness* (Panagiotopoulos *et al*, 2023). In clinical practice, we see that *Emotional Deprivation* and *Unfairness* are also often relevant schemas in people with Obsessive-Compulsive Personality Disorder.

Obsessive-Compulsive personality traits as described in the DSM-5 are examples of surrender to these schemas. For example, surrender to the schema of *Unrelenting Standards* leads these clients to work hard, lose themselves in detail and/or take more time to complete tasks. Some clients with this schema have an Inverted Coping Mode and deal with it differently. These clients struggle to maintain structure in their lives – their sleep/wake rhythm is disrupted, their eating patterns are chaotic, and their household is often a mess. At first glance, such a lifestyle pattern may seem to be a manifestation of the schema *Insufficient Self-control/Self-discipline*, but sometimes it can actually be an inversion of *Unrelenting Standards*. For these clients, inversion has become a survival response – they deal with the constant demands precisely by *not* living according to the schema that dictates hard work and structure.

3.5.2 Modes in Obsessive-Compulsive Personality Disorder

This section describes the possible modes of a client with Obsessive-Compulsive Personality Disorder (see Table 3.11). All modes that may occur are described, but not all clients will develop all these modes. We then describe the relevant modes for John.

Table 3.10: Possible modes in Obsessive-Compulsive-Personality Disorder

Child Modes (with related schemas)	
Disappointing, Underperforming Child (Unrelenting Standards schema. This is not a Vulnerable Child mode when it is assumed that the Vulnerable Child mode represents total surrender to a schema. This secondary schema of Unrelenting Standards is internalized in the Demanding mode. The Disappointing/Underperforming Child is presented as a Child Mode that can be associated with the schema.)	You are disappointed, not primarily in others, but in yourself with regard to your own standards. In this mode, you need reassurance, realistic standards and play.
Lonely, Unloved Child (Emotional Deprivation schema)	You feel like there is no one who really cares about you or understands how you feel. You might also believe that your feelings are too much for others.
Angry Child	You are angry at others when they don't consider your feelings, even if you haven't expressed them.
Over-diligent Child (Unrelenting Standards schema. Again, this is not a Vulnerable Child Mode when it is assumed that the Vulnerable Child Mode represents total surrender to a schema. The Over-diligent Child is presented as a Child Mode that can be associated with the schema.)	You work hard, are obedient and behave well and nicely.

Angry Child	You get angry because of unrealistic or unreasonable demands. These demands are often projected onto others or institutions. You tend to be unaware that this is actually a projection of your own standards. As such, you get angry at others who you think demand too much.
Rebellious Child	A variation of the Angry Child, but you express rebellion in ways other than open anger. This could, for example, be by intentionally doing things badly, obstruction, etc.
Sulking Child	You protest in a passive way against excessive demands and expectations, characterized by resistance and expressing irritation non-verbally.
Parentified Child (Self-sacrifice schema)	You firmly believe that you need to care for others, ignoring whether this is needed or refused.
Angry Child	You have outbursts of angry accusations that you have to constantly sacrifice yourself and that others do not acknowledge your care.
Aggrieved Child	You experience the imbalance between giving and receiving care as unfair. You feel you have been wronged and that you are treated unfairly.
Pessimistic Child (Negativity/Pessimism schema)	You tend to interpret situations in a negative, pessimistic way. You expect that things will go wrong. The future is dark, and disasters are likely. Hopelessness and dejection are the prominent feelings.
Angry Child	You get very angry when others are optimistic, or even realistic, because you genuinely believe your own pessimistic and gloomy expectations.
Bad Child (Punitiveness)	You feel bad, guilty, and think you deserve punishment.
Angry Child: Protesting Child	You protest emotionally against the punishment imposed by the Punitive mode. You usually direct your anger at others who you perceive as critical.
Sulking Child	You react passive-aggressively in protest against excessive punishments, accusations and restrictions. You sense resistance and convey it non-verbally with irritation.

	Critical Modes
Demanding Mode (Unrelenting Standards schema)	You are critical of your performance and think you need to do better: 'You'd better do your best, or else it will go badly.'
	Avoidant Coping Modes
Detached Self-Soother	You avoid lingering on your feelings by constantly engaging in activities that distract you from your feelings.
Detached Protector	You either ignore your feelings or switch off your feelings by rationalization.
	Inverted Coping Modes
Perfectionistic Overcontroller	You try very hard and make as few mistakes as possible to disguise the fact that you are a failure or lack self-discipline. You try to keep your feelings and needs under control.
Self-aggrandiser	You place yourself above others to make sure the rules are followed.

The Demanding Mode and the Perfectionistic Overcontroller are typical modes of clients with Obsessive-Compulsive Personality Disorder. The Demanding Mode results from internalized (perceived) messages about productivity, efficiency and high standards. In this state, your client evaluates their own performance critically. From this mode, there is therefore an urge to work better and harder.

Example of John's Demanding Mode

John is resting on the sofa after a hard day at the office. Watching the news, he has the satisfied feeling of having done a good day's work and crossed many items off his to-do list. He is now enjoying a well-deserved rest and a cup of tea.

When the news ends, his thoughts drift a bit during the commercial break. Thoughts of tasks that have not been ticked off yet begin to take hold of him. At first, he doesn't feel like doing anything more; he just wants to enjoy relaxing there. But the thoughts keep coming: 'Those things have to be done anyway. You've put it off before and if you don't do it now, the chances are it won't get done tomorrow either. Just do it now, then it's done. You still have some time, and you can deal with this first and then rest more, instead of lazing around now. Come on, just grit your teeth and get it over with!'

And with those oppressive, compelling words reverberating in his head, John drags himself off the sofa and starts walking towards his study. He takes the half-empty cup of tea with him, because if he leaves it there, the house will soon be a mess again…

The Demanding Mode has given John clear behavioural instructions to work hard. The condition of hard work that includes an eye for detail and 'odd jobs' yet to be done can be seen as the Perfectionistic Overcontroller. This Perfectionistic Overcontroller is an inverted mode with a protective function. You can work with your client to choose other, more personal names for their own Perfectionistic Overcontroller. Examples might be the Charger, the Controlling Side, the Foreman or Speedy Gonzales.

The core function of this mode is to avoid experiencing underlying feelings of restlessness, emptiness, failure or inadequacy. But for some clients, it is about more than just avoiding unpleasant emotions. For them, working hard feels so pleasant that this mode can be seen as a Detached Self-Soother – covering unwanted feelings of failure with a pleasant feeling of being useful and doing well. Hard work almost seems like a form of addiction for these clients. They do not feel compelled to work hard; instead, they crave it, like craving the effects of an addictive drug.

Distinguishing between the Demanding Mode and the Perfectionistic Overcontroller

It can be difficult to distinguish the Demanding Mode from the Perfectionistic Overcontroller. Both believe in the benefits of hard work, and that makes them seem like two peas in a pod – best friends forever. The key to differentiating between them involves differentiating a Coping Mode from a Critical Mode. A Critical Mode is a self-reflective state in which the client is critical of themselves and their own performance or actions. A Coping Mode is characterized less by critical self-reflection, and more by a functional focus on work and tasks. The two modes are therefore best distinguished by what they talk about.

The tone of voice will also be different according to which mode is active. The Demanding Mode will sound critical, while the Perfectionistic Overcontroller will sound rather flat and emotionless. Your own emotional reaction will also tend to vary depending on which mode is active. With a Demanding Mode, you may be more inclined to push back because the criticism can sound unfairly harsh. You may feel a bit more detached, or less engaged, with a Perfectionistic Overcontroller.

Metaphorically, the Demanding Mode can be seen as an overly anxious contractor who feels responsible for a task, with all the risks associated with not doing it properly. Meanwhile, the Perfectionistic Overcontroller can be seen as the workplace foreman. Urged on by the contractor, the foreman is hard at work getting the job done. In some cases, this Coping Mode is a 'robotic' state, an engine that is running continuously to perform an incessant stream of chores that are picked up by the sensors.

Example of John's Perfectionistic Overcontroller

John walks to the kitchen with the half-empty cup of tea, sees a plate on the table that had been overlooked by his wife and takes it in passing: 'It needs to be put in the dishwasher anyway, and there's no time like the present.' Arriving in the kitchen, he puts the cup and plate in the dishwasher and also immediately turns it on: 'It needs to be done anyway, and I might as well do that right now.'

On his way upstairs to his study, he takes the dishcloth from the kitchen because 'it's good to change those cloths every day, and this one can go in the wash'. Some of his wife's papers have been on the stairs for a day, and John takes them without much thought: 'It needs to be done anyway, and I might just as well do it now.'

Arriving upstairs, he puts the dishcloth in the washing machine on his way to his office, immediately grabs other items that need washing, and, in passing, cleans up the bathroom briefly and puts the bin by the stairs ('Empty it now and change the bag; the rubbish will be collected tomorrow.'). By the time he sits at his desk, he has done ten tasks in five minutes and experiences the familiar, pleasant feeling of his work mode.

The problems of Obsessive-Compulsive Personality Disorder are primarily characterized by the Demanding Mode and the Perfectionistic Overcontroller. The Vulnerable Child is not a mode that a client with Obsessive-Compulsive Personality Disorder often enters. In fact, in some clients with Obsessive-Compulsive Personality Disorder, it seems as if this emotional side of them is completely absent. This can raises doubts about whether these clients might be diagnostically more likely to have autism (see Chapter 1). However, the difficulty that these clients have in feeling emotions other than irritation or frustration can be explained psychologically by the emotional deprivation in their childhood. In the absence of emotional attention and care from the people who raised them, they have not learned to make/maintain contact with their emotions and needs themselves.

Because they do not recognize this vulnerability in their own daily lives, some clients may resist placing a 'Vulnerable Child' in their mode model. If you do include this Child Mode, that might be one of the first treatment interventions. With the rationale that every human being has this kind of emotional mode, you can place an important focus of therapy on the map. The Happy Child should also be included in the model. The fact that some clients have difficulty connecting with this source of spontaneity and joy from their past does not mean that the Happy Child Mode is absent or does not exist. It just means that the client has difficulty connecting with a mode that we all possess. Every child has a need and predisposition to play, and to enjoy things that are not solely efficient and productive.

3.5.3 Gathering information for the case conceptualization

3.5.3.1 Listing the current problems

John is in therapy at the insistence of his wife Laura. She has made it known that she is no longer happy with their marriage and is considering divorce. She is particularly bothered by the fact that John seems to be interested only in work and does not pay attention to her or engage in any relaxing activities. Laura's comments have made John more aware that he often feels tired and rather gloomy when he is not at work. This is especially noticeable on Sundays or during holidays, when the day is not filled with tasks. Work itself also seems a bit harder to him than before. He mostly notices this in the difficulty he has getting started, and the fact that he is more easily irritated when things don't go the way he wants. He often experiences these irritations when confronted with other people, such as colleagues who he finds to be less conscientious than him.

John works for the city council, checking that planning applications in the city centre comply with laws and regulations. In the course of his work, he regularly comes into conflict with contractors and homeowners on construction sites – such as when he notices construction faults, sometimes halting construction or demanding modifications as a result. In these situations, it usually seems to him that others are at fault; he gets annoyed that they do not see that rules are simply there to be followed.

Laura wanted children, but John wasn't interested. He ultimately convinced his wife that wanting children was just a societal expectation, and it would make their lives much more complex. He persuaded her that there were all sorts of potential problems that they would be better off avoiding by remaining childless.

3.5.3.2 Description of life history

By predisposition John is playful, active and open to others and the world, and as a child he could enjoy playing intensely. His parents often said that he was too lively, and that he needed to learn to hold back a bit more and pause to think before doing something (*Emotional Inhibition*).

John grew up as an only child in a family with parents who were both secondary school teachers. His mother was a maths teacher and his father taught history. Both parents were caring in a practical sense, helping him with homework and organizing all kinds of activities such as music and chess lessons (Demanding Mode). However, there was no warm attention (*Emotional Deprivation*). They both remained rather distant and were constantly preoccupied with their work and daily tasks. In fact, John never saw his parents completely relaxed doing nothing; there was always something to do (*Unrelenting Standards*).

Emotions such as anger in an argument were always discussed rationally. Both parents often used family expressions and sayings: 'Work first, then rest', 'The devil finds work for idle hands to do' and 'If a job's worth doing, it's worth doing well' (Demanding Mode).

3.5.3.3 Questionnaires

The questionnaires are returned completed on the same day you asked for them to be done. John has added a few comments. Some relate to examples of the items in the questionnaire; however, there are also comments on apparent inconsistencies in the questions. You feel some minor irritation when reading those corrective remarks, but then realize that this is a typical example of John's patterns. This is the side of John that is not only focused on hard work, but that can also be critical of others. In those moments, he gives the impression of being a know-it-all. You realize that John is probably unaware of this, and you make a note to explore this a bit more in subsequent conversations.

It is also notable that John scores high on the *Insufficient Self-control / Self-discipline* schema on the YSQ (see Table 3.11). In the conversation that follows, you discuss the items for this schema. It soon becomes apparent that the high scores are better explained by the schema *Unrelenting Standards*. If John has not done a task perfectly, he feels as if he has cut corners. In this context, it is not *Insufficient Self-control / Self-discipline* that is in play but *Unrelenting Standards*.

It is also notable that John scores low on the *Emotional Deprivation* schema. Based on the life history description, you had formed an impression that there was a lack of warmth and care in his past. Given the low scores on this schema, you discuss this hypothesis with John. John does not recognize any lack of warmth or care. However, when you tell him what a normal parenting style is, he acknowledges that his parents did not provide emotional care. He then agrees, with some difficulty, to include *Emotional Deprivation* in the list of his schemas. He does ask for a question mark to be added to it though, because he is not yet completely sure that it applies to him.

Finally, you discuss the scores on the SMI (see Table 3.12). You focus on the Detached Protector and the Detached Self-Soother at some length, despite the relatively low scores on those modes. John seems to have misunderstood the questions about the Detached Protector. He did not recognize 'feeling flat' when he completed the questionnaire. However, in your discussion, he does acknowledge that he is often unsure of his emotions. This has become so normal for him that he struggled with the questions about it in the questionnaire. He had a similar pattern when filling in items for the Detached Self-Soother. He did not recognize questions like, 'I work or play sports intensively so that I don't have to think about upsetting things.' He does recognize the enjoyment of hard work, and, indeed, he does almost nothing else. However, he did not recognize the function of this when completing the questionnaire. In talking about this with you, it emerges that working is indeed a refuge that John is quick to turn to when his wife comes to him with difficult questions about feelings. Because of this, you and John decide that this is a side of him that can be included in the list after all.

Table 3.11 John's scores on the YSQ	
Emotional Deprivation	1.6?
Failure	2.5
Unrelenting Standards	4.1
Punitiveness	3.8
Emotional Inhibition	2.7

Table 3.12 John's scores on the SMI	
Vulnerable Child	1.3
Happy Child	2.3
Angry Child	2.9
Detached Protector	2.6
Detached Self-Soother (Stupefier)	2.2?
Self-Aggrandizer	3.6
Demanding Mode	4.5
Healthy Adult	5.2

3.5.3.4 Childhood photos

When asked for childhood photos, John brings two neatly mounted photo albums full of pictures. These mostly show cultural outings to museums, cities and churches. In the photos, his parents often have a serious look or expression. There are no pictures showing the family members laughing exuberantly or having fun. John is neatly dressed in all the photos, and he looks a bit lonely. When he hears you say that you think the images are somewhat sad and lonely, and that they lack colour and vibrancy, John has to think for a moment and then says: 'Well, that's the way it was… I didn't mind or anything…'

In response to that comment, you pause to talk about children's basic needs. You explain that, while every child needs a sense of security and stability, they also need play, spontaneity, and self-expression. This sounds less relevant to John at first, but over the course of the conversation he does seem to acknowledge that sometimes he was a bit bored, being alone in a house with parents who were constantly working.

3.5.3.5 The downward arrow technique

Prompted by a conflict at work, the downward arrow technique is chosen to explore this situation. It quickly becomes apparent how important work and performance are to John, and it emerges that he feels a very strong responsibility not to make mistakes.

Example of the downward arrow technique

>>John: "And no matter what I say, they don't seem to be interested. I've explained to them that there are rules and regulations, but they just don't care. It's so frustrating!"

>>Therapist: "You got irritated by that?"

>>John: "Yes, of course! Those rules are there for a reason! If everyone just kind of did what suited them, it would be a mess!"

>>Therapist: "So that's your irritation, and perhaps also your fear – that if they don't stick to the regulations, everything will become a mess?"

>>John: "Yes!"

>>Therapist: "And suppose that was true, that you're right and everything did become a mess, what would bother you about that?"

>>John: "That it could have been prevented so easily…"

>>Therapist: "They could have prevented it, or you could have prevented it?"

>>John: "Both, I think… but yes, I could have prevented it. That's why I worry about it so much…"

>>Therapist: "And let's suppose that everything has become a mess, and that means you failed to prevent it, what would that mean for you?"

>>John: "I don't know… it would feel like I'd failed. I could have done it properly, but I didn't manage…"

>>Therapist: "I'm seeing a very different side of you now. I'm seeing much more of a lonely and somewhat anxious John…"

Arriving at this point, John seems to be in a different state of mind. Instead of his usual irritation and focus on facts and work, now he sounds quieter and more thoughtful. For the first time, he uses the word 'feel'. This is actually very emotional for John.

This contrasts with his usual work mode; the quietness and the use of words like 'feel' seem to signal his vulnerable side. The Vulnerable Child Mode expresses itself differently than it would in a dependent or avoidant client – those clients would express themselves more emotionally. The fact that John becomes more emotional when talking about his underlying sense of failure indicates schema activation. The schema that is identified is *Unrelenting Standards* with the underlying schema *Failure*.

3.5.3.6 Diagnostic imagery

In the second session, John talks about a recent problem at work where a contractor didn't do the things that John had asked him to do. He feels irritated by this. However, he is also irritated with himself for not having been able to prevent it: 'I should have known, this has happened before. If only I'd paid more attention or arranged it myself, we wouldn't be in this situation now.'

According to John, his wife thinks he's making too much fuss about it, which creates an unpleasant atmosphere at home. With the rationale that John's emotional reactions appear stronger than the actual events seem to explain, you decide to do diagnostic imagery. This exercise could help gain a better understanding of why John is deeply affected and upset.

Because John has explained the problem situation so vividly and already feels the irritation with himself and others so strongly, you decide to skip the Good Place exercise (see 3.2.5) and let him go directly to the image of the problem situation and its associated feelings.

> **Example of diagnostic imagery**
>
> **>>Therapist:** "Okay, John, so you feel irritated, angry at this other person for not having done what he should have done, and also irritated with yourself. Where do you feel that irritated feeling in your body?"
>
> **>>John:** "I don't know… I feel tense or something…"
>
> **>>Therapist:** "There's no right or wrong answer. Just stay with that feeling of tension, that irritation… is there a place in your body where you particularly feel it?"
>
> **>>John:** "Maybe here." (*Points to his chest and head.*)
>
> **>>Therapist**: "Okay, so you feel that tension, that irritation that he did something wrong, but actually irritation with yourself as well. And that feeling is in your chest and head… And which feeling is strongest, anger at the other person or at yourself?"
>
> **>>John:** "With myself… I should have known… I shouldn't have left it to others…"
>
> **>>Therapist:** "And that feeling of anger with yourself, that tension, is that a familiar feeling for you? Or are you experiencing it for the first time now?"
>
> **>>John:** "No, I know it very well!"
>
> **>>Therapist:** "Just focus on that feeling… that familiar feeling of anger with yourself, that you should have done better, that you shouldn't have let go or relaxed… and let go of the image of the contractor. It isn't him causing

that feeling, you've known it for longer. Let your thoughts go back to your childhood… What images or memories come to mind that could somehow be related to this feeling?"

>>**John:** "Well… what kind of image would that be?"

>>**Therapist:** "It doesn't matter, there's no 'right' image – we're looking into that feeling of irritation with yourself and just seeing what comes up. Anything is good…"

>>**John:** "Well, something I've often thought back to comes up now. I was about ten at the time… no, nine… or was it ten…?"

>>**Therapist:** "Don't think about it too hard, John, just stay with the feeling. So there's this image, and you're young. Are you looking at that image from a distance, or are you back there now?"

>>**John:** "A bit of both… I see myself, but it's also like I'm there again… and I'm sitting at the kitchen table… my father is next to me and he's helping me with my homework. But it isn't nice or anything… it's more tense. I want to do it right, but I remember I could hear my friends playing outside."

>>**Therapist:** "You can hear them playing now?"

>>**John:** "Yes, shouting and all that… and then I tell my father that I'd like to play too."

>>**Therapist:** "Look at your father; how does he react when you say this?"

>>**John:** "Dismissive… 'That isn't important.' I want to go outside and play with my friends, but that isn't important."

>>**Therapist:** "Okay, let me hear how he reacts. Be your father for a moment, just speak how he speaks when he says this."

>>**John:** (*In a stern tone*) "'You need to finish your homework first. Work first, then play. You've only worked for five minutes, there is no way you're already done. If you don't work, you won't be able to achieve anything in life.'"

>>**Therapist:** "How do you feel?"

>>**John:** "Not good…"

>>**Therapist:** "Do you have a feeling of fear, or sadness?"

>>**John:** "Frustrated… because I want to go outside."

>>**Therapist:** "Choose one or more of the following emotions: sadness, fear, anger."

>>**John:** "It happens all the time, so I feel angry… but I can't say that. I just have to finish my homework."

>>**Therapist:** "How does it feel for you, that you can't say that?"

> **John:** "I'm frustrated that I can't say it."
>
> **Therapist:** "Is that a sad feeling? Fearful?"
>
> **John:** "I'm afraid to say those things. I'm angry that I'm not allowed to go outside, but I'm afraid to say it, to go against my father… he's very strong."

3.5.3.7 Using chairwork to get to know modes

In the fourth session, towards the end of the case conceptualization phase, John is rather tired and irritable when he arrives. He has been working long hours and his wife has commented on that. He does understand that Laura has problems with how hard he works, but he sees no way that he could have done things differently this week. There are deadlines, and the only way to meet them is by putting in more hours – this seems abundantly clear to him. His irritation is that Laura doesn't seem to understand this. You note that John is fully convinced that he must work hard, and you suggest an exercise to better understand what John is experiencing in the work mode that he seems to be in now.

> **Example of chairwork with one of John's Inverted Modes**
>
> **Therapist:** "You seem to be consumed with the need to work hard for long hours. Shall we do an exercise that will help us better understand what is happening with you when you're in your work mode like that? I'll just pull up an extra chair."
>
> *(The therapist stands, takes an extra chair and places it diagonally across from John.)*
>
> **Therapist:** "In a moment, I'll ask you if you'd like to come and sit on this chair. On that chair, I want you to get completely into that need to work that you feel. Then, when you get up from that chair and come and sit here next to me again, we can take some distance together to look at how it works with that Hard Worker of yours."
>
> **John:** "And you think that'll help?"
>
> **Therapist:** "Yes, it does. In my experience, it can be very helpful. And research has also shown that this is an effective way to gain insight into people's problems.
>
> **John:** "Alright then…"
>
> **Therapist:** "It's great that you'll give it a try. So, I'd like to ask you to sit in this chair now." *(Points to new chair.)*
>
> *(John stands up and sits in the chair.)*

>>**Therapist:** "Okay, in this chair, I want you to go completely into that feeling that hard work is necessary. It shouldn't be difficult for you, because I think you were already completely in that experience. Just be that Hard Worker. And I'm going to address you that way, as the Hard Worker… So, Hard Worker, you say you have no option but to work hard, and Laura should just accept that, is that right?"

>>**John:** "Yes, I need to get those jobs done and they won't get done by themselves…"

>>**Therapist:** "Okay, that makes sense… I feel that myself sometimes, that I can't do anything but grit my teeth and keep going to get things done on time. Do you see any other reasons why you must keep working, even if it means seeing Laura much less?"

(*In this way, the therapist explores the various reasons and benefits of working hard.*)

>>**Therapist:** "Okay then, in a moment I'll ask you to come back here, next to me. But when you get up from the chair where you are now, remember to leave the Hard Worker there; that's the chair where you can talk about all the benefits and reasons for hard work. Over here, I want you to turn your attention to other perspectives."

(*John stands up and comes to sit next to the therapist.*)

>>**Therapist:** "Okay, so the Hard Worker is sitting there (*gesturing to the empty chair where the client was just sitting*). And that Hard Worker sees all the reasons why there is no other way but to work long and hard, right?"

(*John nods.*)

>>**Therapist:** "But now you're sitting here, I wonder – how does it feel to have to work so hard and have no time to relax?"

>>**John:** "Well, I don't see how it could be any different, because…"

>>**Therapist:** (*interrupts client*) "Sorry to interrupt you, but I understand that the Hard Worker over there (*gesturing again to the empty chair opposite them*) doesn't see how things could be different. But I didn't ask if he thinks it's right to work hard, I asked you, here, how you feel about all that work. Do you feel rested? Relaxed?"

>>**John:** "Well, no, of course not…"

>>**Therapist:** "No? How do you feel then?"

>>**John:** "Well, tired… the days are quite long…"

>>**Therapist:** "And how do you feel when you hear that Laura is annoyed by that hard work? Do you feel good about it?"

> **John:** "Well, not good, obviously…"
>
> **Therapist:** "Not nice… is that sad, anxious?"
>
> **John:** "Well… uh… not anxious… yeah, maybe a bit nervous or something, because I know she's thinking of divorce…"
>
> **Therapist:** "Okay, well you're experiencing all kinds of things in these chairs. Let's stand for a moment and look at everything you've experienced from a distance."

After exploring the experiences from the different chairs and perspectives, the therapist and client stand up and, with a little distance, the two sides of John are named the Hard Worker and Lonely, Tired John. Following this discussion, an extra chair is added to represent John's Demanding Side and, with the therapist working collaboratively with John, the chairs are rearranged to reveal John's mode model.

3.5.4 John's schemas and modes

As a child, John was deficient in almost all the basic needs relevant to Obsessive-Compulsive Personality Disorder. He was deficient in the basic need for connection and spontaneity and play. His parents were almost compulsively focused on rules, standards and fairness. This left John unprepared as a child for a world that is often not fair or just. As a result, he had an indirect deficiency in the basic need for justice.

From these deficiencies, schemas of *Emotional Deprivation, Emotional Inhibition, Unrelenting Standards* and *Unfairness* have emerged. Because John's parents always worked so hard and had remarks about everything, he also developed the schema *Failure*.

John has internalized the modelled and stated importance of hard work and performing well into a Demanding Mode. He had little to no acknowledgement of his feelings or needs as a child and, as a result, he lost touch with this emotional side to some extent.

However, there is an Inhibited Child who has been called Lonely, Tired John in the conversations. John does acknowledge that this is a state of mind he has fallen into from time to time, but he struggles to connect with that side of himself. He is better able to feel his anger, and that side has been called Angry John (Angry Child Mode). That anger may take the form of sulking and being aggrieved if he has not had enough space to relax for a period of time (Protesting and Sulking Child Mode).

It was also mentioned that, sometimes, for example after drinking a couple of glasses of beer, John gets a bit disinhibited and then can have a lot of fun. However, he almost never drinks, as this would leave him with less energy for work. That more disinhibited side has been called Relaxed, Happy John (Happy Child Mode).

John has maintained himself by developing a Perfectionistic Overcontroller (the Hard Worker). This is a side of himself that works hard for long hours. The hard work also often feels very pleasant for John, as if it is a kind of high where everything disappears because he is completely absorbed in it. He also really likes that high when he has had another difficult conversation with his wife Laura. He calls the state he slips into the Focus (Detached Self-Soother). The Hard Worker and the Focus have made Laura so unhappy that she has threatened to divorce him.

John has also learned to be critical of others' work. That side of him is called the Fusspot (Self-Aggrandising Coping Mode).

Table 3.13: John's modes

Child Modes	
Lonely, Tired John (Inhibited Child)	In this state, John feels tired and empty, lonely. This mode rarely manifests, and then mostly in the evening when he has finally finished work and his wife is already asleep.
Angry John (Angry, Aggrieved Child)	In this mode, John might find it very unfair that his work and efforts do not seem to be sufficiently appreciated and others do not put in as much effort as he does.
Critical Modes	
Demanding Mode	In this mode, John is never satisfied with what he has done and always sees areas for improvement.
Avoidant Coping Modes	
The Focus (Detached Self-Soother)	John gets into his work, feels pleasant and useful, and, with that, worries and irritations fade into the background.

	Inverted Coping Modes
The Hard Worker (Perfectionistic Overcontroller)	John dives into tasks and is focused on efficiency and productivity. He makes lists and schedules and often works longer than others.
The Fusspot (Self-Aggrandizer)	John has difficulty delegating tasks, can get annoyed by mistakes others make, and is then stubborn and obstinate.
	Healthy Modes
The Captain (Healthy Adult)	In this mode, John listened to Laura's concerns and sought help. This is also the mode that makes sure he cooperates in exercises, even if he finds them to be absurd or strange.
Relaxed, Free John (Happy Child)	In this mode, John feels relaxed. The pressure of all the 'musts' is gone, and he can make jokes and imagine more impulsive actions.

3.5.5 John's mode model

The modes above have been put into an organized model to gain insight into the dynamics between them (Figure 3.3).

Figure 3.3 John's mode model

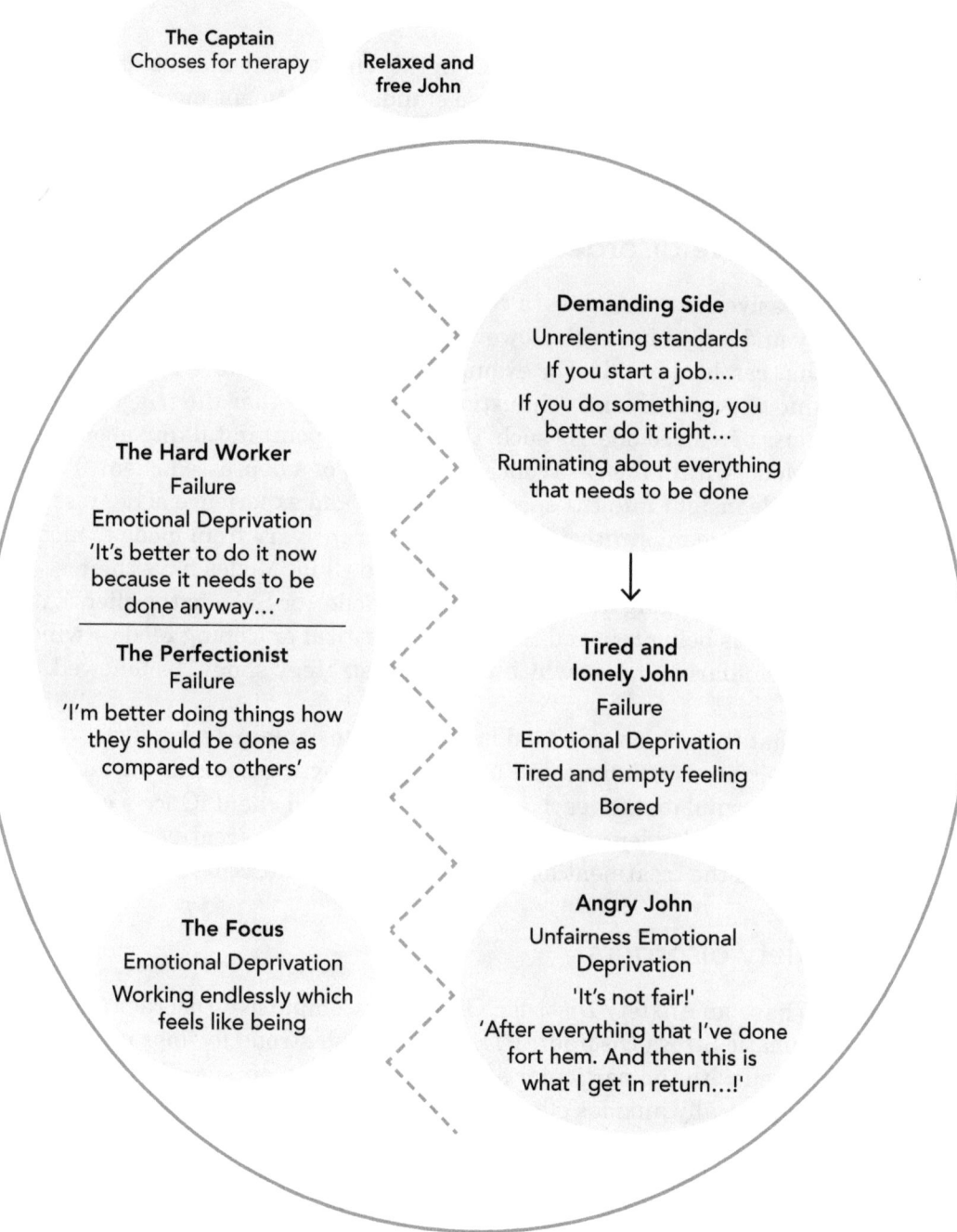

3.6 Mode models for anxiety and mood disorders

As we noted in Chapter 1, the techniques in this chapter can also be used for recurrent anxiety or mood disorders when standard treatment methods do not work adequately. For this reason, we will briefly discuss case conceptualization with these disorders.

3.6.1 Depressive disorders

Several depressive disorders share a common feature of periods of persistent despondency and loss of interest. However, there are many different internal dynamics that can lead to this. For example, one client may have become depressed due to overwork and exhaustion, while for another the trigger may be the loss of a loved one. As such, there is little point in talking about a 'Depressed Mode' within the case conceptualization of a depressed client. That term offers little insight into the specific aetiology and experience of depression. Moreover, the treatment strategies in schema therapy vary from mode to mode. For instance, Critical Modes are contradicted, and Child Modes have their needs validated. By talking about a 'Depressed Mode' (or Side, to the client), it is not clear what is being referred to – a Child, Critical or Coping Mode – which also makes it similarly unclear which treatment strategy should be followed.

This means that there is no standard mode model to explain depression in terms of basic needs, schemas and modes. An idiosyncratic mode model will have to be formulated for each individual depressed client. Once a case conceptualization of the depression is formed, however, the treatment otherwise largely resembles the treatment for cluster C disorders described in this book.

3.6.2 Anxiety disorders

Clients who have an Anxiety Disorder, Obsessive-Compulsive Disorder (OCD) or Post-Traumatic Stress Disorder (PTSD) react with strong feelings of anxiety when confronted with the particular stimuli related to their specific disorder. For instance, a socially anxious client will become extremely fearful when they imagine being present in a group with strangers. In the same way, a client with OCD becomes extremely fearful when they have touched a door handle and cannot wash their hands, and a client with PTSD becomes extremely fearful when they have memories of the trauma.

Within this overwhelming fear, your client is in a Child Mode. The internal or external stimuli have a threatening, negative meaning. This negative assessment of the internal or external stimulus can be seen as a surrender to a disorder-related schema, for example the schema of *Vulnerability to Harm or Illness* in the case of a client with OCD, or the schema of *Defectiveness / Shame* in a client with Social Anxiety Disorder. Characteristics of that negative assessment are overestimating the risk and severity of the danger, combined with underestimating one's own ability to cope with it (Bögels & Van Oppen, 2019).

With this, the state in which that stimulus is rated negatively could be seen as a variant of the Critical Mode – the Warning Critical Mode. In that mode, your client sees a high risk of danger along with the message that they will not be able to handle it. The characteristic avoidance behaviour in anxiety disorders can thus be conceptualized as an Avoidant Coping Mode. In a client with OCD, that Coping Mode might be more an Inverted Coping Mode, in which the client exhibits behaviour that is opposite to the experience of the schema. An example might be performing compulsive rituals such as handwashing when the schema *Vulnerability to Harm or Illness* is activated.

As with the treatment of cluster C personality disorders, schema therapy for anxiety disorders will explicitly work on breaking the avoidance behaviour. With this, schema therapy for anxiety disorders combines cognitive-behavioural elements such as exposure on the one hand, and schema therapy elements such as the use of mode language and chairwork on the other.

3.7 Chapter summary

This chapter has discussed how to structure the case conceptualization phase. The different methods and techniques used in this phase were first discussed in general terms. The way to structure the case conceptualization was then described for the three cluster C personality disorders, each of which involves specific challenges. For example, in Dependent and Avoidant Personality Disorder, it is important to add the Angry Child to the mode model, even if the client appears not to acknowledge anger. The difference between the Compliant Surrenderer and the Dependent Child was also briefly discussed, as well as the difference between the Demanding Mode and the Perfectionistic Overcontroller. The examples of methods and techniques in the case conceptualization that we have included also explain how to deal with specific challenges, such as an avoidant client who does not dare to do diagnostic imagery.

In the therapeutic process, case conceptualization concludes the analysis phase, and the change phase can then begin. The change phase is when active work is done on breaking the client's patterns. In it, Critical Modes are countered, and work is done to get past the Avoidant and Inverted Modes in order to make contact with the unmet basic needs of the Child Mode. Validating these basic needs creates corrective healing experiences that can stimulate emotional growth towards a strong Healthy Adult.

Chapter 4: From case conceptualization to treatment

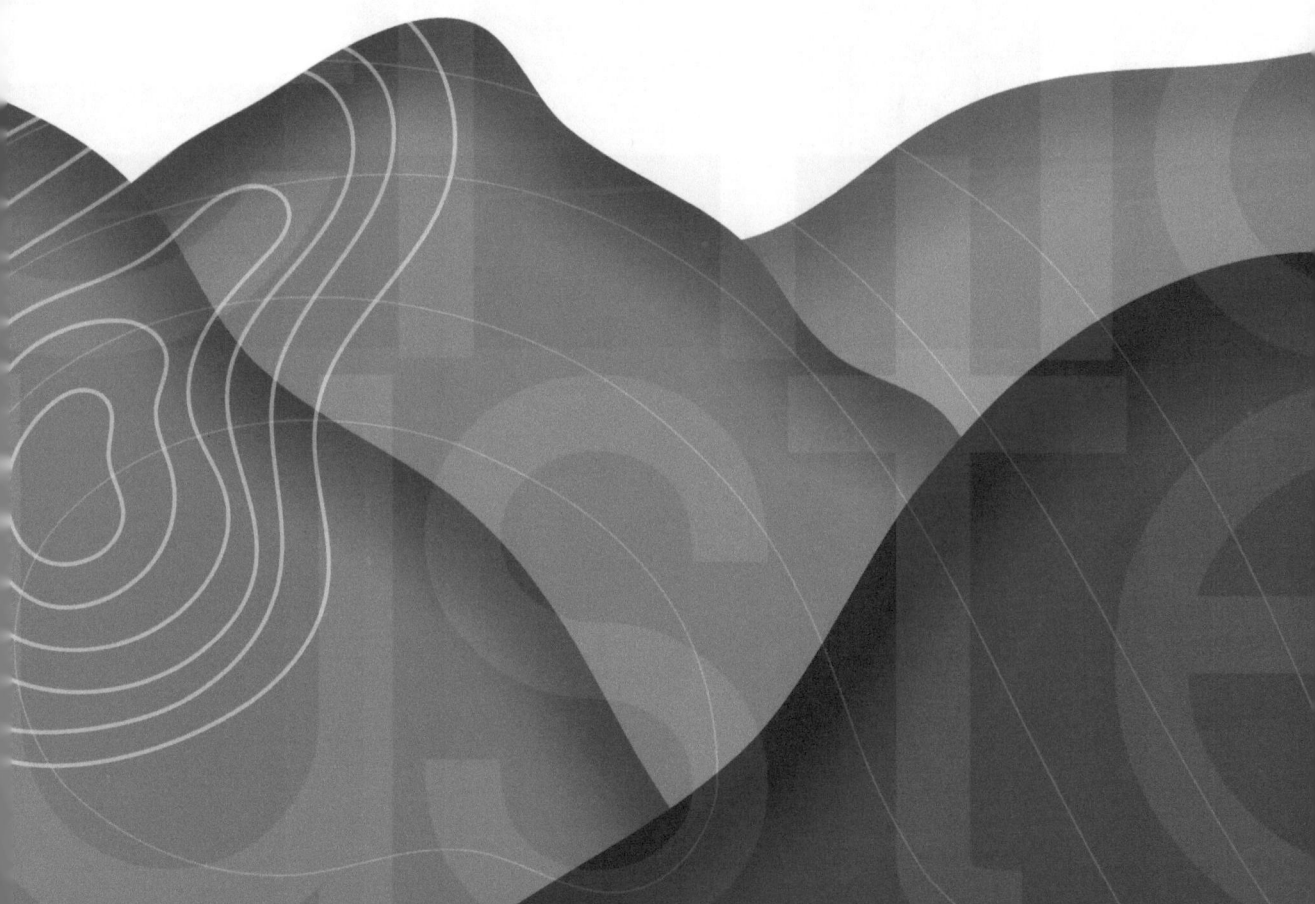

Chapter 4: From case conceptualization to treatment

Chapter map	
4.1	Introduction
4.2	Treatment goals
4.3	Limited reparenting
4.4	Methods and techniques
4.5	Phasing of treatment
4.6	Treatment plans by disorder
4.7	Pause for evaluation
4.8	Chapter summary

4.1 Introduction

In the process of developing the case conceptualization, you will have explained to the client which of their modes ('sides') are causing them problems, and you will probably also have given some broad pointers about treatment. However, after completing the case conceptualization form and the mode model, the final step is to create a treatment plan that is tailored to the client's issues. A treatment plan consists of an explanation of the purpose of treatment, what you want to change, and which techniques will be used. You also describe how long the treatment will take and what its different phases will entail.

4.2 Treatment goals

The ultimate goal of treatment is for the client to no longer meet the criteria for a personality disorder. Research has shown that changes in the Child Modes and the Healthy Adult are the best predictors of a positive therapy outcome

(Yakin *et al*, 2020). The main goal, therefore, is to connect with these modes in each session you conduct with your client. However, in therapy you will often be met with your client's Coping Modes and Critical Modes. One of the goals of therapy is to make the Coping Modes less strong, enabling you to connect with the Child's underlying needs. Another goal is to contradict the Critical Modes, so that your client can learn to internalize healthy messages and replace the unhealthy critical ones.

In clients with a cluster C personality disorder, this generally means working on:

1. Fulfilling the needs of the Child Modes.
2. Combating the Critical Mode(s).
3. Making the Avoidant and Inverted Coping Modes less necessary.
4. Strengthening the Healthy Modes, i.e. developing and strengthening the Healthy Adult and giving the Happy Child much more space.

When formulating these goals, of course, the terms you have entered in the case conceptualization model should be used as much as possible. In the following, we will begin by describing general aspects of a treatment plan. First, we explain the structure and phases of treatment. We will also discuss how to make sure you stay on track during treatment. Then, we will develop the goals specifically by disorder. How these goals can be achieved in practice by adapting treatment techniques for clients with a cluster C personality disorder is described in detail in Chapters 6 to 9.

4.3 Limited reparenting

Fulfilling the client's basic needs means that you offer them corrective emotional experiences. Limited reparenting is the most important instrument with which you generate these experiences. We describe the basic strategy to generate corrective emotional experiences during therapy below.

4.3.1 Schema activation

As we noted in Chapter 2, a corrective emotional experience must first be an emotional experience, and some schema activation is therefore necessary for them to be beneficial to the client. This emotional arousal must be carefully managed. Too little and there will be no benefit, but too much and the client may fall back on entrenched coping styles – surrender, avoidance or inversion.

Even in the initial phase of treatment, frequent and strong schema activation is necessary. This can sometimes be achieved with little effort – for example, your client may be emotional when they come to a session because of something that occurred outside or within therapy. If spontaneous schema activation does not occur, there are several methods and techniques you can use to generate it. For example, you can use imagery rescripting to have your client visualize meaningful, emotional situations. You can use chairwork to try to get past the protective Coping Mode and make contact with your Vulnerable Child. Or you can do an empathic confrontation, to address the fact that your client seems to be falling completely back into their protective Coping Mode.

4.3.2 Corrective emotional experiences

The corrective emotional experience that you offer is actually the validation of the client's basic needs. The form of this experience will vary by basic need. Providing safe connectedness will look different than encouraging independent behaviour. Whatever the basic need is, as a therapist, you show explicit compassion for what your client is lacking. You also work on a cognitive restructuring of the assumptions that ensue from the activated schemas. The compassion and cognitive restructuring shown often lead to an awkward but therapeutic experience for your client. This new experience does need to be consolidated to contribute to the formation of new, more healthy schemas.

4.3.3 Consolidation

A first form of consolidation is to pay explicit attention to the experience that takes place during a session. Ask the client to take time to reflect on the different modalities of this new experience. What is the pleasant feeling? Where do they feel it in their body? Questions like 'What colour or temperature is this feeling?' can also help your client to linger on a new experience and become aware of all the different aspects of it.

Consolidation also means keeping this experience 'alive' using homework. Ask your client to take notes of the experience and what it means. Record an audio flashcard so they can hear the messages you gave during the session again.

With these strategies, your client learns to internalize positive new experiences that can serve as a foundation for developing their Healthy Adult during the course of treatment.

4.4 Methods and techniques

Try to describe the ways in which you intend to influence the client's patterns as concretely as possible, and to use simple terms rather than jargon where possible. You might recommend purchasing *Breaking Negative Thinking Patterns: A Schema Therapy Self-Help and Support Book*, as it describes in detail not only the different steps, but also the techniques. Explain in broad terms that, in the early stages of therapy especially, you will use a lot of experiential techniques such as imagery rescripting and chairwork exercises in order to get to know the various dysfunctional parts of the client better, but more importantly also to work on them. Also briefly explain the cognitive techniques you will use and emphasize the importance of behavioural change in the second half of therapy.

Next, give a brief overview of the techniques themselves. Do not go into too much depth at this point; each of the different techniques should be explained in detail to the client at the point when you come to actually apply them.

For clients with a cluster C personality disorder, the behavioural change component in particular is likely to provoke resistance or even fear. As a therapist, you must therefore stress the importance of this on the one hand, but also reassure the client that it will happen step-by-step on the other. Motivate them to stick with therapy and to discuss any obstacles with you. Explain that it will sometimes be difficult in the short term, but that in the long-term they will become more independent, less avoidant and more relaxed.

A warm, encouraging style of limited reparenting, focused from the first conversation on fulfilling the needs of the client's Child Mode, is essential to keeping clients with cluster C personality disorders motivated to stick with therapy and achieve lasting results.

4.5 Phasing of treatment

The phases of treatment and the goals for each phase have already been briefly covered in Chapter 2 (see 2.7). The first phase consists of the case conceptualization (Chapter 3) and the treatment plan (Chapter 4). While discussing the treatment plan, you will explain to the client that the therapy takes two years and there are three phases:

- Initial phase (20 weekly sessions).
- Middle phase (20 weekly sessions).
- Final phase (10 monthly sessions).

At the end of each phase, there is a moment for evaluation to discuss which goals have already been achieved and the goals that are still to be worked on.

In the first two phases, you have a very active role as the therapist, but from the middle phase onwards, you take more of a coaching approach and your client will increasingly have to direct the process of change themselves. In the final phase, you gradually create still more distance, coaching the client 'from the sidelines.' You are still actively involved and encouraging, but your client will have to apply what they have learned in their life themselves.

The process of change, and the shifting role of the therapist within it, can be compared to a child growing up (Farrell *et al*, 2014; Reubsaet, 2018; Brockman *et al*, 2023). When children are very young, the parent still has an active, leading role. In adolescence, this will (necessarily) change to a more coaching, encouraging role. In the final phase of treatment, the therapist must increasingly relinquish control and let go, like the parents of an older adolescent or young adult who can give active encouragement from the sidelines but can no longer take over to ensure that things work out as they hope.

The different phases of schema therapy treatment are described in more detail below.

4.5.1 The initial phase

In the initial phase of treatment, you provide psychoeducation on basic needs, schemas and modes and the role of parenting in them. The emphasis in this phase is on experiential techniques, but cognitive techniques can also be initiated. As the therapist you play an active role (see 2.5). This means that in experiential techniques, you are the one who takes the lead in fighting the Critical Mode and reducing the Coping Modes. When applying cognitive techniques, you also play an active role in completing the self-enquiry circle and making a start on the cognitive diary. And when implementing cognitive challenge techniques, you will still have to be quite active in coming up with counterarguments, because your client is likely to find it difficult to do this.

Chapters 5 to 7 describe how these techniques can be adapted specifically for Dependent, Avoidant and Obsessive-Compulsive Personality Disorder, respectively.

By the end of this phase, the following objectives should have been achieved:

- Your client can apply the key concepts from schema therapy.
- You are able to do experiential exercises.
- There have been corrective emotional experiences.
- They are largely able to retain the experiences they have gained in the session until the next session.
- Your client can cooperate well with the cognitive techniques.
- Some effect is visible in the results of the questionnaires.

4.5.2 The middle phase

In the middle phase of treatment, experiential techniques remain very important, but cognitive and behavioural techniques also become more central. Your client begins to try out new behaviours, first in the session and then increasingly in the outside world. The dependent client will have to learn to ask for advice from the therapist and people around them less often; the avoidant client must learn to express themselves more and do new things. The obsessive-compulsive client must practice doing less than their best and allowing themselves to making mistakes.

In this phase, the client increasingly takes on the role of the therapist during imagery rescripting and chairwork exercises. You then assume much more of a coaching and encouraging role. This phase also explicitly works on strengthening the Healthy Adult, expressing anger, and stimulating the Happy Child.

By the end of the middle phase, the following objectives should have been achieved:

- Looking back at problem situations, your client can recognize modes at work.
- Your client is able to visualize the Healthy Adult.
- Your client is able to use the Healthy Adult in experiential techniques.
- Your client is able to have compassion for their Vulnerable Child.
- Your client understands why the Critical and Coping Modes are not correct.
- Your client can already display different behaviour in the session.

4.5.3 The final phase

In the final phase of treatment, the main goal is for the client to become more self-directed in the techniques you use within sessions. The aim in this phase is also to break the client's behavioural patterns so that they behave differently in everyday situations. This is more easily said than done. As we pointed out in the behavioural techniques, it is very difficult for cluster C clients in particular to try out new things. Changing behaviour will arouse resistance in your client. A further complicating factor may be your client discovering that behavioural change sometimes has far-reaching consequences for relationships, work and other activities. Important people in your client's life will see them change, and there may not be unanimous agreement that it is a positive thing. What you think is a healthy change, such as a dependent client standing up more for their own opinions, might not always be appreciated by their family or friends.

As a therapist, you have an increasingly stimulating role with regard to your client's goals. You will encourage them not only to change their behaviour, but also to make important choices about relationships and work or other pursuits. Your encouragement sometimes needs to take a somewhat forceful form, otherwise your client will not get moving.

You may also get discouraged at times if your client does not take new steps. In the final phase of treatment especially, support from a peer supervision group can be very important to help you keep your client moving forward. But if all goes well, change will happen. The dependent client will be able to decide whether a more equal relationship with their partner is possible; the avoidant client might decide to change jobs because their current position is secure but not challenging; and the obsessive-compulsive client may decide to allocate their time very differently and make much more room for relaxation and fun. The focus remains on optimal fulfilment of basic needs, taking into account capabilities and circumstances.

By the end of this phase, the following goals should have been achieved:

- Your client can recognize their modes in problem situations and switch back to the Healthy Adult.
- Your client can look back at problem situations and independently make arguments against the Coping and Critical Modes.
- Your client is able to display different behaviours outside the sessions.
- Your client can make significant changes in their life if necessary.

4.6 Treatment plans by disorder

Using the mode model you created, you will tailor the treatment plan specifically to your client. Examples of treatment plans for Dependent, Avoidant and Obsessive-Compulsive Personality Disorder are given below, described as you would explain it to a client. As before, we will use our three case studies of Claire (dependent), Jenny (avoidant) and John (obsessive-compulsive) to represent the three cluster C personality disorders.

4.6.1 Dependent Personality Disorder

Treatment plan: Claire

Your treatment aims to support Subordinate Claire to increase her autonomy and independence. As a result, she will discover that she can do much more for herself than she currently thinks. Under the influence of the Strict One, you have come to think you are worthless and stupid, but that is not true at all. We will fight this Punitive Side of you, the Strict One, until she gives up. At the same time, we will be speaking to the Clown and the Pleaser because they are still very active in helping you avoid bad feelings. During your childhood, you learned that these were the best ways to satisfy your parents. But now that you're an adult, those same sides of you often get in the way of you going your own way or discovering what you want and are able to do.

Those sides of you say you may never get angry either, because that would only scare off other people. I have said before that anger is a normal, human emotion and that it is very healthy to be able to get angry. In the second half of your therapy, you will learn that anger is also a normal part of being human, and how and when to express it.

We are going to strengthen the Healthy Adult so that it can help you get better and better at making your own choices in life and supporting Little Claire when she is struggling. Happy Claire will also get much more space. When you know what you want and what you like better, you can also enjoy your happy and creative side more.

These are our objectives. The therapy will take two years: forty weekly sessions in the first year and ten monthly sessions in the second. In the first twenty or so sessions, we will focus on the childhood causes of the Strict One, the Clown and the Pleaser as we described them in your case conceptualization. The main emphasis will be on having you experience now what you missed then. To do that, we will often use imagery exercises to go back to the past and make →

sure that what you lacked as a child is recognized and validated. We will also use chairs to address different sides of you and to do roleplay, and we will explore and change your thought processes. You don't know how to do that yet, so I will take an active role in the initial phase.

The middle phase consists of twenty sessions, also once a week. In this phase, I will coach you to play an increasingly active role in the exercises I mentioned before. You will slowly take over full control, but I will keep giving you tips along the way. In this phase, we will also actively work on behavioural change; after all, for the therapy to work you will eventually have to do things differently in your everyday life. You will learn step-by-step how your Healthy Adult can tackle things in an independent way.

In the final phase, which is in the second year, you will mostly work independently on change; and you will come and discuss how things are going with me once a month for ten sessions.

4.6.2 Avoidant Personality Disorder

Treatment plan: Jenny

Your treatment is designed to let Lonely, Shy Jenny discover her needs. At this point, you don't really know what you want and think because you've always had to suppress your own feelings, needs and opinions. You've often felt lonely because others always demanded a great deal of attention for their complaints and problems, and there was no attention left for you. We're going to make sure that you start fulfilling your needs much better without feeling guilty. This will help you feel less gloomy and anxious.

The Prosecutor always makes you think that it's your fault if others don't feel good, and that you're a burden to others if you ask for something for yourself. That isn't true, and we're going to fight the Prosecutor's ideas until you get enough space for yourself – space to discover what you need, what you think, and what you want for yourself. You are a sensitive woman who quickly picks up signals from others that things are going badly for them. That's why we're also going to work on making you less quick to act on that, and to start to understand more what your boundaries are.

We will ask the sides of you that protect you from the Prosecutor – the Silent One and the Cocoon – to step aside. You used to really need those sides to cope with your insecure mother and sick father. But now they're getting in the way of social contact with other people and preventing you from feeling or expressing your own needs.

→

The Cocoon does make you feel good in the short term, but it has also led to drinking too much alcohol in the past. Fortunately, that's no longer the case, but you do have other ways to get that feeling, like watching TV series late into the night. With this, the Cocoon continues to keep you away from other activities and also from other people.

The Silent One tries to prevent other people from finding out that you're awkward or even self-centred. It does this by making you stand out as little as possible and avoiding social situations. Because of this, you're now often literally silent – you hardly even dare to speak to me or ask me for anything. The Silent One also prevents me from discovering what is going on inside you, so I will ask the Silent One to give you more space to talk about your feelings. The Silent One may also try to cancel our appointments at times, but I want to encourage you to come to every session.

The Prosecutor, the Silent One and the Cocoon were all created in your childhood because you grew up in circumstances where your basic needs were not met.

Finally, there is also Grumpy Jenny, who is irritated but never dares to really get angry, because then the Blaming Side immediately becomes active. In the second half of treatment, you will learn how to deal with anger. We will strengthen your Healthy Adult side so she can help you get better and better at expressing yourself, standing up for your opinions and making sure your needs are met. That side will also help Little Jenny become less lonely, because she gets to know new people and learns to manage friendships better. Happy Jenny will also be encouraged to start experimenting with new things to discover what suits her and what she enjoys. You will only realize what enjoyment and fun are once you start doing that more often.

These are our objectives. The therapy will take two years: forty weekly sessions in the first year and ten monthly sessions in the second. In the first twenty or so sessions, we will focus on the childhood causes of the Prosecutor, the Silent One and the Cocoon as we described them in your case conceptualization. The main emphasis will be on having you experience now what you missed then. To do that, we will often use imagination exercises to go back to the past and make sure that what you lacked is recognized and validated. We will also use chairs to address different sides of you and to do roleplay, and we will explore and change your thought processes. You don't know how to do that yet, so I will take an active role in the initial phase.

The middle phase consists of twenty sessions, also once a week. In this phase, I will coach you to play an increasingly active role in the exercises I mentioned before. You will slowly take over full control, but I will keep giving you tips along the way. In this phase, we will also actively work on behavioural change; after all, for the therapy to work you will eventually have to do things differently in your everyday life. You will learn step-by-step how your Healthy Adult can tackle things in an independent way.

In the final phase, which is in the second year, you will mostly work independently on change; and you will come and discuss how things are going with me once a month.

4.6.3 Obsessive-Compulsive-Personality Disorder

Treatment plan: John

Your treatment is designed to let Little John discover what he needs. You are always so hard at work and busy making sure you do everything perfectly that you hardly ever relax. You get tired and you can no longer feel clearly what your real needs are. You also notice in your relationship with your wife Laura and with others that it bothers them that you pay so little attention to feelings. This often leaves you alone. In fact, you feel lonely; you just don't notice it very often because you're constantly busy.

Your Demanding Side plays a major role in this. He says that you always have to do everything perfectly, and finishing the work always takes priority over everything else. He sets the bar way too high, and he is never really satisfied with what you do. There is no room at all for relaxation or fun. Because of this, we're going to make sure that this side of you is restrained, and that you learn to set realistic goals for yourself.

There are three sides of you that help make sure you aren't on the receiving end of demands and admonishments from the Demanding Side, and that you don't feel how tired you are sometimes. They are the Perfectionist and the Fusspot on one hand, and the Focus on the other. We'll engage with those sides to make sure they work less hard.

We'll say to the Perfectionist that in reality it isn't possible to do everything perfectly your whole life – if you try, you'll end up burned out and divorced. The Fusspot might know all the rules inside out, but that's no reason to criticize or look down on those who don't. That often comes across as arrogant or pedantic, which can offend people.

The Focus does give you a good feeling in the short term. He distracts you from unpleasant feelings by working even harder, but as a result, you don't notice how lonely you are. It's no surprise that you think this is normal, because you haven't learned to pay attention to feelings or that there is a place for relaxation and fun. After all, there was none of this in your childhood home. Your parents' lives consisted only of hard work, doing everything right and always being reasonable →

and fair. You were their only child, so they put all their energy into teaching you the same philosophy. And if you didn't succeed, they criticized you, which can sometimes make you feel like a failure.

This also sometimes makes you angry when you feel that too much is asked of you and others don't always follow the rules. That's Angry John. But it seems unreasonable to you to get really angry, so you end up swallowing your anger but continuing to sulk.

We will strengthen the Healthy Adult so he can help you get better and better at setting realistic goals and having time for relaxation and fun. That means we will also make room for Relaxed, Free John. The Healthy Adult can also make sure that your needs for more and better contact with other people are met. We will also invite your wife a few times, if you consent, to discuss how you can improve your relationship.

These are our objectives. The therapy will take two years: forty weekly sessions in the first year and ten monthly sessions in the second. In the first twenty or so sessions, we will focus on the childhood causes of your Demanding Side, the Perfectionist, The Fusspot and the Focus as we described them in your case conceptualization. The main emphasis will be on having you experience now what you missed then. To do that, we will often use imagination exercises to go back to the past and make sure that what you lacked is recognized and validated. We will also use chairs to address different sides of you and to do roleplay, and we will explore and change your thought processes. You don't know how to do that yet, so I will take an active role in the initial phase.

The middle phase consists of twenty sessions, also once a week. In this phase, I will coach you to play an increasingly active role in the exercises I mentioned before. You will slowly take over full control, but I will keep giving you tips along the way. In this phase, we will also actively work on behavioural change; after all, for the therapy to work you will eventually have to do things differently in your everyday life. You will learn step-by-step how your Healthy Adult can tackle things in an independent way.

In the final phase, which is in the second year, you will mostly work independently on change; and you will come and discuss how things are going with me once a month.

4.7 Pause for evaluation

The period of transition from case conceptualization plus treatment plan to actually beginning the therapy is a good time to discuss again with your client what will change and what effort it will take. It is also important to reiterate the benefits of this change.

Clients who are very dependent on others sometimes cannot imagine life as a Healthy Adult, in which they decide important things for themselves. In particular, this tends to cause anxiety when it comes to functioning independently and changing behaviour. There may also be a fear of how others will react. If this is the case, you can revisit the reasons why the client sought help and reiterate the choice of schema therapy. There will sometimes be people around your client who actually benefit from their dependent behaviour, and who may therefore try to sabotage your efforts, consciously or otherwise. You can invite such people (often family members) to a conversation with the client to investigate where their resistance lies. Try to explain the client's problem to them, and why change not only means an improvement for the client but also for them.

Clients who are very avoidant will often feel inferior or unsuccessful and don't want to say what is going on within them. They are afraid that you, like others, will judge or reject them. This not infrequently leads to cancelling or coming late to meetings, so it is important to stimulate clients to always come to sessions. Explain that they can always discuss with you why they found something difficult or what made them anxious. Often, avoidant clients do not really know what their feelings and needs are, because they have never had space to discover them. Getting in touch with their feelings and needs can be stressful and frightening, so it is important to explain that it will be done in small steps.

Obsessive-compulsive clients often tend to elaborate on all topics in detail. You will have noticed this in the case conceptualization phase. This is the time to explain to the client that you will often interrupt them, because the process of therapy is not about them doing everything perfectly. You predict that they will find it very difficult to work less hard while also not yet having a very good sense of what to do instead. Indeed, they will have to learn to do nothing useful once in a while and, at first, they are likely to experience this as unpleasant. Explain that they will only learn to appreciate this gradually.

Discussing the treatment plan and taking a moment for evaluation is not a requirement, but is an important aspect of therapy because this is when you make clear what is going to change and how much time the client has available to do it. This is important not only for your client but also for you as the therapist, because clients with a cluster C disorder tend to delay change. Some therapists even have cluster C traits themselves, which can lead to treatments sometimes going on endlessly without meaningful results. Because of this, it is important that you too, as the therapist, commit to the treatment plan.

4.8 Chapter summary

This chapter has described how to make the transition from the diagnostic phase to the treatment phase. A treatment plan should describe both the goals of the treatment (the 'what') and the techniques (the 'how'). For cluster C clients in particular, it is important also to include the treatment duration and what is involved in each phase (the 'when'). Finally, using the case studies of Claire (dependent), Jenny (avoidant) and John (obsessive-compulsive), we have briefly explored what an individualized treatment plan looks like.

Chapter 5: Dependent Personality Disorder

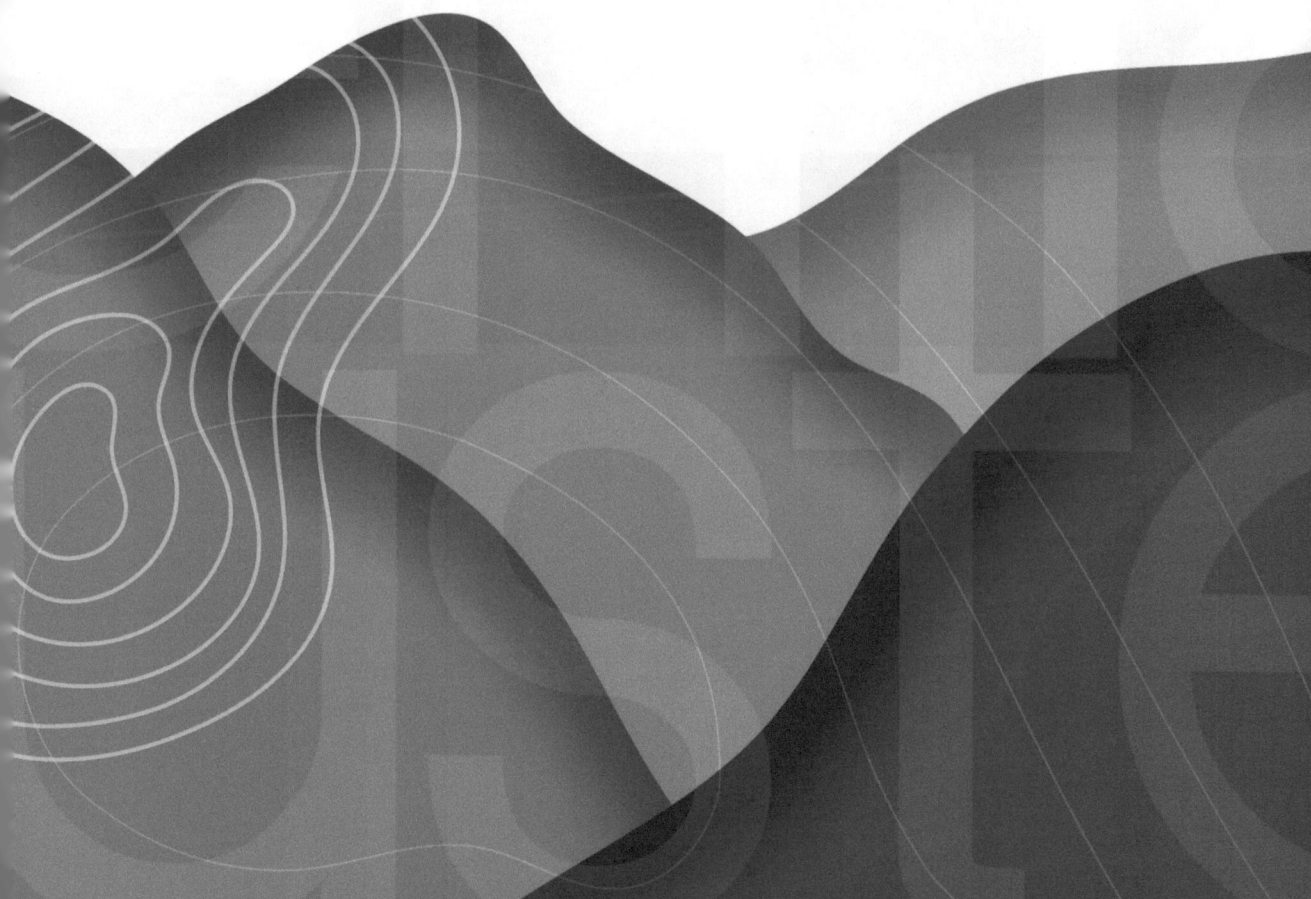

Chapter 5: Dependent Personality Disorder

Chapter map
5.1 Introduction
5.2 The Punitive Mode
5.3 Imagery rescripting with the Punitive Mode
5.4 Coping Modes
5.5 Historical roleplay with the Compliant Surrenderer
5.6 Sticking points in historical roleplay
5.7 The Dependent Child
5.8 Stimulating anger in the Dependent Child
5.9 Chapter summary

5.1 Introduction

This chapter describes the objectives of the treatment of Dependent Personality Disorder – which, in short, is to encourage dependent clients to increase their autonomy and independence. To achieve this, it is necessary to silence the client's Punitive Mode, which will be undermining any attempt at autonomy. At the same time, the client's Coping Modes (in Claire, our case study of Dependent Personality Disorder, these are the Clown and the Pleaser) will have to become less active, as these modes hinder the development of self-identity, independence and self-confidence.

In Chapter 4 we described Claire's treatment plan. We will now describe how we work towards establishing treatment goals for Claire in the initial phase of therapy.

5.2 The Punitive Mode

Claire has a Punitive Mode, the Strict One. This is the result of a childhood in which her father often criticized her and was very strict. When Claire is in her Punitive Mode, she believes she is stupid and ugly and does everything wrong. Furthermore, she thinks she is unable to cope with the world, which is full of dangers, and where something bad can easily happen – people getting angry, falling sick or having accidents. She got that idea from her mother, who was herself always extremely afraid of diseases and accidents.

One of the goals of therapy is to fight the Punitive Mode. As the therapist, you will have to take the lead in the early stages of treatment. You cannot yet assume that there is a Healthy Adult who is able to do that on their own. Schema therapy offers you various methods and techniques to counter the client's internalized punitive messages.

> **Methods and techniques to tackle the Punitive Mode**
> - Imagery rescripting, in which you use imagination to confront the antagonists who gave your client these messages.
> - Chairwork, in which you put the Punitive Mode on a separate chair and contradict it.
> - Historical roleplay, in which you re-enact significant situations from the client's past that contributed to forming the Punitive Mode, and demonstrate healthy parenting.
> - Cognitive techniques, in which you explore and adjust the client's negative self-image.

In the next section, we will describe how you can use imagery rescripting when dealing with the Punitive Mode.

5.3 Imagery rescripting with the Punitive Mode

The core of imagery rescripting is visualizing and processing significant events to generate corrective emotional experiences. There are different ways in which you can arrive at those meaningful images or memories. Sometimes, your client will spontaneously talk about such memories, in which case you can ask them to close their eyes and describe a memory as if they were reliving it. At other times, it is more difficult to access these meaningful memories.

Dependent clients sometimes find it very difficult to visualize memories from their childhood in which they lacked something, feeling a strong loyalty to their parents or even a sense of guilt when doing so. In such cases, a clear rationale for and structure of the exercise can help to reach those images.

Imagery rescripting step-by-step
Step 1: Introduce imagery rescripting and negotiate with the Coping Mode.
Step 2: Imagine a 'Good Place'.
Step 3: Unpleasant situation in the present.
Step 4: Affect bridge to the past.
Step 5: Explore meaningful experiences in the past.
Step 6: Rescript these meaningful images.
Step 7: Return to the 'Good Place' (if desired).
Step 8: Review and homework.

This step-by-step plan is not a mandatory script. It is more of a suggestion for how you can find your way in this experiential exercise. We explain these steps in more detail below.

5.3.1 Step 1: Introduce imagery rescripting and negotiate with the Coping Mode

You have already done diagnostic imagery work in the case conceptualization phase. As a result, you will not be introducing the idea of an imagery exercise for the first time. Still, a brief introduction is important to give an anxious client a sense of safety and predictability. You should also give an idea of approximately how long the exercise will take, as while clients clearly do find value in such exercises, research has shown that an unpredictable duration can be stressful (Ten Napel-Schutz et al, 2011). When explaining the exercise, don't forget to include a message of hope for the client's recovery. Explain that the aim of this exercise is not to ruminate on unpleasant experiences, but to use them to generate a healing experience that will make your client feel better.

Example of introducing imagery rescripting

Claire has an appointment with the dentist. Normally, her boyfriend would accompany her because Claire often has panic attacks in these kinds of situations. However, he has his own problems and is not always available. He has said that he will not go this time, and because of this Claire is very anxious about the appointment. She has just told you that she really doesn't think she can go alone and is considering cancelling it.

>>**Therapist:** "I can hear how out of sorts you are. You really are very scared to go to the dentist now that your boyfriend can't come along, aren't you?"

>>**Claire:** "Yeah, I really don't think I can do it… What if something goes wrong, or I'm in a lot of pain? Would I still be able to get home safely? And if something does end up going wrong, I really won't know what to do…"

>>**Therapist:** "I can imagine how uncomfortable you'll feel without your boyfriend coming with you when you wanted him to. And I can see that you're very upset about this. That's why I'd like to do an exercise. It will help us understand what is affecting you so much, but it will also allow me to help you feel a bit better, too."

>>**Claire:** "Oh, what is it?"

>>**Therapist:** "Well, I'd like to do an imagination exercise with you. We already did this during one of our first conversations, do you remember? I asked you to keep your eyes closed for ten minutes."

>>**Claire:** "Oh yes, I remember, but that was quite stressful at the time. I don't know if I can take that on top of everything now. It's already so much."

>>**Therapist:** "I hear your tension and stress. But I'd like to emphasize again that this exercise will really benefit you – not only by helping you to better understand what's going on, but also by actually making you feel better. Maybe I should start by explaining a bit about what we'll do next. I think it's nice to know what to expect."

Because you will now be processing and rescripting the images, rather than just exploring them as you did in the diagnostic phase, it is important to explain the procedure briefly before you start. Most clients will welcome an exercise in which you appear confident, but some will have doubts and may require a bit more explanation. These doubts are often about whether the exercise will trigger negative emotions for them, or whether it is possible for an imagery exercise about past events to have a healing effect in the present. This doubt and resistance is an expression of the client's Coping Mode, and you will have to negotiate with it to perform the exercise.

Arguments in the negotiation with the Coping Mode
- Research has shown that this is an effective method.
- We have all had the experience that it's nice to fantasize about how things might have worked out differently.
- Your head is filled with unpleasant experiences, and, with this exercise, we will be able to replace them with healthier, more pleasant experiences.
- I know the idea sounds strange – but I would rather do something that can help you than avoid it just because you think it's unlikely to work. I think you and your symptoms are much too important to neglect anything that might be helpful.

Example of negotiation about imagery rescripting

>>Therapist: "In a moment, I'll ask you to keep your eyes closed for about ten minutes. It isn't hypnosis – you'll stay completely in control, and you can open your eyes at any time if you want to. Keeping your eyes closed is only a way to concentrate better on what you're feeling and what images come up. I'd like to start with the dentist situation, because I can hear how much it bothers you. But I think it isn't the only situation that's bothering you. I think this fear might also have something to do with previous experiences in your life. And because of this, I'll ask you during the exercise to concentrate mainly on the feeling you had in the situation regarding the dentist, and to look at what images or memories from your past come to mind."

>>Claire: "Oh no, so I also have to think back to unpleasant events? I really don't want to do that. I'll completely panic, and I already feel really bad."

>>Therapist: "It's true that I'll ask you to let images come up from your past, yes. But it's not only to understand where those fears come from. With this exercise, I actually want to change those images. To make it into a positive, enjoyable experience."

>>Claire: "But surely that isn't realistic?! I mean, I know what actually happened, and that can't be changed."

>>Therapist: "I know it might sound strange if you haven't experienced it yet. But research has shown that this really is a very effective technique. It's understandable that you wonder how it can help, because, of course, you can't change the past..."

(Claire nods.)

>>Therapist: "But when you imagine something very vividly, it isn't just a thought, it's a real experience. You must have had this sort of experience before, of thinking back to a situation earlier in the day and imagining what you might have done differently, or what you should have said. And maybe having that vivid fantasy made you feel just a bit like you really had done things differently. Does that sound reasonable?"

> **Claire:** (*hesitantly*) "Yes, maybe sometimes…"
>
> **Therapist:** "Look, your head is full of events and experiences of feeling bad, anxious, insecure or criticized. With this exercise, we can give you some different experiences – experiences that can actually make you feel stronger, more powerful. And you can then carry that feeling with you for a while after the exercise. How does that sound?"
>
> **Claire:** "Yeah, it sounds all right, but it still sounds very strange. And I don't know if I can handle it."
>
> **Therapist:** "Well, I think you can handle it easily, but I also want you to know that you don't have to do it all by yourself. I'm going to help you. I'll guide you through the exercise. Shall we just give it a try? Then we can see afterwards how you felt about it."
>
> **Claire:** "Yes, okay then. But what do I have to do?"

5.3.2 Step 2: Imagine a 'Good Place'

It isn't absolutely necessary to start the exercise by finding a 'Good Place' – a memory that is comforting for the client. The essence of imagery rescripting is in processing significant, sometimes traumatic, memories. Nevertheless, using a Good Place to start from can help make the exercise a success. Firstly, visualizing a Good Place is a way to 'warm up' and ease into the exercise. Your client gets a chance to practise evoking images before they need to specifically evoke traumatic images. The image of a Good Place also gives an opportunity to regulate the emotions that come up in a healthy way.

You may have noticed that we are talking about a 'Good Place' and not the 'Safe Place' often mentioned in other literature (van Genderen & Arntz, 2021). Asking to visualize a Safe Place focuses the exercise mainly on the basic need for safety. A Good Place, however, can provide space for images that meet the client's basic needs other than safety. For Claire, safety may be a relevant basic need, but connectedness might be a much more important one. Similarly, for an obsessive-compulsive client like John, an image of freedom, with room for relaxation, might be more appropriate.

Help the client to make the image as realistic as possible. To do this, take the time to have them insert themselves into the image. As therapists, we sometimes go a bit faster than ideal, and in doing so we don't give clients the time that they really need. To avoid this, ask in detail about sensory information, such as what your client sees, what sounds they hear and what smells they notice. You can also ask them to physically turn their head a little and, during that movement, to 'look around' the space they are visualizing.

Example of imagining a 'Good Place'

>>Therapist: "First, just assume a calm, relaxed posture, so you're not too distracted by being uncomfortable or the position of your body during the exercise."

(Claire sits up a little straighter.)

>>Therapist: "Now I'd like to ask you to close your eyes and keep them closed for the next ten to fifteen minutes."

(Claire closes her eyes.)

>>Therapist: "Take a deep breath, and just take a moment to be aware of your feet on the ground… the chair beneath you, and your breathing. You don't have to change anything about it, just notice that your breathing has its own rhythm. Sometimes a little faster, sometimes a little slower. And from this position, I'd like to ask you to let the image of a Good Place come to mind. This can be any place, as long as you feel comfortable there. And once you have an image, can you tell me what you see?"

>>Claire: "At home on the sofa."

>>Therapist: "Okay, just take a moment to look around calmly. Or maybe turn your head a little from left to right, and with your mind's eye, look around the room where you're sitting. What do you see now?"

>>Claire: "The sofa, with some soft cushions snuggled comfortably against me. The cat is on my lap. The TV is on. The curtains are closed, and some candles are lit. *(While describing the image, Claire turns her head, as if looking around the room.)*

>>Therapist: "And are you there alone or do you see anyone else?"

>>Claire: "No, my boyfriend is there too."

>>Therapist: "And where is he sitting? Is he to your left or your right?"

>>Claire: "He's sitting to my right, nice and close to me, and holding my hand."

>>Therapist: "Are there any particular sounds that come to you now that you're here?"

>>Claire: "Yes, maybe the sounds of the TV, some adverts or something…"

>>Therapist: "And how do you feel now, sitting here on the sofa, with your boyfriend holding your hand, the cat on your lap and the candles lit?"

>>Claire: "Nice and relaxed, nice and safe."

>>**Therapist:** "Just enjoy this feeling. Where exactly do you feel it in your body, that relaxed, safe feeling?"

>>**Claire:** "Here… (*puts her hands on her belly.*) In my belly."

>>**Therapist:** "Good, just keep your hand there for a while and enjoy that nice feeling."

5.3.3 Step 3: Unpleasant situation in the present

Next, make the transition to the recent, schema-activating event. Take time for the transition and to build the visual image of that event. Visual images bring up emotional responses (Holmes, 2010), and carefully building these visual images will increase the emotional impact of the exercise, which is ultimately what you want to achieve.

Example of visualizing an unpleasant situation in the present

>>**Therapist:** "Okay, so I want to ask you to let go of this image now. Let it fade a bit. We'll get back to it in a moment, but right now I'd like you to make some space for other images. I want to ask you to focus your thoughts on the situation we were just talking about, the dentist. And the moment when your boyfriend said that he isn't feeling well so he can't go with you. Think about that scenario – do you see it now?"

(*Claire nods.*)

>>**Therapist:** "Just pause the picture for a moment, and describe what you see, so I can have a look at it too."

>>**Claire:** "He says that he's not going along."

>>**Therapist:** "Where do you see him now? To your left, or to your right? Or is he right in front of you?"

>>**Claire:** "To the left, in front of me."

>>**Therapist:** "Turn your head so you can look straight at him now."

(*Claire turns her head slightly to the left.*)

>>**Therapist:** "And now just look at his face when he says he isn't coming along. What do you see?"

>>**Claire:** "I see that he isn't feeling quite right, he looks so worried."

>>**Therapist:** "What about him shows you that? Is it his eyes? Or something else?"

>>**Claire:** "He looks tired – he has bags under his eyes, and he looks a bit dull. I immediately worry about him, but I also feel the panic rising in myself."

>>**Therapist:** "And where do you feel that panic in your body?"

(Claire clutches at her chest.)

>>**Therapist:** "So your boyfriend sees you now, and he says to you that he isn't coming, and you feel panic rising in your chest. And what's going through your mind? What is it that you are so afraid of?"

>>**Claire:** "That it will all go completely wrong. That I won't know what to do. That I won't be able to handle it."

5.3.4 Step 4: Affect bridge to the past

Visualizing a recent unpleasant situation in this way is intended to re-trigger the schema activation that took place at the time. The experience of that schema activation, with all its cognitive, emotional and physiological components, can create a bridge to the original events that led to the formation of the schema(s).

Your goal in visualizing the recent unpleasant situation is not yet to offer a corrective, healing experience. Don't be too afraid to make your client emotional, as it is precisely these emotions that will contribute to a successful exercise.

Example of affect bridge to the past

>>**Therapist:** "I hear that you're feeling very miserable when you imagine this situation, but I still want you to stay in touch with it for a moment. And check with yourself: is this the first time you've had this feeling, or do you recognize it from before? Is there something familiar about it?"

>>**Claire:** "Yes, I know it very well. I've always felt that…"

>>**Therapist:** "Okay, then it's not just this situation with the dentist and your boyfriend not coming with you that makes you feel this way – it's also an old feeling from the past. Let the image fade a little now and concentrate on the feeling. And just let images or memories come up of situations from your past in which you experienced the same feeling in one way or another."

>>**Claire:** "Well, I can't think of anything now."

>>**Therapist:** "Do you mean it's hard for you to think back on it because you think it won't be much fun to do it?"

(Claire nods.)

Clients sometimes struggle to let images from the past arise. This can be because the emotions associated with them are too intense. The difficulty in bringing such images to mind is therefore due to a form of avoidance behaviour, conscious or otherwise. One possible strategy to gain access to those images is to start with more neutral, less triggering images and to gradually make them more emotional. For example, you can first ask your client to visualize one of the childhood photos that they brought in during the case conceptualization phase. With this done, it then becomes possible to place the parents or other significant attachment figures into the picture with the child that your client now sees, and to being to trigger the emotional interactions in this way.

> **Example of visualizing a neutral situation**
>
> **>>Therapist:** "First just think about that photo of the little girl you used to be. Remember, the picture that we looked at together here?"
>
> *(Claire nods.)*
>
> **>>Therapist:** "Just take a look at that picture in your mind's eye and describe it for me. Describe the girl for me that you see in that picture…"
>
> **>>Claire:** "Well… She's about six years old, she's wearing a dress…"
>
> **>>Therapist:** "And how does she look, is she happy or not?"
>
> **>>Claire:** "No, she is not happy, she seems a bit sad…"
>
> **>>Therapist:** "And do you understand why she's sad?"
>
> **>>Claire:** "Yes, it could be something to do with Mum… That Mum feels bad or something…"
>
> **>>Therapist:** "So can you put your mother there now, with that girl?"
>
> *(Claire nods.)*

5.3.5 Step 5: Explore meaningful experiences in the past

Again, take your time to let the image build up. Even if your client is already emotional when the image is mentioned, it is still important to take the time to have them describe the image. For instance, you can ask to 'pause' the image, creating some time for the image to be described. In the example, Claire has an observer perspective, meaning that she is looking at the little girl and her mother like an outside observer. This perspective is useful in order to easily get some information about the context. 'How old is the child you see there?', you might ask. 'Where do you see them standing?'

Example of exploring meaningful experiences in the past

>>**Therapist:** "So now you see that little girl and your mother opposite her. Where are they? What do you see around them?"

>>**Claire:** "They are in the living room. Mum is sitting on the sofa, and I'm standing there in front of her like this."

>>**Therapist:** "Can you point them out, so I know where you see them?"

(*Claire gestures to a spot in front of her.*)

>>**Therapist:** "And what kind of light is it, is it daytime?"

>>**Claire:** "Yes, daytime, it is light."

>>**Therapist:** "And what does your mother say now, or what does she do that makes that girl so sad? What do you see happening?"

>>**Claire:** "Mum is scared."

>>**Therapist:** "How can you tell she is scared?"

>>**Claire:** "Her eyes look so, so scared. And she is nervous."

>>**Therapist:** "And what is Mum afraid of?"

>>**Claire:** "Mum is afraid that something will happen to me."

Ultimately, you want the client to place themselves into the perspective of the child they see in front of them. That first-person perspective, from the child's point of view, will provoke a stronger emotional experience.

Example of exploring meaningful experiences in the past – continued

>>**Therapist:** (*in a slightly softer voice, as if talking to a little girl*) "Just be that little girl now. Hey, Claire, Mum is afraid that something might happen to you. But why is she so afraid of that now?"

>>**Claire:** "I actually want to go play with my friend. And I said that too, but then Mum got all scared and now she is talking about all the things that could go wrong."

>>**Therapist:** "How does her voice sound as she says that?"

>>**Claire:** "She sounds very tense, very worried. And she says she doesn't want anything to happen to me, and that my friend lives so far away and anything could happen."

In the exercise, there is now an image of Claire as a little girl together with her overprotective mother. The mother in the picture is a punitive antagonist. She may not be as angry as Claire's father could have been, but, through her overprotectiveness, her mother does punish Claire's need for autonomy. There is a clear message in her over-anxiety, which Claire hears: 'The world is full of dangers, and you can't handle them.'

5.3.6 Step 6: Rescript these meaningful images

The aim of the exercise from here is to change the visualized events into a healthier, healing experience. As such, you must make a choice as to when to step into the picture. What is the best point in the visualized events for you to intervene? One study has shown that late intervention, just before the most traumatic parts of the memory, is more effective than early intervention (Dibbets & Arntz, 2016). This indicates that we should not be too afraid of the emotions evoked when visualizing traumatic events, and the right moment for intervention is best determined by your client's level of emotional arousal and their Window of Tolerance. You should therefore aim to make the image as emotional as possible so that it can generate a corrective, healing experience; but at the same time, you must ensure that the emotions evoked are still (just) tolerable for the client. For example, regularly ask the client how they are feeling and note any non-verbal emotional signals. While they may be emotional, all the time they are still responding to your questions they are still in touch with you and they are still (just) within their Window of Tolerance (Krans, 2022, personal communication).

> **Example of rescripting meaningful images**
>
> **>>Therapist:** "How is it for you to hear all that?"
>
> **>>Claire:** "Not great." (*Voice begins to quiver a little and she bows her head.*)
>
> **>>Therapist:** "And what is that 'not-great' feeling?"
>
> (*Claire starts crying.*)
>
> **>>Therapist:** "Claire, what is that not-great feeling? Is it sadness?"
>
> **>>Claire:** "What?"
>
> **>>Therapist:** "Okay, I don't think that's a good situation for a six-year-old girl. I want to step in to help you. Can you put me there now? Ideally, I'd like to stand between you and Mum. Do you see me?"
>
> **>>Claire:** "I don't know... maybe... I don't know."

If the emotions evoked are too strong, the client may move outside their Window of Tolerance. Then it becomes difficult, if not impossible, for them to experience the rescripting. In such situations, the emotions evoked will need to become a little less intense. Ask the client to focus on sensory experiences – hearing your voice, feeling the chair beneath them the ground under their feet. You could also ask them to open their eyes for a moment so they can see you and the space around them.

> ### Example of making emotions less intense
>
> **>>Therapist:** "No problem. Just listen to my voice, and while you're listening to my voice, try to remember what I look like. Do you see me now, as you hear my voice?"
>
> **>>Claire:** "A little… maybe…"
>
> **>>Therapist:** "Otherwise, just open your eyes."
>
> (*Claire opens her eyes.*)
>
> **>>Therapist:** "Just look at me for a moment. Do you see my face, my eyes?"
>
> **>>Claire:** "Yes."
>
> **>>Therapist:** "And what do you see when you look at me like that? How do I look? Do I look angry, or do I look understanding. Do I look hard, or do I look soft?"
>
> **>>Claire:** "Soft. As if you want to help me. Sympathetic."
>
> **>>Therapist:** "Great! Because that's what I feel too, I sympathize very much. That's why I want to help you. Look at my face again for a moment, and now close your eyes again. Take the image of me, with that soft look on my face, with you. Do you see me now, between you and Mum?"
>
> (*Claire nods.*)

There are no set rules for rescripting the image. You can address the antagonist first, or the child. You decide whether to choose one or the other based on the relevant basic needs and the client's level of emotional arousal, and whether your client tolerates your intervention. When there is serious insecurity, it is preferable to provide safety first and to address the antagonist. However, if your client is already very tense but there is no immediate threat of insecurity, it is preferable to start by thinking of the child's emotions in the image. In Claire's example, there is no direct lack of safety from the mother's side. Claire is very tense and anxious, though, and she has already had difficulty placing the therapist into the picture. In this case, you may therefore choose to dwell on the emotions evoked first and calm Claire down a little with compassion and understanding. You will also help to adjust the activated schemas by offering realistic considerations.

Example of rescripting aimed at the child

>>Therapist: "Hey Claire, I'm here now because I can see you're sad when your Mum talks about everything that could go wrong, about all the risks. And I don't think that's a good thing for anyone, and certainly not for you. Of course, her worries make you sad and anxious. I'd feel that way too, if I was you. You want to go play with a friend, and Mum starts talking about all the dangers out there. And then she says you can't go. It seems quite normal to feel anxious and sad about that. Does that make sense at all?

>>Claire: "Yes."

>>Therapist: "I understand all of that very well, Claire. And that's why I also want to say something to your mother."

Try to make your interventions as realistic as possible. By turning away from the client in the direction of the visualized antagonist, your client will hear from the change in your voice that you are no longer speaking to them but to the antagonist. If you also try to use a different tone of voice when you do this, the experience that you are addressing someone else becomes even more realistic. You will speak more clearly, perhaps more firmly, to the antagonist, than when you turn back to your client in the role of the child.

Example of rescripting aimed at the antagonist

(The therapist now turns away from Claire and talks towards the place where Claire's mother is standing in the image, opposite Claire, using a reasonable but clear tone.)

>>Therapist: "Claire's mother, I hear that you're doing your best to take very good care of Claire. You're trying to make sure nothing happens to her, is that right?"

(The therapist now turns back to Claire.)

>>Therapist: *(in a soft tone)* "And what does Mum say?"

>>Claire: "Mum says that yes, she's trying very hard. She is very afraid that something will happen to me and she would feel terrible about it, and that's why she's trying to be so careful."

>>Therapist: *(turns back to Claire's mother, again using a clear tone)* "And I think that's really very nice and sweet of you. But you know, you are caring so hard that there's actually no room left at all for Claire and what she really needs. Of course she needs to be safe, but she also needs room to discover the world and all the fun things there are in it. My concern is that you are so focused on safety that there is no room left for a bit of independence. Claire needs to learn that she can already do quite a lot herself, and that she can learn to rely on herself and not just on you."

(The therapist turns back towards Claire.)

> **Therapist:** "How does Mum react to what I'm saying now? Does she understand it a little bit when I talk about those needs other than safety?"
>
> **Claire:** "Yes, I think she would get that... yes, she does."
>
> **Therapist:** "And how do you feel when you hear me speak like this? Does it all make a bit of sense?"
>
> **Claire:** "Yes, I get it. It's kind of crazy how you stand up for me. But it's also great..."

5.3.7 Step 7: Return to the 'Good Place' (if desired)

Before asking the client to let go of the image, allow some time for this corrective experience to have its full effect. If the client has indicated that they like how you stand up for them, ask about all the aspects of that experience. Where do they feel that pleasant sensation in their body? What words fit that feeling? Which part of the rescripting mainly gave them that pleasant feeling? The time and attention you spend on the healing experience helps to consolidate the experience, and it also helps them to remember it.

Depending on how the rescripting goes, you may now decide to recall the image of the Good Place from the start of the exercise. If the imagery rescripting was successful, and the client resolved the unpleasant situation you were working with, then there is no need to do this – the situation itself has been rescripted into a Good Place, and it is enough to gently bring the exercise to an end. However, this did not happen in Claire's example, and she is still in the original situation. An important part of therapy, and of this exercise, is to teach your client a healthy way to regulate emotions. They need to learn the simple lesson that, after stress and tension, there must be some relaxation time to recover.

Another important lesson is that the client can not only bring up unpleasant feelings, but also release them. This is important for some clients, because they are afraid that if they allow painful emotions to come through, they will be unable to let go of them again.

> ### Example of returning to the Good Place
> **Therapist:** "Okay, I want to ask you to let go of this image now. Just let it float away. I want to create some space to go back to that Good Place from just now. What was that Good Place again?"
>
> **Claire:** "You mean at home on the sofa?"

> **Therapist:** "Yes, exactly, at home on the sofa. I want you to think back to that situation and the image of your living room, the sofa, the cat on your lap, your boyfriend just to your right. I want you to imagine that image again."
>
> **Claire:** "I can't stop thinking of my mother…"
>
> **Therapist:** "I understand it's hard to get back to your Good Place, so take your time. Turn your head to your right for a moment; your boyfriend is there. Do you see him?"
>
> **Claire:** "Yes…"
>
> **Therapist:** "Do you feel him sitting close to you? He's holding your hand, isn't he?"
>
> **Claire:** (*smiling*) "Yes."

Using the visual cues you noted at the start of the exercise (Claire's boyfriend to her right, the cat on her lap), you can help your client get back to their Good place. Don't move too quickly to the point at which they open their eyes again and you start the review. Calming down after the intervention is an important part of the exercise, so take some time for it.

5.3.8 Step 8: Review and homework

The review is an important part of the exercise. The client's attention, and yours as the therapist, is often primarily focused on the visualization and the experiences being evoked. Training courses and the literature also focus on the visualization itself. However, visualization and the rescripting of images is primarily intended to generate a corrective emotional experience, and if that experience is to contribute to meaningful change in the future, then it must be consolidated. Discussing the experience and giving meaning to the lessons learned are important ways to achieve this. Not only do you want to provide a healthy and positive experience, but you also want your client to understand what was experienced, its significance and its meaning.

Kick off the review by reminding the client of the reason for doing this exercise, namely that there was a recent situation in which schemas were activated. You now understand much better why the situation was so difficult for the client. No wonder they felt very emotional: not only was it a difficult situation at the time, but on top of that they have just relived it as well as re-experiencing the anguish of the little child they once were.

Your client must learn to look at themselves with more understanding and compassion as a first step towards building a healthier self-image that can counter the image offered by the Punitive Mode. Furthermore, they will have to learn to increasingly internalize the realistic arguments against the Punitive Mode that you have provided. That is why it is important to reiterate those counterarguments in the review, and to make your client aware of the positive emotions that are evoked by this.

These experiences can be further consolidated by giving homework. In this way, you can put the main conclusions you discussed down on paper, like a flashcard. A flashcard such as this could also be a recorded message, an audio flashcard. The advantage of this is that the client hears not only the content, but also hears your voice. If the goal is for your voice and words to become more internalized by the client as a counterpoint to their Punitive Mode, then it is important for that voice and those words to be heard often.

5.4 Coping Modes

One of Claire's Coping Modes is the Pleaser. That is the name given to her Compliant Surrenderer. In this mode, Claire conforms to the wants and needs of others instead of listening to what she needs herself. This is a consequence of a childhood in which she conformed to her critical father, who disapproved of what she did and who she was. It is also a result of the concern she had from a young age for her anxious and worried mother.

One of the goals of Claire's therapy will be to make the Pleaser less strong, so that Claire is better able to feel her own wants and needs. Unlike her Punitive Mode, the Pleaser does not have to be eliminated altogether – after all, there is nothing wrong with caring for significant others or being considerate of their feelings. However, Claire focuses on other people too often and too much, and weakening the Pleaser is therefore important.

Schema therapy offers various methods and techniques to reduce Coping Modes, and to connect with Child Modes.

> **Methods and techniques to address Coping Modes**
> *Experiential techniques:*
> - Chairwork in which the Coping Mode is put on a separate chair.
> - Imagery rescripting in which contact is made directly with the Child Mode.
> - Historical roleplay.

Cognitive techniques:
- Naming the Coping Mode and investigating its advantages and disadvantages.

Therapeutic relationship:
- Directly asking about the feelings of the Child Modes.
- Empathic confrontation with the disadvantages of Coping Modes in the contact.

In the section below, we will describe how to conduct a historical roleplay using the same situation we used for imagery rescripting. In this way, we aim to show that you can use either technique for these kinds of topics and situations.

5.5 Historical roleplay with the Compliant Surrenderer

Historical roleplay is an experiential technique with multiple objectives. First, this technique can provide more insight into the past formation of schemas. The cognitive aspects of these schemas can be identified, and their credibility can be scored. Furthermore, roleplaying provides the client with insight into the interactions between the antagonist and the client as a child. Because you too will participate in the roleplay, you can also gain insights into past interactions between the client and key attachment figures. Finally, roleplaying also offers the opportunity to explore a different course of events. With this, you can offer your client a corrective emotional experience.

In the initial phase of therapy, the client's Healthy Adult is not yet sufficiently developed to generate this experience itself. As a therapist, you will therefore have to stand up for your client's needs, just as you did in imagery rescripting. In the middle and final phases of therapy, your client will learn to stand up for their needs themselves (see Chapter 8).

The historical roleplay technique comprises a number of different elements and steps, and it is therefore quite technically challenging for therapists. Below is an overview of steps you can follow when using it in clinical practice.

Step-by-step plan for historical roleplay in the initial phase
Step 1: Introduce historical roleplay and explore current symptom patterns.
Step 2: Identify a meaningful related event from the past.
Step 3: Re-enact event: client as child; therapist as antagonist.
Step 4: Review first roleplay and identify schemas formed.
Step 5: Re-enact event: client as antagonist; therapist as child.
Step 6: Review second roleplay and identify any schema-refuting information.
Step 7: Re-enact event: client as child; therapist as 'good-enough' parent.
Step 8: Review third roleplay and formation of healthy schemas.
Step 9: Review whole roleplay, consolidation and homework.

5.5.1 Step 1: Introduce historical roleplay and explore current symptom patterns

There are a number of ways to introduce historical roleplay. The simplest way is to announce at the beginning of a session that you will be doing such an exercise at some point within that session. Alternatively, you might choose to weave the exercise into the session more organically, according to what the client brings up.

You might also ask your client a week in advance if they would like to think about a past situation that (partly) led to a particular schema or mode. In Claire's case, the triggers that she often talks about are situations in which she adapted to others' needs or wants, rather than expressing herself. However, the trigger events your client talks about may not only relate to Coping Modes. They might also talk about the feeling of activated Child Modes again, or describe a situation involving experiences related to their Critical Modes.

> **Example of exploring current symptom patterns**
>
> *Claire talks about her boyfriend wanting to visit his family last weekend. Claire didn't much want to do that; she really needed some peace and quiet. When she started to explain that to Jonas, he was clearly disappointed, so she quickly relented and went with him. She was afraid that he would get angry if she had stuck to her preference.*

>>**Therapist:** "So you conformed to what your boyfriend wanted, even though in this situation that meant doing something you didn't want to do. Is that what happened?"

>>**Claire:** "Yes, but I didn't mind, actually! I quite like his family, and we hadn't seen them for a while so…"

>>**Therapist:** "But you said you were looking forward to a quiet weekend, right?"

>>**Claire:** "Yes, that's true, but I mean it wasn't so bad that I went along either."

>>**Therapist:** "Okay, I believe you – that you were fine with it in the end. But I do hear that this was another situation where you let your own needs be pushed aside. And that certainly sounds familiar to me – it's the Claire who is mainly concerned with what others need. (*Now, the therapist gestures to a spot next to Claire.*) So, who am I hearing, when it comes to focusing on what others need? Even when that is at the expense of your own needs?" (*Here, the therapist points to Claire's belly.*)

In the early stages of therapy, you will actively help the client to recognize their different modes. However, if your client lacks autonomy, you might choose occasions from their past about which they can independently contribute ideas and thoughts, without necessarily creating the expectation that they should already have all the answers. In this way, you encourage self-expression and autonomy.

Example of exploring current symptom patterns – continued

>>**Claire:** "I think that myself, don't I?"

>>**Therapist:** "Yes, I understand that you really believe so. But I mean more: which side of you is always trying to please others to avoid them getting angry or otherwise feeling bad? For myself, I think this is the Pleaser. Could that be true?"

>>**Claire:** "Yeah, it could be, yes."

>>**Therapist:** "Yes? Where do you recognize the Pleaser in what happened this week?"

>>**Claire:** "Well, I actually wanted to stay home, but went along anyway."

>>**Therapist:** "Yes, that does indeed sound like the Pleaser, doesn't it?"

5.5.2 Step 2: Identify a meaningful related event from the past

During the case conceptualization, you will have worked with the client to relate their current symptoms to significant experiences in their childhood.

You should therefore be able to refer to an example that was explored during that phase. If the client can think of an alternative example themselves then it would be preferable to use that, as this is another opportunity to encourage self-expression and autonomy.

> ### Example of identifying a meaningful related event from the past
>
> **>>Therapist:** "We've already talked about how the Pleaser emerged early in your childhood under the influence of your father's critical attitude and the concerns you had about your mother. Can you remember a typical situation where you just adapted, even if you found it difficult?"
>
> **>>Claire:** (*thinking for a long time*) "I can think of a situation, but my mother often had difficulties herself, so I don't know if it's a good example."
>
> **>>Therapist:** "Tell me about it, and together we'll see if it's a good example to practice with."
>
> **>>Claire:** "Well, I was never allowed to play with children from school who didn't live on our street. My mother thought it was dangerous."
>
> **>>Therapist:** "That does sound like a good example. Why did your mother think it was dangerous?"
>
> **>>Claire:** "She thought it was too far, and she worried that if something happened then she wouldn't be able to get to me."
>
> **>>Therapist:** "Okay, it seems your mother was a bit too concerned. Let's act that out."

5.5.3 Step 3: Re-enact event: client as child; therapist as antagonist

The historical roleplay is conducted in three rounds. The first round is to re-enact the event as it actually happened in the past. The main purpose of this round is to gain more insight into the formation of the client's schema(s) and patterns of behaviour. However, explain that you not only want to use this technique to gain insight, but also to offer the client a healing experience. The hope that you offer to the client in this way is needed to motivate them to engage with the technique. With some clients, you will have to negotiate with the resistant Coping Mode. The advantage of the Compliant Surrender (the coping mode used by Claire) is that this resistance is not present, or is much less present, and you can therefore start the technique more easily.

Example of introducing the first round of roleplay

>>Therapist: "I think the fact that your mother was overly concerned is a good example of how a past event is connected to what happened last week in the situation with your boyfriend. It seems that you learned something in that situation, or in similar situations, which still plays out in the present. So, let's act out this scenario so we can take a closer look at exactly what happened. Agreed?"

>>Claire: "What do you mean, act out?"

>>Therapist: "Well, literally that we act out that scene from your past here and now. We'll bring that scene into the present and into this room, and first we'll just re-enact exactly what happened. Afterwards, I'll look more closely at the situation with you, so we can understand together what that girl from back then learned at that time."

>>Claire: "So we're going to perform some kind of play?"

>>Therapist: "Yes, a roleplay. And you seem to find that a bit odd?"

(*Claire nods.*)

>>Therapist: "I understand that. Perhaps it does seem a bit strange that we're not going to talk about what happened, but instead re-enact it, like a play. But you know, I'd rather do something that seems odd but can help us move forward, than avoid it just because it seems odd. I think that you, and the problems that brought you here, are much too important to just rule out anything without giving it a try. How about we just have a go, and then afterwards we'll think together about what it achieved?"

>>Claire: "Alright then." (*Nods hesitantly.*)

The biggest pitfall for the therapist here is that you will keep talking with your client about the event for too long. In these conversations, you can easily be drawn into exploring the meaning of events. However, the aim of this exercise is not to discuss events in words, but instead to gain insight into schemas by reliving a situation through roleplay. A good tip is to get up from your chair fairly quickly and start preparing the roleplay with your client, rather than staying seated and exploring the event too deeply.

Example of setting up the first round of roleplay

>>Therapist: "Good! First, then, I'd like you to come and stand with me for a moment."

(*The therapist stands, and Claire follows so they are standing next to each other in the room. The therapist gestures to a side of the room that will become the roleplay area.*) →

>>**Therapist:** "Let's bring that scene from the past to life here. So, we'll re-enact that situation with you and your mother. Take me with you for a moment: where did this happen – was it in the living room at home perhaps?"

>>**Claire:** "Yes, in the living room, and if this is the living room, then the lounge area is over there."

>>**Therapist:** "And your mother is standing where?"

>>**Claire:** "She's standing there… (*pointing to a spot in the roleplay area.*) And then I'm standing here." (*Claire points to a spot near her mother.*)

Make sure you get a good briefing from your client beforehand on how to play the role of the antagonist. The aim is to make the roleplay as lifelike as you can, and as close to your client's real-life experience as possible. Ask for some instructions about posture, manner of speech, movements and so on. But again, be careful that this does not take up too much time or distract from the roleplay itself.

Example of preparing to play the antagonist

>>**Therapist:** "Okay, so you tell your mother about the plan to go and play at your friend's house. Now I'm about to play the part of your mother, so can you tell me how she behaves? How exactly does she talk about everything that could go wrong?"

>>**Claire:** "Well, very tense and nervous. She starts hesitantly at first as if the realization dawns, and then she starts chattering a bit. Yes, she rattles on a bit, about all the things that could go wrong."

>>**Therapist:** "So she sounds nervous and tense, and she talks fast?"

>>**Claire:** "Yes, exactly."

>>**Therapist:** "And does she have any particular gestures that are typical of her?"

>>**Claire:** "Well, she can stand like this fidgeting with her hands and rocking a bit from one foot to the other."

>>**Therapist:** "Good, so I'm getting a bit of a picture. Now, you'll be playing yourself as a child in the roleplay. How old were you again in this situation?"

>>**Claire:** (*having to think about it*) "I think this was something that happened when I was about six."

Your client will also have to get into the role they are playing – that of the child – as best they can. For Claire, you might ask how old she is and which friend she wanted to play with.

> **Example of re-enacting event: client as child, therapist as antagonist**
>
> **>>Therapist:** "So, now be that six-year-old girl, and start asking if you can go and play at your friend's house."
>
> **>>Claire:** (*in the role of the six-year-old child*) "Mummy, I want to go and play at Miriam's this afternoon."
>
> **>>Therapist:** (*trying to look nervous and worried as per Claire's guidance, rocking from one foot to the other and fidgeting with his hands*): "No, Claire, you can't. Miriam lives all the way across town, doesn't she? What if something happens? I won't be able to be with you right away to help. And you've never been there before, so I have no idea if it's safe or if her Mummy or Daddy will be there."
>
> **>>Claire:** "Yes, but Mummy…"
>
> **>>Therapist:** "No, Claire, I really don't think it's safe…"
>
> (*Claire is silent.*)
>
> **>>Therapist:** (*makes a time-out sign*) "Okay, let's just stop here."

Roleplaying these situations often does not take long. They are usually short interactions of no more than a minute.

5.5.4 Step 4: Review first roleplay and identify schemas formed

The first question to ask after the first round is complete is whether the re-enacted situation resembled your client's memory of it. If not, you may need to re-enact the situation with some direction from your client to make the roleplay more realistic.

Then, together with your client, you can try to identify the schemas that were formed at that time. This is a somewhat more cognitive element of the exercise, in which the client seeks to identify implicit assumptions about themselves and others. You might have to do some investigating to discover these core beliefs, because your client may find it very difficult to put the basic feelings of the schemas into words. Still, it is worthwhile identifying them. These core beliefs are scored on their credibility at key points during the exercise. In this way, you some feedback about the effectiveness of the technique.

Example of identifying schemas formed

>>**Therapist:** "Okay, let's just stop here. First, I have a question: was that similar to how it really was? Is that basically how you remember it?"

>>**Claire:** "Yes, it definitely was like that. Maybe my mother would have been even more nervous, but it really did feel as it was back then, yes."

>>**Therapist:** "Even more nervous? Wow. Stay in this experience for another moment, keep being that six-year-old girl for a little longer. How do you feel now?"

>>**Claire:** "I don't know, anxious and sad maybe."

>>**Therapist:** "Anxious and sad, anything else?"

>>**Claire:** "Well, I don't like my wanting to play being immediately brushed aside."

>>**Therapist:** "You don't like it in the sense of being frustrated? A sort of irritation?"

>>**Claire:** "Well, I don't know about irritation… but I don't like it, no…"

>>**Therapist:** "Okay, sad and also a feeling of not liking it. Let's just step out of this situation for a moment and look at what happened from a distance."

Each roleplay is followed by a review in which you and the client investigate what conclusions the client drew about themselves and the other person at that time.

Example of reviewing first roleplay

(The therapist walks over to the place where they first discussed the exercise and, with the client next to him, looks back on the roleplay.)

>>**Therapist:** "Okay, now if we just look back at what took place over there, what do you think that six-year-old girl learned?"

>>**Claire:** "Well, that it doesn't matter that much what you want, because Mummy is way too anxious for something like that?"

>>**Therapist:** "Yes, that sounds right. And what was more important in that situation, that the little girl wanted to play, or that Mummy was anxious?"

>>**Claire:** "Yeah, that Mum got anxious, of course…"

>>**Therapist:** "Exactly. So, what did that girl learn about her needs, and about standing up for what she wants?"

>>**Claire:** "That those things don't matter very much."

>>**Therapist:** "So the little girl actually learned: 'What I feel, what I want, that's not important'?"

>>**Claire:** "Yes, I suppose that's right."

>>**Therapist:** "And from that experience as that six-year-old girl, how true is that thought? How credible is it?"

>>**Claire:** "As that six-year-old girl?"

>>**Therapist:** "Yeah, how did the little girl experience that? Did she think it was a hundred per cent true that what she wanted for herself didn't matter much? Or less?"

>>**Claire:** "Well… It wasn't completely unimportant, but it very often was less important than other things, as it also is now… ninety-five percent?"

>>**Therapist:** "Okay. And what does the little girl learn about others from this interaction? How does she look at the mother she sees before her?"

>>**Claire:** "That's a difficult question. Mum's just very scared."

>>**Therapist:** "And what scared her in this situation?"

>>**Claire:** "Well, that I said I wanted to play with Miriam."

>>**Therapist:** "Okay, so you said what you want, and then you notice that your Mum gets very scared. Is that something you recognize? Had it happened before?"

>>**Claire:** "Yes, it was always like that. I also learned that I shouldn't just come ourt and ask things like that – she just can't handle it."

>>**Therapist:** "It sounds like you learned that your mother gets scared when you speak up about what you want?"

>>**Claire:** "Yes."

>>**Therapist:** "So: 'The other person can't handle it when I say what I want, and they will get scared'?"

>>**Claire:** "Yes – scared or angry, but that was more my father."

>>**Therapist:** "'The other person can't handle it when I say what I want, and they will get scared or angry'? How does that sound?"

>>**Claire:** "Yes, that's true, yes, that's about right."

>>**Therapist:** "And how believable is that for the six-year-old girl? That 'The other person can't handle it when I say what I want, and they will get scared or angry'?"

>>**Claire:** "Yes, that is a hundred per cent true."

Write down the client's statements, and also note the credibility of the self-image they have just identified and the image of others and the world around them.

5.5.5 Step 5: Re-enact event: client as antagonist, therapist as child

The next step is to re-enact the event again, but now with the roles reversed. This time you, the therapist, play the client as a child, and the client plays the antagonist. Explain that this will help you understand what happened in that past situation even better. Introduce the roleplay by asking the client to inhabit the role of the antagonist as much as possible. Ask how old the antagonist was at that time, and what the circumstances of their life were. This is often relevant if the antagonist would react very differently today. For example, it may be that the client's mother had just got divorced and had to take care of three young children, so she was struggling to handle the pressures in her life.

> **Example of re-enacting event: client as antagonist, therapist as child**
>
> **>>Therapist:** "We'll now act out the same scene again, but this time we'll switch roles. So we're in the same situation, but now you're Mum and I'm you as a six-year-old girl."
>
> **>>Claire:** "Okay, but why do we have to do that?"
>
> **>>Therapist:** "Well, we don't have to, but it seems like a good idea to me. Something happened in that situation that you're still encountering today. So let's take another good look at it to get a better understanding of what happened. And by switching roles so you look at it from your mother's point of view, maybe that will give us some additional information. Shall we just give it a try?"
>
> *(Claire nods.)*
>
> **>>Therapist:** "So, you'll play Mum now. That means I'll ask you to empathize as much as you can with your mother. You are six, so how old is your mother?"
>
> **>>Claire:** "Whew, that's a tough one… I'll have to do the maths… Maybe forty or so?"
>
> **>>Therapist:** "Okay, so your mother is about forty then. So just be your mother now. What does your life look like?"
>
> **>>Claire:** "Well, I'm married to my father (*has to laugh at this*) and he's away a lot. And when he's around, he's angry, and I'm often afraid of something bad happening, especially with Claire."
>
> **>>Therapist:** "Now let's step back into the past again."
>
> *(The therapist walks to the side of the room where the roleplay is being performed, but now stands where the six-year-old girl was.)*

>>Therapist: "You are your mother… So, you're standing in the living room now, and there's your six-year-old daughter, Claire. Okay, let's start…"

>>Therapist: (*playing the role of the little girl as well as possible, and speaking in a childlike voice as Claire did*): "Mummy, I want to play with Miriam right now."

>>Claire: (*acting very nervously, rocking and fidgeting with her hands*) "No, that isn't possible, because she lives all the way across town! And what if you get sick, or something bad happens? You might fall and hurt yourself! And how would I get to you?"

>>Therapist: (*makes a time-out gesture*) "Okay, let's just stop here. You've played your mother – can you keep being her for a bit? Just stand here for a moment, and I'll speak to you as your mother, okay?"

(*Claire nods.*)

>>Therapist: "Claire's Mum, I heard you say that you won't let Claire go to play with Miriam. Can you tell me again why you're not letting her go?"

>>Claire: "Well, I'm afraid that something will go wrong. And then I won't be able to be there for her."

>>Therapist: "Yes, I do understand that sometimes things can go wrong in life. But Claire is only six, and it doesn't seem to matter at all to you what she wants."

>>Claire: "But I just don't want anything to happen to her, I really couldn't handle that! (*As Claire:*) Yes, I think she would say that, that she wouldn't be able to handle it, she said that a lot."

>>Therapist: "Phew. I now understand a bit better what you meant when you described your mother. She really is very anxious and nervous, isn't she?"

>>Claire: "Yes, it was like that a lot, yes."

>>Therapist: "I notice that I felt all kinds of things about that. I still feel it in fact. It was dreadful to see your mother so nervous, but the fact that my wanting to play was just brushed aside so quickly immediately seemed wrong. I also have some of that feeling of not liking it that you just mentioned. For me, it's more clearly irritation. And some of that sadness too – the sadness that what I say doesn't seem to matter at all."

>>Claire: (*looking at the therapist enquiringly*) "Do you really mean that?"

>>Therapist: "Yes, I definitely mean it! I can perfectly well understand that it really isn't nice for a six-year-old girl. How is it for you to hear that?"

>>Claire: "Quite good, actually. It's nice that you see and experience it the same way, that it's not completely my fault."

>>**Therapist:** "No, it definitely isn't your fault! Okay, let's stop here. Let's step away from this past scene for a moment, and let's go back to the place where we can think about everything that happened."

(The therapist and Claire walk back to the original position to discuss the roleplay.)

5.5.6 Step 6: Review second roleplay and identify any schema-refuting information

Reversing roles in this way may create new insights for your client. However, it may also simply confirm what they already assumed. For example, Claire was able to experience, while in the role of her mother, that what she, Claire, wanted for herself as a child didn't matter much. Still, role reversal in roleplay can have an effect on the credibility of the schemas. For example, your client may come to realize that the antagonist's behaviour was mainly a manifestation of their own inability to be mindful of what a child needs. This might seem a minor nuance, but it is significant: the overall situation hasn't changed, but the source of the problem has moved from the client to the antagonist.

Example of reviewing second roleplay and identifying any schema-refuting information

>>**Therapist:** "Okay, well let's take a quick look at what we just learned. What did you take away from this roleplay?"

>>**Claire:** "Yeah, I don't really know. Well, maybe that my mother was mostly concerned with keeping things safe for me."

>>**Therapist:** "Yes, that struck me as well when I was just talking to her about what happened. I also noticed how she was completely consumed by those worries and fears. It seemed to be about you, but she was actually concerned most with her own worries. Is that relevant to the thought of 'What I feel and what I want don't matter'? How do you look at that now?"

>>**Claire:** "Now? How do I look at it now?"

>>**Therapist:** "Yes, having just empathized with your mother so much, and having noticed how scared she was of all risks and dangers. So how do you look at the idea that your feelings and wants don't matter?"

>>**Claire:** "Well, for my mother, it really didn't matter that much; I mean, she wasn't concerned with that. She was just concerned with keeping me safe. Talking about it like that now, it does feel different, that my needs and what I want are important, but she just wasn't concerned with that."

>>**Therapist:** "So how credible does that thought feel to you now then, the thought that 'What I need, the fact that I want something, is not important'?

>>**Claire:** "Yes, a little less. Fifty percent or so?"

>>**Therapist:** "Great. And then the thought 'The other person can't handle it when I say what I want, and they will get scared or angry'... How do you look at that now?"

>>**Claire:** (*looking thoughtful in silence*) "Well, that's true, that she couldn't handle it, but that didn't actually have that much to do with me; for her, everything was just dangerous. And that was really how she was. I mean, of course it isn't necessarily true that everyone is that scared, or that they'll get scared when I say something."

>>**Therapist:** "So you can see that this is how your mother experiences things - that what you want makes her anxious. However, you can also see that for her *everything* is a source of anxiety – but this doesn't have to apply to everyone. How true does that thought 'The other person can't handle it when I say what I want, and they will get scared or angry' feel now?"

>>**Claire:** "Yeah, less. Something like fifty percent again?"

>>**Therapist:** "That's great, it's not about right or wrong, it's just about taking a measurement of how it feels for you now, with all the information we're discussing."

5.5.7 Step 7: Re-enact event: client as child; therapist as 'good-enough' parent

In the final round of the historical roleplay, you offer the client a corrective emotional experience by responding in the role of a 'good-enough' parent. In this initial phase of therapy, you cannot expect your client to be able to figure out how to defy their mother's wishes – their Healthy Adult is not yet sufficiently well-developed. This will, however, become possible in the middle and final phases. That is why, in this step, you act out the event again, but this time you change the ending of the interaction by modelling what a 'good-enough' parent would say or do in such a situation. In this regard the technique resembles imagery rescripting, in which you also act as a 'good-enough' parent. The major difference here is that someone standing up for the client's needs it is not only imagined – they actually see you doing it. The physical presence of the therapist makes historical roleplay a different experience from imagery rescripting.

Example of introducing the third round of roleplay

>>Therapist: "Good, then there's one last round I'd like to do with you. We've now re-enacted the situation as it really occurred, with you as the child. Then we reversed the roles, and that gave us more information. So now we realize that your needs, the things you want, actually do matter, but that you were unlucky that your mother – and indeed your father, you said – didn't provide space for that. This was mostly due to your mother's own fears and the fact that she was only occupied with that. In this last roleplay, I'd like to re-enact the situation one more time, but this time I want you to experience how things should have gone, and how that feels."

>>Claire: "I don't understand."

>>Therapist: "I mean that in this last roleplay, you're six-year-old Claire again, but now I'm playing the parent that I would have liked you to have."

>>Claire: "Yes, but that makes it look like Mum did it all wrong. She was also a very kind person, you know."

>>Therapist: "I'm glad you've pointed that out. But that isn't what I mean. I'm not saying your mother did it all wrong. I know she did a lot of good. And what I hear from her is that, above all, she wanted things to be safe and good for you. But despite that, her fears were so great that there was no room left for you – and that isn't good. So I want you to experience what you really should have experienced at the time – what it's like to have a mother who isn't always anxious, and who does know what you need."

If your client seems to have a conflict of loyalties, explain to them why you think good care was not provided, without passing judgement on the antagonist. An important tip is to pull the focus away from the antagonist and to focus more on your client's needs. Your aim for this last round is mainly to help your client learn that the negative experience of the past event was due to the fact that something was missing, and now you want to offer them a corrective emotional experience by providing them with the missing ingredient.

Example of re-enacting event: client as child, therapist as 'good-enough' parent

>>Therapist: "Are you wondering how it feels when your needs are listened to? When there is space for that?"

>>Claire: "Yes, I am actually."

>>Therapist: "Then let's re-enact it again, but this time with me answering you – not your mother, who was preoccupied with her own worries. Come, let's go back in time for a moment…"

(The therapist and Claire walk to the roleplay area.)

>>**Therapist:** "Good, Claire, so I want to ask you to put yourself back into the same place. You're six again, and you want to have fun playing with your friend Miriam. Okay, start when you're ready."

>>**Claire:** "Mummy, I played with Miriam at school today and it was a lot of fun. And I want to go and play at her house this afternoon."

>>**Therapist:** (*briefly as himself*) "Nicely done! Well, I think it's a great idea for you to meet up this afternoon. I think Miriam does live a bit further away, so I'll have to sort out dropping you off and picking you up, but we'll arrange it. It's nice to play at someone else's house occasionally, right? Miriam will have toys and games you don't know."

(*Claire smiles a little at that last comment.*)

>>**Therapist:** (*makes a time-out sign*) "Good, let's leave it there, shall we?"

(*Claire nods.*)

>>**Therapist:** "Well, how was that for you?"

>>**Claire:** "Well, my mother would never talk like that. She would start saying that…"

>>**Therapist:** "Sorry to interrupt, but I'd like to know how you felt about it. I know your mother wouldn't react like that, but this time you were hearing me. And I think that genuinely would be a normal reaction for a parent in such a situation. In any case, that's how I would and did react with my own children. How did it feel for you?"

>>**Claire:** "Yes, well, nice… It was just nice and pleasant that you were so positive."

>>**Therapist:** "Although I did say something about Miriam living so far away, right?"

>>**Claire:** "Yes, but it wasn't an issue, you just had to arrange a drop-off and pick-up."

>>**Therapist:** "Yes, exactly. I think that your mother sees many dangers in life and in the world, but often they're just practical things that can easily be worked around or solved. And that's also what a child needs to learn, that it's good to explore the world and that while you do need to plan properly, in the end you're perfectly capable of that."

5.5.8 Step 8: Review third roleplay and formation of healthy schemas

In the final phase of the exercise, reflect on the credibility of the client's core thoughts. Remember to remind the client of the reason for doing the historical roleplay in this session. Your client has fallen back into old patterns in the past week, for example, and has now had a corrective experience from the healthy response you have modelled.

Example of reviewing the third roleplay and formation of healthy schemas

(The therapist and Claire have returned to their chairs to discuss the exercise further.)

>>Therapist: "I'm curious – now that you've just had this new experience, with a different parenting response, how do you look at the thought that 'What I feel and what I want don't matter'? Just now, it was fifty percent credible. Has that changed?"

>>Claire: "Yes, it has, yes. I really liked that you were so nice and that you didn't think it was crazy that I wanted something."

>>Therapist: "And does that make it less credible that your needs don't matter?"

>>Claire: "Yes, exactly… and also because I now think even more that it was actually my mother who was so full of her own worries, and it didn't really say much about me at all…"

>>Therapist: "That it didn't mean that you weren't important?"

>>Claire: "Yes…"

>>Therapist: "How credible do you find it now, after that new experience, that your feelings and needs don't matter?"

>>Claire: "Ten percent, maybe? Something like that?"

>>Therapist: "It's up to you. And this isn't about right or wrong, it's just about how you experience that thought now."

>>Claire: "Yes, ten percent then."

>>Therapist: "Okay, and what about that other thought: 'The other person can't handle it when I say what I want, and they will get scared or angry?' That one was also something like fifty percent credible just now. Has anything changed in that?"

>>Claire: "I don't know… yes, I think so."

>>Therapist: "I'm curious to hear about it."

>>Claire: "Well, I still do think that Mum couldn't handle it if it was possible that something dangerous could happen. But now I do think that it could well be that other people would react the same way you did. So normal, let's say."

>>Therapist: "So that thought is less credible?"

>>Claire: "Yes… but I still find it stressful… Maybe thirty percent still…"

>>Therapist: "Totally fine! Again, this is not about right or wrong."

5.5.9 Step 9: Review whole roleplay, consolidation and homework

Finally, evaluate the whole roleplay and compliment your client for participating so well.

> ### Example of reviewing historical roleplay
>
> **>>Therapist:** "We're slowly getting to the end of the session. And we sure have done a lot today! Congratulations, Claire – well done! I really think it's so great how you're thinking and collaborating so actively to explore all this and gain new experiences."
>
> (*Claire smiles a little shyly.*)
>
> **>>Therapist:** "You seem to feel awkward hearing this, or maybe you kind of like it?"
>
> **>>Claire:** "Yes, it's nice, yes – but also I don't quite know what to do with myself."
>
> **>>Therapist:** "Well, I would mostly just try to take it in and enjoy it. Compliments are nice, but I think maybe you aren't used to hearing that you can do things well. I think it's very good that you're starting to get used to that, because you really can do a lot!"

To further consolidate the therapeutic experience, ask the client to write something about it themselves, or make a recording for them. Give the client some homework so that they re-read the text or listen to the recording regularly. You can also give them an audio flashcard in which you repeat the main conclusions.

> ### Example of consolidating the experience
>
> **>>Therapist:** "I think it would be good to be able to come back to this a bit more often. You do need repetition to get used to it. For my part, I'll make another recording like this for you. What do you think?"
>
> **>>Claire:** "Yes, I'd like that. The recordings do help, especially as it's you speaking."
>
> **>>Therapist:** "And I'll be happy to do that. Look, at some point, you'll start making your own recordings. Or maybe there will come a time when it's no longer necessary to work with recordings at all. But for now, I'm happy to help you with that, because then my words can gradually start to become your words. Do you have your mobile with you?"
>
> (*Claire nods and takes her mobile phone from her purse.*)

>>**Therapist:** "Now, if you could just set it to record audio?"

(*Claire is busy with her mobile for a moment, then she hands it to the therapist.*)

>>**Therapist:** "Good. Claire, if you're listening now, I want to start by paying you a compliment. It's great that you've taken the time to listen to this recording. It can help remind you of what you've learned and experienced. It's very difficult for you to say what you want, what you want to do, or what you need. Most of the time you tend to adapt to other people. That's the Pleaser side of you. Of course, it's hard for you to speak up for what you need. This can be tough for everyone at times, but you never actually learned in your childhood that it's okay to say what you want. When you did say what you wanted, your mother immediately got scared. This happened so many times that it made you believe that your feelings, what you want, wouldn't matter.

(*Claire is listening intently.*)

>>**Therapist:** "You came to believe that others get scared or angry when you said what you did or didn't want for yourself. But your needs do matter, Claire. Your mother was so consumed by all the dangers she feared that she had no room left for your feelings and needs. But that is her problem, and those are her fears. You aren't being difficult if you want something or don't want something. I like to hear what you think, what you want. I also want you to keep telling me what you do and don't want. That's how you get to know about the world, and about life. And you'll find that there is a lot of beauty to discover in your life. Of course, sometimes you need to plan in advance to do that, but that's no problem. And if it's still stressful sometimes, you can learn, and I'll help you with that. I'll help you learn to do it yourself, and to live your own life."

(*The therapist stops the recording and hands the phone back to Claire.*)

>>**Therapist:** "How does it feel to hear that message?"

>>**Claire:** "Good. Yes, very good."

5.6 Sticking points in historical roleplay

5.6.1 What if the client cannot think of a meaningful related event from the past?

If your client is not able to provide examples for historical roleplay, you can use diagnostic imagery to link a recent event to a significant event in the past.

Example of identifying a meaningful related event from the past

>>Therapist: "I think the Pleaser is there for a reason. So, I suggest we do an exercise that helps us understand how the Pleaser came into being. Is that okay with you?"

>>Claire: "What kind of exercise do you mean?"

>>Therapist: "An imagination exercise, like we've done before. In a moment, I'll ask you to close your eyes for a few minutes and think back to the situation last week when your boyfriend said he wanted to visit his family. First, I'll ask you to focus on the feeling you had in that moment. Next, I'll ask you to think back to memories from your past that might somehow be related to this. That way, we might be able to understand a little better what experiences from your past led to the Pleaser being so active last week."

(*Claire nods.*)

>>Therapist: "Okay, if you can close your eyes now, we'll get started."

(*Claire closes her eyes.*)

>>Therapist: "Take your thoughts back to that conversation with your boyfriend. That conversation where he says he wants to visit his family. And you said that you would really prefer to stay home. Do you see the situation in front of you again?"

(*Claire nods.*)

>>Therapist: "Can you tell me what you see now?"

>>Claire: "He says: 'Yes, but we haven't seen them for a while, and I'd really like to visit them. We already missed Mum's birthday, and I don't want to miss anything else.'"

>>Therapist: "And how does his voice sound as he says that?"

>>Claire: "Definite. As if no discussion about it is possible."

>>Therapist: "And how do you feel while he says that?"

>>Claire: "Tense. A little bit insecure and tense, because I don't know if he'll get angry if I keep saying that I really don't want to go with him."

>>Therapist: "And where do you feel that tension in your body?"

(*Claire points to her chest.*)

>>Therapist: "So you hear his firm voice, and he says he really doesn't want to miss out on anything else, and at this you feel a tension in your chest. An anxious tension because you're afraid he might get angry. And what do you want to do now?"

>>Claire: "I want to reassure him. I want to tell him not to worry – that we'll go to see his family together, and that I'm totally fine with that."

>>**Therapist:** "So you feel very much inclined to go along with his wishes?"

(*Claire nods.*)

>>**Therapist:** "Do you feel that somewhere in your body as well?"

>>**Claire:** "Well, a little bit like I want to lean forward."

(*Claire leans forward a little and extends her arms a little.*)

>>**Therapist:** "Now concentrate on that feeling of fear in your chest, the fear that the other person might get angry. But also, that feeling of leaning forward and wanting to reassure the other person. Is this the first time you've felt this, or do you recognize it?"

>>**Claire:** "Yes, I definitely recognize this feeling."

>>**Therapist:** "Okay. Then the feeling you're having now isn't only related to this situation but perhaps also to past events. Now concentrate on that feeling, the sense of anxiety and of wanting to reassure the other person. That feeling you experience as if you want to lean forward a bit. And let the image of your boyfriend fade; it's not just about that situation last week, but the feeling. Let images come up from your past, images that could somehow be connected to this feeling. What do you see now?"

>>**Claire:** "Mum. I see Mum."

>>**Therapist:** "And where do you see her? Can you point to her?"

(*Claire points to a spot to the right in front of her.*)

>>**Therapist:** "Just look at your mother, how does she feel?"

>>**Claire:** "She is afraid…"

>>**Therapist:** "And do you have any idea what is making her afraid?"

>>**Claire:** "I asked if I could play at a friend's house. But that friend lives on the other side of town, and now Mum is all worried and scared."

>>**Therapist:** "Does your mother say anything about her concerns?"

>>**Claire:** "Yes, she's talking about everything that could go wrong and that it's not at all safe when I'm so far away, because she wouldn't know how to reach me quickly if something was wrong."

>>**Therapist:** "Just be that little girl now. How old are you?"

>>**Claire:** "I don't know… About six, maybe?"

>>**Therapist:** "Then just be that six-year-old girl. And your mum is telling you about all the dangers that exist if you were to go and play at your friend's house. And you see her fear. How do you feel now?"

> **Claire:** "Afraid. Sad, too."
>
> **Therapist:** "And what makes you so sad, Claire?"
>
> **Claire:** "I'd actually like to go and play at my friend's house, but I'm not going to, I really can't do that to Mummy."
>
> **Therapist:** "You feel that you need to take care of her?"
>
> **Claire:** "Yes..."
>
> **Therapist:** "Where do you feel that in your body?"
>
> **Claire:** "I don't know... A bit like I want to go to her. As if I want to hold her, and tell her that it will all be fine."
>
> (*Claire leans forward slightly as she says this.*)
>
> **Therapist:** "Okay. Now let the image of your mother fade. Just let it go. And come back to this room. Move your hands and feet for a moment. And then, when you're ready, you can open your eyes again."
>
> (*Claire opens her eyes.*)

The visualization is interrupted here in order to continue as planned with the roleplay exercise. Of course, you could equally continue working with the visualized situation, but then it becomes an exercise in imagery rescripting rather than historical roleplay.

5.6.2 What if the client cannot imagine themselves as a child or antagonist?

When introducing historical roleplay for the first time, your client might find it uncomfortable to play themselves as a child or to play their own father or mother. In such situations, you can make things easier by first inserting a brief visualization. Ask the client to close their eyes and imagine the child of that age or an antagonist in that situation. Once that is successful, then ask them to represent that person in the roleplay.

5.7 The Dependent Child

Limited reparenting aims to encourage self-expression and autonomy. In the role of a healthy parent, you naturally provide the safety the client needs to be able to relax. However, you also need to remain firm enough to encourage your client to speak up and do more things independently. Safety in the form of warm care and support alone, however, is not enough to break the schemas of *Dependence/Incompetence* and *Subjugation*. So do adopt the attitude of a warm, validating parent, but make sure it is also one who encourages their child to speak up and do things independently.

A dependent client's greatest fear is that standing up for their own opinions might hurt or anger other people and lead them to abandon their emotionally or physically. This makes them afraid to speak their mind on small, everyday matters. Expressing anger is therefore completely unthinkable for many dependent clients. We noted in Chapter 3 that many dependent clients can barely recognize their own anger. We also indicated that placing anger in the mode model is one of your first therapeutic interventions with clients who have this level of inhibition. The rationale here is that anger is a normal human reaction, and it is also a source of strength that can help us to break persistent patterns.

In the initial phase of therapy, you are a role model for expressing anger in a healthy way. In your actions against Punitive Modes, you demonstrate that anger can be an important tool to stop negative expressions. A dependent client, who has always associated anger with misery, may find that anger from you, as a therapist, helps them in this initial phase. They feel more seen and valued because the therapist is angry with the Punitive Mode. These are corrective emotional experiences that will help your client to recognize and express their own anger. We describe how to help the client in this process below.

5.8 Stimulating anger in the Dependent Child

As we have seen, dependent clients have negative thoughts about the consequences of expressing anger. You will therefore need to examine these ideas critically, and adjust them if necessary, before your client is able to express anger in a healthy way.

You can achieve this cognitive restructuring of the client's assumptions about anger by identifying the benefits of anger, practicing expressing anger with a complaint exercise in a safe environment, using cognitive diaries, and expressing anger in practice. This last suggestion is only possible in the middle or end phase of therapy, but you can do the following exercises from the beginning of treatment.

5.8.1 Listing the benefits of anger

Reflect together on the question 'What is good about anger?' and write down all the arguments that you come up with (see the box below). If your client is more aware of the positive aspects of anger, the next step of expressing anger is likely to be more attainable.

> **What is good about anger?**
> - Anger helps us to feel and set boundaries.
>   *If you avoid anger, you will sense much too late that people are overstepping your boundaries, and as a result you might get hurt or even abused.*
> - Anger helps us stand up for our needs.
>   *As with setting boundaries, anger helps you feel what you need. By feeling what you don't want, you can also find out what you do want or need.*
> - Anger has a connective effect.
>   *Arguments happen in every relationship. During those arguments, you express your feelings and needs, showing yourself as raw and honest to the other person. If that argument is properly resolved, the relationship bonds can become stronger.*
> - Anger is a source of strength and energy.
>   *Anger gives a lot of energy. You don't fall asleep easily when you are angry, because of the adrenaline coursing through your body. That energy also gives you the power to break patterns of thinking and behaving that are persistent. For example, it gives you the power to say: 'I've had enough of always having to conform to others. Now I'm going to do what I want for once!'*
> - Anger can also give us pleasure.
>   *We often laugh at comedians and other performers because of how they express anger about other people, politics or something else. So apparently, getting worked up about something can also be a source of positive emotions!*
> - Anger helps us to release tension.
>   *Venting anger can literally have a 'pressure valve' function – it allows you to release built-up tension, after which you feel relief.*

Investigating your client's assumptions about anger does not need to be completed in one go, and you will often spread it over a few sessions. Once you have spent sufficient time on the positive aspects of anger, you can start to practice expressing anger with your client. Encouraging them to express more anger is a form of counter-conditioning. For the client, anger is associated with negative feelings, and now you want to associate expressing anger with positive experiences. One way to make that positive association within a session is by stimulating anger in the form of a game: the 'complaint exercise'.

5.8.2 Stimulating expression of anger with the 'complaint exercise'

With the complaint exercise, your client can learn to express anger in a playful way. Introduce the exercise as a good way for your client to learn that expressing anger can be pleasant. As the therapist, you participate in the exercise and take turns with the client to talk about things about which you've recently felt irritation or frustration. Initially, these should be impersonal things like an alarm going off early, bad weather or traffic. As the exercise progresses, some irritations related to other people can also be expressed.

> **Example of the 'complaint exercise'**
>
> **>>Therapist:** "Well, Claire, we've come a long way with your treatment, and I want to say that you're doing very well."
>
> **>>Claire:** (*smiling a little uncertainly*) "Yes, do you really think so?"
>
> **>>Therapist:** "Definitely! You're much more aware of your different sides, like the Pleaser. You're also doing well participating in the exercises. And now you're also well on way to learning that anger isn't necessarily something bad or dangerous."
>
> **>>Claire:** "Yes, although I still find that difficult…"
>
> **>>Therapist:** "Yes, and that's what I want to discuss today. You're aware now that your ideas about anger aren't quite right, but you're still learning and finding your way when it comes to actually feeling and expressing anger. Can I put it that way?"
>
> **>>Claire:** "No, that's right, yes… sorry…"
>
> **>>Therapist:** "You don't have to say sorry! Of course you aren't great at it yet – how could you be, with what you went through? You were never set examples of a healthy way to express anger. In fact, you've actually had very unpleasant experiences with anger, especially with your father who could get so unreasonably angry."
>
> **>>Claire:** "Yes…"
>
> **>>Therapist:** "That's why we're going to practice teaching you how to express anger today. This will be an exercise in which you find that expressing anger can also be fun and enjoyable. We did discuss that, but I saw you looking very sceptical, didn't I?"
>
> **>>Claire:** "Yes, you did say that, but I can't imagine it…"
>
> **>>Therapist:** "That's why we're going to do an exercise today where you'll find that it's really true. We're about to do an exercise where we'll take turns talking about something we're angry or irritated about."
>
> **>>Claire:** "But I never have anything like that. I'm never angry or anything."

>>**Therapist:** "Well, as I said before – you're human, after all. And humans feel angry at times. So that anger is there, even if you might not always recognize it yet. But surely you experience situations sometimes that you're not very comfortable with?"

>>**Claire:** "Yes, of course, I do..."

>>**Therapist:** "Okay, then we'll do an exercise where we take turns talking about a situation where we didn't feel very comfortable, Okay?"

>>**Claire:** "..."

Your client may have a very distorted view of anger, such as that it always means shouting. They won't (yet) be able to recognize such an intense form of anger in themselves. Because of this, when introducing the exercise, try to find words that are more in line with what they can recognize. 'A rather unpleasant feeling of "I would rather that had been different"' can be excellent wording to get the client to engage with this exercise.

Example of the 'complaint exercise' – continued

>>**Therapist:** "Then I'll start... let me think... Well, I was travelling by train the other day and I had a few minutes to change, but then my first train was delayed so I missed the connection. I wasn't too pleased about that, as you can probably imagine."

>>**Claire:** "Yes, I can imagine that! That's so annoying!"

>>**Therapist:** "Well, it's not super-annoying, but it's certainly not very pleasant either. Do you have any examples like that?"

>>**Claire:** "Well... when I came here this morning, I got all wet in the rain, even though the weather forecast had said it would stay dry. I didn't enjoy that very much..."

>>**Therapist:** "No, I can imagine! What did you think this morning when that happened – when you got wet, having been told it would stay dry?"

>>**Claire:** "Well, at the time I was like 'Ugh!'" (*pulling a dirty face.*)

>>**Therapist:** "I see you pulling a face when you say that, it really wasn't nice, was it?"

>>**Claire:** "No, it really sucked..."

The aim of this exercise is not only to express angry words, but also to make the client more aware of the experience of anger. As a therapist, you can model some experiential aspects of this process of gaining awareness in order to help your client. Actively participate to encourage your client – by doing so, you will lower the threshold of shame and embarrassment that makes it difficult for the client to accept and express their anger.

> ### Example of the 'complaint exercise' – continued
>
> **>>Therapist:** "I had that myself this week – I got caught in the rain too. I was really like 'Yuck!'" (*The therapist pulls an irritated facial expression, eyebrows furrowed.*)
>
> (*Claire laughs a little at this.*)
>
> **>>Therapist:** (*laughing a little himself*) "You have to laugh, don't you?"
>
> **>>Claire:** "Oh, sorry! I'm not making fun of you or anything!"
>
> **>>Therapist:** "Don't worry, I didn't think so! I just notice that it also makes us laugh when we talk about this – about things that irritate us or have irritated us. And I was reminded of what we just said – that anger can also be funny. Do you remember?"
>
> **>>Claire:** "Yes..."
>
> **>>Therapist:** "Well, this is an example of that, I think..."

Not only do you make your client aware of the experiential aspects of anger – the various emotional, physiological and behavioural aspects of it – but you also help them become aware that expressing anger can also be pleasant, as you discussed before the exercise.

> ### Example of the 'complaint exercise' – continued
>
> **>>Therapist:** "Anyway, let's keep going. What are some other examples of 'ugh' moments you've had?"
>
> **>>Claire:** "That the roads were busy and I hit a long traffic jam. On a Saturday evening!"
>
> **>>Therapist:** "Oh, that's irritating! Or that people drive too slowly in the fast lane!"

Once the client has demonstrated the ability to express irritation about situations or events that did not directly involve another person, you can move to the next step in which you practice expressing anger about other people. For a dependent client, this may be a somewhat more difficult step, because a person might be hurt by that anger – or because they fear that, as a therapist, you might think it silly to be angry with someone.

Example of the 'complaint exercise' – continued

>>**Claire:** "Yes, or tailgating!"

>>**Therapist:** "Indeed! Have you ever experienced that?"

>>**Claire:** "Yes! That same night, there was a really annoying guy who was really pushing while I was driving at the speed limit."

>>**Therapist:** "What do you think at a moment like that?"

>>**Claire:** "Well, I'd rather not say…"

>>**Therapist:** "Ah, come on, just say it! No one will hear but us."

>>**Claire:** (*in a soft tone*): "Well, a jerk or something…"

>>**Therapist:** "Say it again, but this time twenty percent louder."

>>**Claire:** (*slightly louder*) "Jerk!"

>>**Therapist:** "Come on, say it again, another twenty percent louder, and now like you could have said it in the car. Throw yourself into it!"

>>**Claire:** (*now in a firmer voice*) "Jerk!"

>>**Therapist:** "Well done! How do you feel now?"

>>**Claire:** "A bit strange…"

>>**Therapist:** "Bad-strange, or good-strange?"

>>**Claire:** "A bit of both… I'm a bit embarrassed, but it also feels good to say…"

>>**Therapist:** "Yeah, right?! It's good to say something like that loudly and forcefully, isn't it? And where do you feel that good feeling in your body?"

(*Claire gestures to her chest with both hands.*)

>>**Therapist:** "In your chest like that, yes? Think back to the moment, with him tailgating you, and say it again – 'Jerk!'"

>>**Claire:** "Jerk!"

>>**Therapist:** "What do you feel in your chest now?"

>>**Claire:** "A free feeling… open or something… strong…" (*At this she smiles.*)

>>**Therapist:** (*also smiling*) "I can see that smile on your face again, and it's nice to see. Do you feel more or less energy than before this exercise?"

>>**Claire:** "More! Much more!"

>>**Therapist:** "Yeah, right? I notice that about you too, you seem much more lively. And that's what I meant when I talked about how anger can give you energy."

In this way, the 'complaint exercise' creates a situation where you can encourage or coach the client to say something again or more loudly, and to become aware of the experience of anger. Then, you can link that awareness back to the cognitive restructuring of thoughts about anger. In this way, the exercise can be full of corrective experiences that your client gains by expressing anger. In a relaxed and cheerful atmosphere, anger is shared, and examples are laughed at. In this way, the client learns to become aware of all the experiential aspects of anger.

At the end of the exercise, however, it is important to consolidate these new learning experiences. You can do this by taking time in the session to reflect on the experiences and by asking questions such as 'What did you learn in the exercise?' or 'What do you want to take away from this exercise?' Finally, give the client some homework to consolidate the experience. This might be to encourage them to write down some things that annoyed them that day, and each day until the next session, for example.

5.9 Chapter summary

In the first phase of treatment for clients with Dependent Personality Disorder, the focus is on combating their Punitive Mode and Coping Mode, and the therapist will play an active role in this. The Punitive Mode can be combated using various techniques, but we have described here how it can be done with imagery rescripting. You can also use this method for the Demanding or the Blaming Modes. The same applies to the historical roleplay that was used in this chapter to process an Avoidant Coping Mode.

The ways in which clients can learn to deal with anger in the first phase of therapy include listing the benefits of anger and doing a 'complaint exercise'. These exercises can also be relevant for clients with Obsessive-Compulsive Personality Disorder.

Chapter 6:
Avoidant Personality Disorder

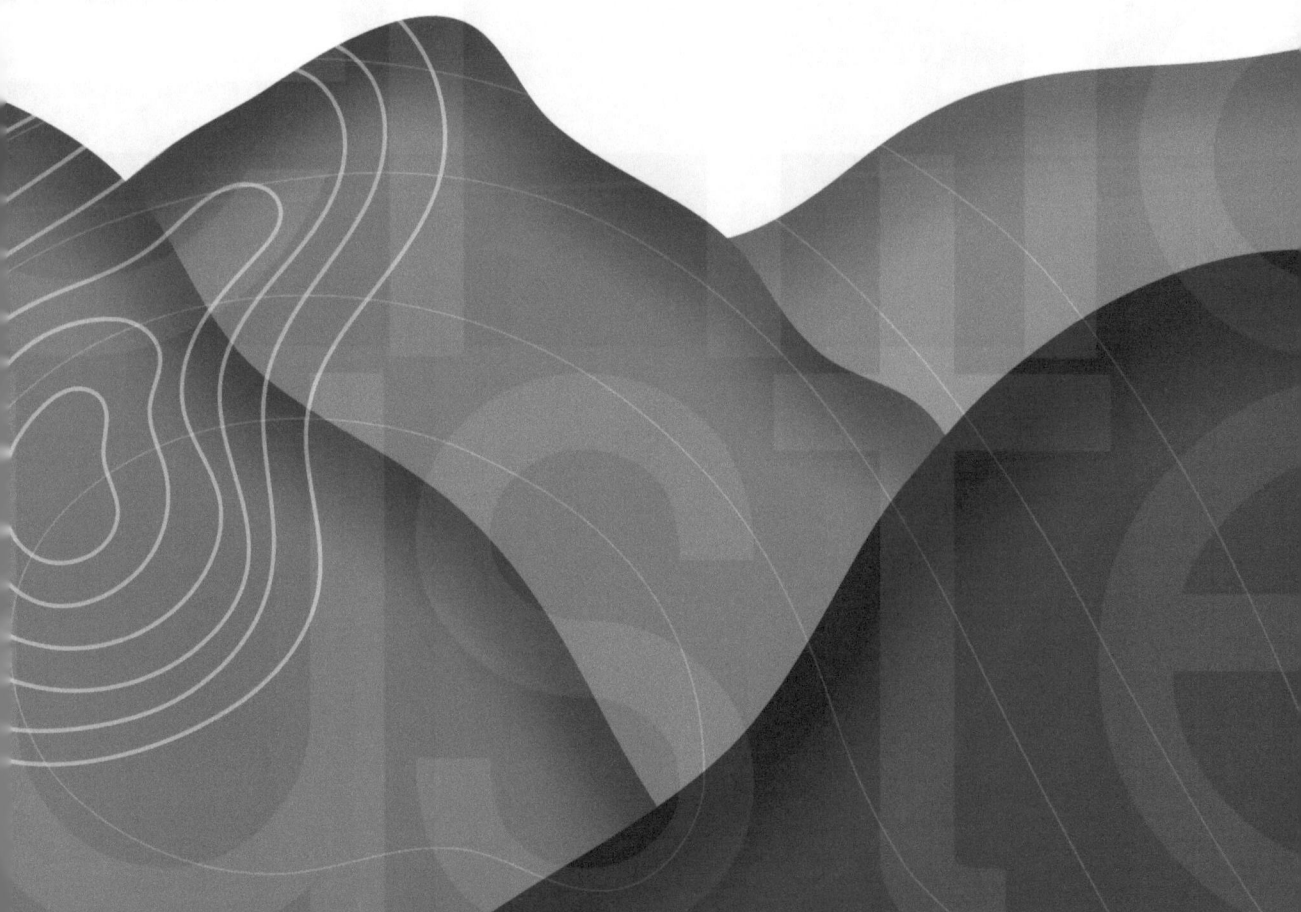

Chapter 6: Avoidant Personality Disorder

Chapter map	
6.1	Introduction
6.2	The Blaming Mode
6.3	Imagery rescripting with the Blaming Mode
6.4	The Avoidant Protector
6.5	Empathic confrontation with the Avoidant Protector
6.6	Child Modes in Avoidant Personality Disorder
6.7	Stimulating self-expression with the Inferior and Ashamed Child
6.8	Sticking points in stimulating self-expression
6.9	Chapter summary

6.1 Introduction

This chapter describes the general objectives of the treatment of Avoidant Personality Disorder – which are ultimately to get clients more in touch with their emotions and their basic unmet needs for emotional connection and self-expression. To achieve that goal, the Critical Mode will have to be combated, which in avoidant clients can often be a Blaming Mode. Finally, clients will have to learn to reduce their Avoidant Protector and engage in more interpersonal contact in which they express themselves.

In practice, it can often prove difficult to achieve these goals. Avoidant clients feel inadequate, and recognizing or expressing their feelings or needs evokes strong feelings of guilt. Furthermore, the Avoidance coping style is persistent, which makes it difficult to achieve (sufficient) behavioural change. Therapists often avoid empathic confrontations with these Avoidant Coping Modes because they do not want to appear too critical of the client, since clients with Avoidant Personality Disorder already feel so deficient.

In this chapter, we describe how to handle these challenges and problems. For each mode, a specific technique is highlighted and discussed in more detail. These techniques may also be suitable for clients with Dependent or Obsessive-Compulsive Personality Disorder. Table 1.1 shows the chapters in which you can find different methods and techniques for each mode.

6.2 The Blaming Mode

Clients with Avoidant Personality Disorder feel guilty quickly and often. Interventions designed to generate positive, corrective emotional experiences sometimes seem to be counterproductive. For example, clients sometimes do not feel relieved when the therapist addresses the Critical Mode in imagery rescripting or chairwork, but instead feel guilty. These clients often learned in childhood that standing up for their own feelings or needs is a burden to others, including significant others such as parents or siblings. Such key attachment figures will have frequently displayed a sad, tired, insecure or disappointed reaction when the client expressed their feelings or needs in childhood.

> **Example of explicit and implicit messaging**
>
> As a seven-year-old, Jenny asks her parents to play a game because she is bored. Her father looks at her, weary and depressed, and does not respond further. Her mother reacts with tearful eyes: 'Oh, I've already worked so hard to provide you with every amusement and convenience, and now you come and criticize me that you're bored. I really don't know how I'm supposed to take care of everything anymore.'

In this example, an accusatory message – that Jenny is a burden on others – can either be communicated literally, as it was by her mother, or conveyed more implicitly, as it was by her father. He may not have said anything in words, but in his gloomy, depressed demeanour and gaze gave a clear, unspoken message: 'I'm already having a tough time, and if I have to take your needs into account, I'll feel even worse.' It is often implicit messages like these that make avoidant client feel guilty, anxious and sad.

Over the years, these accusatory messages are internalized into a Blaming Mode. Without the other person even having to be present, the avoidant client can slip into their Blaming Mode. In that mode, their attention is focused on the other person's (imagined) suffering, and again that unspoken message can be read – that this suffering is a result of what the client has done or failed to do, or because of who they are. As a result, the client falls into the Inferior/Ashamed Child Mode in which they feel guilty, sad and anxious.

The objective of treatment is to reduce this Blaming Mode. In the initial phase, as a therapist, take a clear stand against the Critical Modes in order to have your client clearly and unambiguously experience a different, healthier message. However, fighting a Blaming Mode is different from fighting a Punitive Mode. A Punitive Mode is very harsh and forceful in its critical messages. To negate these messages, you will therefore have to take strong and sometimes harsh action against it. A Blaming Mode, however, gives its critical messages in a softer, more indirect way by focusing on the suffering of others. Acting forcefully or harshly against such messages does not sit well with clients who may already feel guilty. If your client feels guilty, they have not yet realized that this Blaming Mode is the main problem rather than their own behaviour and needs.

A better strategy for combating the Blaming Mode is to first make these implicit messages more explicit. By 'reading the implied accusatory messages out loud', the client is made more aware of these accusatory assumptions. You will then have to help them understand why these perceived accusations are not as realistic as they believe. Your active help as a therapist is needed to help your client realize that standing up for their needs and feelings is not the same as doing something to the other person.

As a final step, help the client to draw attention away from the other person's perceived suffering, and to focus more on their own feelings and needs. As long as your client's attention remains focused on others, the Blaming Mode can easily be activated.

Strategy with the Blaming Mode
1. Make implicitly communicated accusatory messages explicit.
2. Cognitive restructuring of the accusatory assumptions.
3. Focus attention on own needs rather than the other person's.

An imagery rescripting exercise with Jenny that executes this strategy is described in the next section. For a detailed description of imagery rescripting in the initial phase of treatment, please refer to Van der Wijngaart (2020). The strategy can also be achieved using other techniques, such as chairwork and historical roleplay.

6.3 Imagery rescripting with the Blaming Mode

This section provides step-by-step guidance for using imagery rescripting with the Blaming Mode. The full process of imagery rescripting has already been described in detail in Chapter 5, so we will not repeat it here. Instead, we will take a 'close-up' look at the latter part of the process, beginning with linking an unpleasant situation in the present to a meaningful event in the past. As before, this is not a mandatory script that must be followed; it is a framework to assist you in finding the best way to help your client through this experiential exercise.

Close-up process for imagery rescripting with the Blaming Mode
Step 1: Unpleasant situation in the present.
Step 2: Affect bridge to the past.
Step 3: Rescript these meaningful images.
Step 4: Strengthen the Happy Child.

6.3.1 Step 1: Unpleasant situation in the present

When you ask Jenny to describe a recent situation in which she felt bad, she initially talks about the actual moment itself. Specifically, this is when she is sitting at home after visiting her friend Eline, and not during the visit.

However, clients' feelings of guilt often do not have much to do with the actual context they were in at the time. At your request, Jenny visualizes a situation where she felt bad. Normally, you would process that image yourself to change the unpleasant feeling. However, the situation Jenny visualizes is not actually the one that made her feel bad. Within the situation that she has visualized, she (the Jenny in the visualization) is feeling bad because she is thinking about something else. To solve this problem, you need to ask her to visualize those secondary thoughts, and then those are the images that you process and rescript – a visualization within a visualization, as it were.*

---

* This is known as the '*Inception* technique', referring to the film *Inception* (2010), in which characters within a dream can end up in another dream. Hence the name: an image (the thought that is the actual reason they feel bad) within an image (the first image, of the context/situation in which they felt bad).

Example of visualizing a recent unpleasant event

Jenny visited a good friend with whom she feels able to relax a bit more. She spoke enthusiastically about a film she had seen that touched her. Back at home, she thinks back and realizes that her friend didn't say much, and it was mostly she herself who talked. Jenny worries about the possibility that her friend may have found this boring and thought that Jenny talked too much. She feels guilty for letting herself go like this. You suggest an exercise to understand this feeling better, but also to help her.

>>Therapist: "Just try to imagine yourself sitting there again, when you've just returned from the visit… how do you feel now?"

>>Jenny: "Really very, very bad… horrible… I'm thinking about Eline, and how she must have felt…"

>>Therapist: "Okay, so as you sit there, your thoughts drift to Eline, and if you put yourself into those thoughts now, what do you see?"

>>Jenny: "How do you mean?"

>>Therapist: "Well, it sounds like you're sitting in your room, but a not-very-nice movie is playing in your head about Eline and how she feels. Can you describe that movie you're seeing, almost as if you are literally watching Eline and how she feels?"

>>Jenny: "Well, then I see me sitting and talking again…"

>>Therapist: "Are you looking at yourself now or are you there, talking again?"

>>Jenny: "Well, I'm kind of looking at the situation, but mostly at Eline…"

>>Therapist: "And describe Eline as you see her now?"

>>Jenny: "She looks bored … but also sad … as if she actually wanted to talk about something else, but now she has to listen to this stupid story of mine…"

>>Therapist: "Do you see that in her eyes, or in her face or posture?"

>>Jenny: "In her face, she looks tired, unhappy…"

6.3.2 Step 2: Affect bridge to the past

So, Jenny's recent unpleasant event was not so much an actual event, but more her visualization of someone else feeling unhappy. It is these mental images that have activated the schemas that now make her feel so guilty. The next step is to gain more insight into the original significant events, usually from the client's childhood, that led to the formation of these schemas.

Example of affect bridge to the past

>>Therapist: "And what kind of bad feeling is that? Is it sadness, fear, anger, or guilt? Don't think too hccard about it, just experience the feeling…"

>>Jenny: "Guilty … sad … also kind of afraid that now she won't want to hang out with me anymore…"

>>Therapist: "So you're afraid she won't want to hang out with you anymore? And what do you feel guilty about?"

>>Jenny: "That I was just talking all that time, that I wasn't paying attention to her at all… Maybe she was struggling with something and she couldn't talk about it because I was just chattering…"

>>Therapist: "So you feel guilty for short-changing her by talking about your own experiences? As if by doing that, you've done something to her?"

(Jenny nods sadly.)

>>Therapist: "And where do you feel that guilty, fearful and sad feeling in your body?"

(Jenny points to her chest.)

>>Therapist: "In your chest, okay… I understand this is a very unpleasant feeling, but I still want to ask you to keep in touch with it. Just put a hand on your chest and focus on that feeling… Is this the first time you've had this feeling, or is it familiar at all?"

>>Jenny: "I have it very often… always…"

>>Therapist: "Then focus your attention on the feeling and let the image of Eline fade away. This feeling isn't just from the situation with her… What images or memories from the past come to mind when you stay in this feeling of guilt, fear and sadness?"

You make original, early-childhood memories easily accessible to your client by not only asking about the emotions they experienced in the recent situation, but also paying attention to the physiological and cognitive components of the schema activation.

Example of affect bridge to the past – continued

>>Jenny: "I don't know… I'm reminded of my father… he too could look like that… so absent, as if something was bothering him…"

>>Therapist: "So you're seeing your father now? Can you describe what you see, so I can look at it with you?"

>>**Jenny:** "Well, he was always in his room, lying there on the bed…"

>>**Therapist:** "So you see him lying on the bed now?"

>>**Jenny:** "Yes…"

>>**Therapist:** "What else do you see? Is it bright in the room?"

>>**Jenny:** "He has the curtains closed, and it's daytime but it's dark in the room because of the curtains… I don't feel comfortable with that."

>>**Therapist:** "Do you see yourself as well? Or are you there as Little Jenny?"

>>**Jenny:** "A little bit of both…"

(*Here, the therapist chooses to get more information about the context of the visualized event from Jenny's observer perspective.*)

>>**Therapist:** "Just look at your father and Little Jenny. How old do you think Jenny is when you see her standing like that?"

>>**Jenny:** "Maybe seven… or eight?"

>>**Therapist:** "And how does she seem to feel in this situation? Can you describe her for me?"

>>**Jenny:** "Well, she's standing there, looking a bit … cautious, maybe? She just came in, said she's a bit bored and asked if he wants to play a game. But he just looks at her, tired … gloomy … and she isn't sure how he feels or whether it's good that she's there."

>>**Therapist:** "I think you can already feel a bit of her tension?"

(*Jenny nods.*)

>>**Therapist:** "Put yourself into her place, just be her… (*From now on, the therapist speaks a little softer, almost as if talking to a seven-year-old.*) Tell me, what's going through your mind now you're standing here with your dad lying in this dark room?"

>>**Jenny:** "I'm a bit scared… he's feeling bad, and now I'm bothering him too…"

>>**Therapist:** "And you feel afraid?"

>>**Jenny:** "Yes, I'm scared, but mostly I feel guilty… now he feels even worse because of all my questions."

6.3.3 Step 3: Rescript these meaningful images

At this point, you decide to step into the picture and directly address the father. The decision to step in now is primarily determined by the client's emotional arousal (see 5.2.6). The intervention is intended to provide a corrective emotional experience, and this requires some schema activation. However, the emotions evoked should still be bearable for the client. You notice that Jenny is clearly emotional from having put herself into the situation being discussed. Her voice sounds sad, and she seems completely absorbed in the image, so her reactions to your questions are somewhat delayed.

Example of rescripting meaningful images

>>Therapist: "Then I would like to come in now, with you and your Dad. I'd like to help you. Can you see me?"

>>Jenny: "I don't know… he already feels so bad, and I don't want to make it worse."

>>Therapist: "You're afraid that things will be even harder for him if I join?"

(Jenny nods.)

>>Therapist: "Well, it's true that I do want to say something to him. And yes, it's possible that he may not appreciate everything about it. But not coming in to help you when you feel so anxious and guilty – that doesn't seem right either. It feels like I'm letting you down, like it's not important how you feel, and I don't want that. I don't want to be one of those people in your life who gave you the idea that your feelings don't matter. They do. So, I'd still like to come in. But maybe it will help you to know that I want to help your father too. That I want to arrange help for him if it is needed?"

>>Jenny: "Yes, I'd like that…"

>>Therapist: "Good, I'm coming in then. Where do you see me now? Ideally, I'd like to stand between you and your father, just diagonally in front of you… can you see me?"

(Jenny nods.)

>>Therapist: "Where do you see me, to the left or right of you? Can you point at me?"

>>Jenny: "There, a bit to the right in front of me." *(She points to a spot in front of her to the right.)*

>>Therapist: "Good, then I want to say something to your father first."

Arriving at this point, as the therapist, turn in the direction where the client has identified the antagonist, in Jenny's case her father. Addressing the antagonist 'physically' in this way makes the rescripting more realistic for the client.

Example of rescripting meaningful images – continued

>>Therapist: (*in a calm, reasonable tone*) "Jenny's father, I get the idea you're not feeling well. I can see because you're lying here in the dark during the day, and I can also see it in the tired, gloomy look in your eyes. I can see this, but Jenny sees it even more clearly than me. She's a sensitive child, and she can see immediately that you don't feel well. And for Jenny, who just asked if you wanted to play a game, this look in your eye is a clear message. It's like reading a caption that says 'I'm already feeling so bad, and now you're bothering me too. Your questions are making me feel even worse.'"

>>Therapist: (*turns to Jenny and asks softly*): "Is that right, Jenny?"

(*Jenny nods slowly.*)

After expressing the implicitly communicated accusatory messages out loud, you will need to help the client with the cognitive restructuring of them.

Example of rescripting meaningful images – continued

>>Therapist: (*turning to father*) "I'm sorry that you're not feeling good, and I think it would be wise for us to investigate what kind of help you need. However, for now, the most important thing is to tell Jenny that she did nothing wrong. She asked if you wanted to play a game. That's a very normal question for a child. And it's a good thing – good that she's telling you what she thinks, and what she wants and needs! I understand that it's irritating for you – that this question seems to be just one more burden to bear – but that's your problem and not something Jenny needs to be confronted with. She can't help it that you feel bad, and it certainly isn't her fault. In my world, parents take care of children, not the other way around. Your job as a father is to teach her that it's good to feel what she needs and good to express it. By doing that, you'll actually help her to avoid becoming depressed and unhappy in life."

>>Therapist: (*turning towards Jenny*) "How is for you to hear that?"

>>Jenny: "Two sided... it's good on one side ... but my Dad really is trying to do his best... I feel so sad for him." (*Jenny begins to cry softly.*)

At this point, it is important to help your client experience the healthy, new messages and their healing effect more fully. For Jenny, this requires her to pull her attention away from her visualized father and focus more on her own feelings and needs. At the same time, her mounting sense of guilt may also be the result of her visualization of her father's suffering. You may wish to repeat the first steps of your strategy, especially if this is one of the first occasions on which the Blaming Mode has been addressed this way.

Example of rescripting meaningful images – continued

>>Therapist: "Do you feel sad now because your Dad doesn't like what I'm saying?"

(*Jenny nods slowly.*)

>>Therapist: "And how can you see that, that he doesn't like how I address him?"

>>Jenny: "He looks dejectedly at the floor… and I think he would say something like: 'I know, I'm not a good father to her at all… I ruin everything…'"

>>Therapist: (*turns back in the direction of the visualized father*) "Sorry, but I'm intervening for a moment because it's happening again. I know you find this very difficult – you're looking at the floor, saying that you're ruining everything, and clearly struggling. But what you're really doing is sending another message to Jenny that she is troublesome, that she's the one to blame for you having such a hard time. And that isn't true! Your struggles aren't down to Jenny, and she can't help it if you find it hard to be spoken to like this. And she certainly shouldn't start thinking that it's better to push her needs and feelings aside. Now, if you're struggling so much, I'll refer you to a very knowledgeable colleague who can help. But for now, you need to hold back your sadness; and if that doesn't work, just go outside for a while so Jenny doesn't have to see it. (*Therapist turns to Jenny.*) And I'd like to ask you to look at me and listen to me. See me crouching in front of you, listen to my voice. Can you see me, hear me?"

(*Jenny nods.*)

>>Therapist: "You haven't done anything wrong, Jenny, in fact, it's a very, very good thing that you're telling us what you want and need! I think it's important to know that. Your father will get help, you don't have to worry about him. My eyes and my attention are focused on you… how does that feel?"

>>Jenny: "It's nice… yes… kind of warm, relaxed…"

>>Therapist: "And where do you feel that warm, calm feeling in your body?"

(*Jenny points to her chest again.*)

>>Therapist: "Then put your hand on the spot with that nice feeling… just enjoy it. And perhaps now it would be good for us to get out of this dark room for a while. Where would you rather be?" (*Here the therapist starts talking in a bit more lively and cheerful way, as if to appeal to the Playful, Free Child in Jenny.*)

>>Jenny: "I want to go outside … maybe play a game…"

6.3.4 Step 4: Strengthen the Happy Child

Take your time with this part of the exercise, which not only addresses the antagonist, but also the client's spontaneous and playful side. This is an important corrective experience for clients with Avoidant Personality Disorder. Pay attention to the different modalities of this playful piece of visualization, because it helps to consolidate the experience.

> **Example of strengthening the Happy Child**
>
> **>>Therapist:** "A game? How nice! What would you like to play?"
>
> **>>Jenny:** "I want to play football…"
>
> **>>Therapist:** "Oh, it's great that you like playing football! Can I play too?"
>
> **>>Jenny:** (*smiling*) "Yes, of course…"
>
> **>>Therapist:** "I'm not as good as I'd like to be, but I still enjoy it. Can you see me fumbling with the ball?"
>
> **>>Jenny:** "Yes, you're trying to do tricks, but they're not working out well." (*Laughs*.)
>
> **>>Therapist:** (*laughing too*) "Yes, I know, I'm trying hard, but it's not really working out, is it? I do like to see you laugh, though. How do you feel when you see me fumbling with the ball and laughing about it like that?"
>
> **>>Jenny:** "Yeah, good… happy."
>
> **>>Therapist:** "And where do you feel that nice, happy feeling?"
>
> **>>Jenny:** "Here." (*Puts a hand on her stomach*.)
>
> **>>Therapist:** "Just keep your hand there, and enjoy that nice, happy feeling. After all the tension, it's good just to enjoy feeling free and playing. Just watch me fumble with the ball and, if you want, I think you could take from me in no time."
>
> **>>Jenny:** "Yes, I think so too." (*Has to laugh out loud at this*.)
>
> **>>Therapist:** "It's so nice to see and hear you enjoying yourself like that, Jenny!"

6.4 The Avoidant Protector

The Avoidant Protector may cause your client to not show up to a session, to arrive late, not to do homework, or to cancel other appointments. Within the sessions themselves, the Avoidant Protector may cause the client to talk softly or not to answer at all. These are all forms of avoidance, with the function that the underlying feelings of failure or inadequacy are not felt by the client, or at least are not visible to the therapist.

The aim of treatment is to lessen the influence of the Avoidant Protector so that you and your client can better connect with their underlying feelings and needs. To achieve this, it will be necessary to 'negotiate' with the Avoidant Protector in order to get past the client's avoidance. There are several methods and techniques for doing this, and for connecting with the Inferior/Ashamed Child (see box below).

> **Methods and techniques for overcoming the Avoidant Protector**
>
> *Experiential techniques:*
> - Imagery rescripting
> - Chairwork
> - Historical roleplay
> - Empathic confrontation
> - Using crisis
>
> *Cognitive techniques:*
> - Discussing advantages and disadvantages
> - Calculating the probability of dreaded disasters if avoidance is stopped
>
> *Behavioural techniques:*
> - Behavioural experiments
> - Stimulating self-expression (see below in this chapter)

In the section below, we will describe how you can conduct an empathic confrontation with the Avoidant Protector in the initial phase of therapy.

6.5 Empathic confrontation with the Avoidant Protector

Empathic confrontation can easily trigger feelings of failure and inadequacy in a client with Avoidant Personality Disorder. The client will have a strong Blaming Mode, which is quickly activated when you say in the empathic confrontation how difficult you find their avoidance. In that moment, your client sees this as confirmation of their longstanding self-image of failure and inadequacy. With so much schema activation, they may not be able to hear or process the corrective, healthy messages of your intervention easily.

Furthermore, as a therapist, you will be highly aware of these schemas in your client. That awareness can make it difficult to say something critical when they already feel so bad about themselves. Common schemas among therapists, such as Self-Sacrifice (see Table 2.1), can make confrontation even more difficult. It can feel as if you are harming the client, causing them unnecessary anxiety and distress just as the Blaming Mode does, while they are already having a hard time. This may lead you to delay or avoid empathic confrontation.

An empathic confrontation is therefore not only a matter of handling the client's schemas, but also the schemas activated in yourself. The best way to handle this two-way schema activation (in the client and also in yourself) is described below.

Process for empathic confrontation with the Avoidant Protector
Step 1: Compassion for schema activation in the therapist.
Step 2: Deal with schema activation in the therapist – thinking realistically.
Step 3: Perform empathic confrontation.

6.5.1 Compassion for schema activation in the therapist

In the same way as for clients, you need to start with compassion for the feelings evoked by the schema activation within yourself. It's understandable that you might be apprehensive about saying something that your client will find annoying or hurtful Needless to say, you don't want them to feel bad, so it can be stressful when you're about to confront them with their Avoidant Protector. It's natural to want to avoid that confrontation.

Perhaps confronting others is something that you find difficult at the best of times, and, with your own past history, it might be understandable that you struggle to give another person criticism or negative feedback. It may therefore be completely reasonable that you feel an urge to just postpone the empathic confrontation, or not to do it at all.

6.5.2 Deal with schema activation in the therapist – thinking realistically

If you do find it difficult to engage in a confrontation, take a moment to think calmly about what dangers you fear, and examine for yourself whether they are realistic.

Your client may find the empathic confrontation somewhat unpleasant in the moment, but with it, you offer them the chance to break patterns and become happier in their life. They may confuse the empathic confrontation with the accusatory messages from their childhood. But of course, understanding how to discuss the adverse effects of avoidance is not the same thing as saying that their feelings or needs do not matter.

Another important consideration is the advantages and disadvantages of not doing the empathic confrontation. The advantages will mostly be short-term – you avoid schema activation in the client and yourself for this session. The disadvantages, however, only become apparent over the longer term, when, for example, the client keeps cancelling appointments or arriving late to your sessions, and these patterns do not change.

6.5.3 Perform empathic confrontation

The conclusion, then, is that sooner or later you will have to empathically confront the client. What is the best way to do that with someone who is quick to feel guilty and who firmly believes that they are inadequate?

An empathic confrontation has two elements. On the one hand, you confront the client with a pattern or behaviour that needs to be broken. On the other, you express your understanding of the background and function of that pattern of behaviour. The actual confrontation is often the most schema-activating part of the intervention. However, as we have noted for other exercise, some schema activation is necessary for the intervention to be emotionally significant and to make it a corrective emotional experience.

In clients with Avoidant Personality Disorder, there is often already so much schema activation in the session that it is not necessary to begin with the confrontation. For this reason, start instead with understanding and empathy. This may be different for a client with Obsessive-Compulsive Personality Disorder who is comfortable with their Perfectionistic Overcontroller; here, it may be more effective to start with confrontation and add empathy later. With clients with Dependent Personality Disorder, it is again often best to start with empathy, because they tend already to feel very tense and insecure.

However tactfully you try to apply the intervention, your words will still often activate the client's Blaming Mode. At that point, your healthy feedback is translated into accusatory criticism, leaving your client feeling a familiar sense of failure and inadequacy. Be alert to that, and externalize the Blaming Mode as much as possible with words and gestures – as if you were pointing out a bad translator in the room who is twisting your words.

Tips and tricks for handling schema activation in the therapist

- Keep your speaking pace slow. Schema activation can often lead to an increase in the pace of speech. The increased tension and higher pace of speaking can unnecessarily activate your client's schemas further.
- Keep speaking in terms of modes ('sides', to the client). You aren't criticizing your client as a person, but their Avoidant Protector.
- Look away from the client from time to time, in order to give yourself a break from being confronted with signals of schema activation.
- Make regular summaries to ensure that bother you and client remain aware of the actual message that the exercise is designed to convey.

Example of empathic confrontation

Jenny often arrives late for sessions. When she comes in ten minutes late, she always apologizes profusely and clearly seems to feel very bad about it. However, she keeps doing it, despite the fact that you have discussed it and applied various techniques to reduce her Avoidant Protector. Even though you realize it is the Avoidant Protector causing this behaviour, you do find it annoying. You're a little hesitant to bring it up because you know Jenny already feels so bad about herself. But after consulting your peer group, you decided to confront her anyway. Jenny has just come in late again.

>>Jenny: "I'm so sorry! I know I'm always late… it seems like I can't do anything right, I can't even get here on time."

>>Therapist: "Well, that's actually what I wanted to talk to you about today, about that lateness. If I'm completely honest, I find that I don't much like it."

(Jenny looks anxious and immediately becomes rather quiet.)

>>Therapist: "If it happened once, or if you were just a few minutes late, I wouldn't say anything. But I've noticed that it happens often, and you're ten or even fifteen minutes late. And when that happens, I'm just sat here waiting. I can't do anything else, because I don't know if and when you'll come. Can you understand that?"

>>Jenny: *(in a soft voice)* "I know, it won't happen again, I'm sorry…"

>>Therapist: "Well, I like the fact that you want to change it, but I haven't come to that yet. I wanted to discuss what I notice in you first. When I look and listen to you like this, it seems like you're not listening to me, but to your Blaming →

Side. (*The therapist points to a spot diagonally behind Jenny.*) I'm saying that I don't like having to wait, but it seems like you're hearing something completely different. Is that true?"

>>Jenny: "Yes, but I do understand that you're fed up with me and I'm ruining the therapy."

>>Therapist: "Okay, but now I hear the Blaming Side twisting my words. (*The therapist again points to the Blaming Mode's place.*) Because I'm not fed up with you at all, and I don't think you're ruining the therapy. So, I'd ask you to listen not to her (*pointing to the Blaming Mode's place*) but to me. Can you try looking at me?"

(*Jenny looks up.*)

>>Therapist: "I'm certainly not fed up with you. I think you're important, and I enjoy working with you. I know you're trying your best, really I do. I think it's the Avoidant Side I've been running into a bit lately. And it's not that I think it's stupid or anything, not at all. I'm glad you've had it. With your father so depressed and your mother so anxious and stressed, it helped you get through a difficult time as best you could."

(*Jenny looks slightly more relaxed.*)

>>Therapist: "So I can easily see where it came from. And I also understand that, to your Avoidant Side, it can still seem that avoiding difficult situations and feelings is the best thing to do. But I also think that circumstances have changed. And now, with me, it really is different than it was with your parents. I'm not depressed or stressed, I do think your feelings are important, and I do want to pay attention to them. So it's troublesome when the Avoidant Side makes it so hard to connect with you. Because she keeps you away from sessions, I'm less able to help you and less able to listen to what you feel and need. And I do find that a bit annoying. How does that sound to you?"

>>Jenny: "Yes, I understand that, yes…"

>>Therapist: "Does it still feel like I'm saying I'm fed up with you when I tell you how I experience your Avoidant Side?"

>>Jenny: "No, I know you're talking about my Avoidant Side in particular, and that you think… uh… yes, that you aren't fed up with me, let's say…"

>>Therapist: (*smiling*) "That I think you're important and I enjoy working with you, you mean?"

>>Jenny: "Yes, that, yes…"

6.6 Child Modes in Avoidant Personality Disorder

Limited reparenting aims to encourage self-expression and connection. As the role model of the healthy parent the client should have had, you of course provide the safety they need to be able to relax. However, you must also remain firm enough to encourage them to speak up and sometimes to do things they find uncomfortable. Safety in the form of warm care and support is not enough on its own to break through the schemas of *Defectiveness/Shame* and *Failure*. You therefore need to adopt the attitude of a warm, validating parent who is not afraid to confront the client in an understanding way and encourage them to speak up.

Clients with Avoidant Personality Disorder have often learned that they are not as good, intelligent or attractive as other people (Inferior and Ashamed Child). As a result, they have learned to ignore or suppress their own feelings and needs (Intimidated Child). They have also developed a strong focus on others (Parentified Child), and they are particularly focused on avoiding criticism and condemnation. Consequently, these clients have not learned to recognize and validate their own feelings and needs – they often do not have a good sense of what these needs are and, when they do know, they find it difficult to express them.

6.7 Stimulating self-expression with the Inferior and Ashamed Child

For avoidant clients, a major goal of therapy is therefore to encourage self-expression. But how do you do that? Encourage this self-expression by explaining to your client that they can ask themselves the question often and regularly: 'What do *I* want/need *right now*?'

By emphasizing the 'I' in that question, you ask the client to direct their attention to their own needs and feelings, rather than what others think and want. By emphasizing 'now', you draw their attention to small, concrete needs throughout the day. The advantage of these concrete needs, like 'I need food, drink, a walk', is that they are easy to validate – certainly easier than larger, higher needs like the need for happiness or more freedom.

Example of the client discovering their needs

>>Therapist: "Well, Jenny, if there's one thing we've been working on in your therapy, it's that you learn to listen to your own needs instead of setting them aside because you're afraid that others will think they're strange. Too often in your life, your needs have been pushed aside as if they aren't important. So what you can learn here is to ask yourself 'The Question'. This is the question: 'What do I want/need NOW?'."

(*Jenny looks a little surprised.*)

>>Therapist: "Because that question is all about what you want, what Jenny wants. It's all about what you need. Not what others want, what you think others want from you, or what would be appropriate, but your own needs. And it's also about what you need right now. So the question isn't 'What do you need in your life?', which is way too big. It's small steps: What do *I* want or need *right now*? How does that sound?"

>>Therapist: (*nods somewhat shyly*) "Yes, that does make sense…"

Practicing with this question, and validating the needs that the client mentions, should preferably be done immediately in the session. That way, you can make adjustments if your client is inclined to focus their attention more on the difficulties and impossibilities of fulfilling their needs. As you provide active coaching, strive for small moments of success when your client speaks up about something they want for themselves. Reinforce these moments as much as possible to help consolidate these corrective learning experiences.

Example of the client discovering their own needs – continued

>>Therapist: "Let's just practice that here, in the session. Can you say that question out loud?"

>>Jenny: "What do *I* need?"

>>Therapist: "Exactly! 'What do *I* need or want *right NOW*?' Can you say it again?

>>Jenny: "What do *I* need *now*?"

>>Therapist: "Very good! And what is the answer to that question? What do YOU want RIGHT NOW?"

>>Jenny: "Well, I don't know…"

>>Therapist: "Aha, okay. Well, needs are always there. Sometimes it's hard to connect with them, but they're there. So, let's dig a little deeper. What do you secretly feel like or need? Right now, at this moment?"

>>Jenny: (*starts to laugh a little nervously*) "Now? At this moment?"

(*The therapist nods encouragingly.*)

>>Jenny: "At this moment? Well… I fancy a cup of coffee." (*Laughs a little shyly.*)

>>Therapist: "That's great! You asked the question, and you got an answer too! Very good! Black or with milk? Sugar?"

(*Jenny looks a little surprised.*)

>>Therapist: "Do you want that coffee black, or with milk or sugar?"

>>Jenny: "Uh… just black, that's healthier."

>>Therapist: (*looks at Jenny for a moment*): "What do YOU want NOW?"

>>Jenny: "Uh, yeah, actually with sugar then…"

>>Therapist: "Okay!!

(*The therapist gets up and walks out of the room, returning with a cup of coffee.*)

>>Therapist: "Here you go."

(*Jenny takes a sip.*)

>>Therapist: "Good?"

(*Jenny nods and laughs a little.*)

>>Therapist: "And I see a smile on your face. How does it feel now, with a cup of coffee and a smile on your face?"

>>Jenny: "Yes, it's nice, yes."

>>Therapist: "Better than before, or worse?"

>>Jenny: "No, better."

>>Therapist: "Okay, so now we also have proof that it works. You asked that question, and then you listened to what you need or want right now, and that gave you a good feeling. A better feeling than what you had just before, right?"

(*Jenny nods.*)

Of course, it isn't always possible to fulfil the client's need immediately. You should therefore also encourage them to mention things that can't be done right away. You won't, for example, go to the bakery to get a piece of cake if that's what they want, but daring to feel and express this desire is what is important, whether it can be fulfilled at once or not.

The homework is for the client to ask this question every hour of the day, and to try to fulfil the needs they identify as much as possible. It is important to write this question down on a flashcard or, with your client, think of another way to keep 'The Question' in mind. This could be a symbolic photo, or a message on the home screen of their phone.

6.8 Sticking points in stimulating self-expression

A danger with the self-expression technique that we have described is that clients may quickly perceive problems that could arise. This can lead to awkward answers to the question: 'What do you want/need now?' Some common responses and ways to handle them are set out below.

6.8.1 The client answers: 'I don't know'

Explain to your client that our needs are always there, but they can change – sometimes they are weaker, sometimes stronger. This can make it difficult to recognize them, especially given that the client has not yet learned to recognize even clear needs properly. If this happens, repeat the question, but stimulate their imagination with questions like: 'Imagine you could make a wish, what would it be?' or 'Imagine you were the main guest of a TV programme hosting a perfect day for you, what would that day be like?'"

6.8.2 The client answers with things that are not practical in reality

Sometimes clients will answer the question of what they want or need with things that are not practical to achieve in reality, at least not in the short term. Examples of this might include a relationship, to move to a new house, to go on holiday or to stop working. The practical limitations of such wants and needs can lead the client to feel despondent.

Don't go along with thinking in terms of boundaries and limitations; instead, ask the client to close their eyes and visualize what that relationship, new home or holiday would look like. Have them imagine themselves in this Good Place as well as they can, and then ask how it feels to imagine themselves this way. In this way, even without a move or a holiday, a positive experience can still be generated using the power of imagination.

6.8.3 The client answers with things that are unhealthy forms of the Avoidant Protector

Some clients may answer the question with things like wanting to sleep, watch TV, drink wine or play computer games. These are unhealthy forms of the Avoidant Protector. If you encounter these kinds of responses, explain to the client that needs are not always the same as wishes or desires. So if they say they want to drink wine, what is the underlying need? Rest, relaxation, freedom, fun, spontaneity? Once that underlying need is identified, you can discuss alternative, healthier ways to validate it.

6.9 Chapter summary

This chapter has discussed how to deal with common challenges in treating clients with Avoidant Personality Disorder. Messages of blame can often be communicated between people in indirect, implicit ways, and these can then be internalized by the recipient. By making those implicit messages explicit in therapy, you can help the client to critically examine and adjust their effect, and to lessen the sense of self-blame. Avoidant clients can learn to recognize their own needs better by regularly asking themselves the question 'What do I want/need NOW?' This question shifts the focus from the perceived criticism or suffering of others to the client's own needs, and teaches them to validate them.

We have emphasized the importance of empathic confrontation when the Avoidant Protector remains too active. Confronting clients who already feel inadequate can lead to schema activation in the therapist. It is therefore important to know how to handle both your own schema activation and that of the client during an empathic confrontation.

These strategies are not exclusively used to treat clients with Avoidant Personality Disorder, and stimulating self-expression or fighting a Blaming Mode can also be part of the treatment of other personality disorders or syndromic disorders.

Chapter 7: Obsessive-Compulsive Personality Disorder

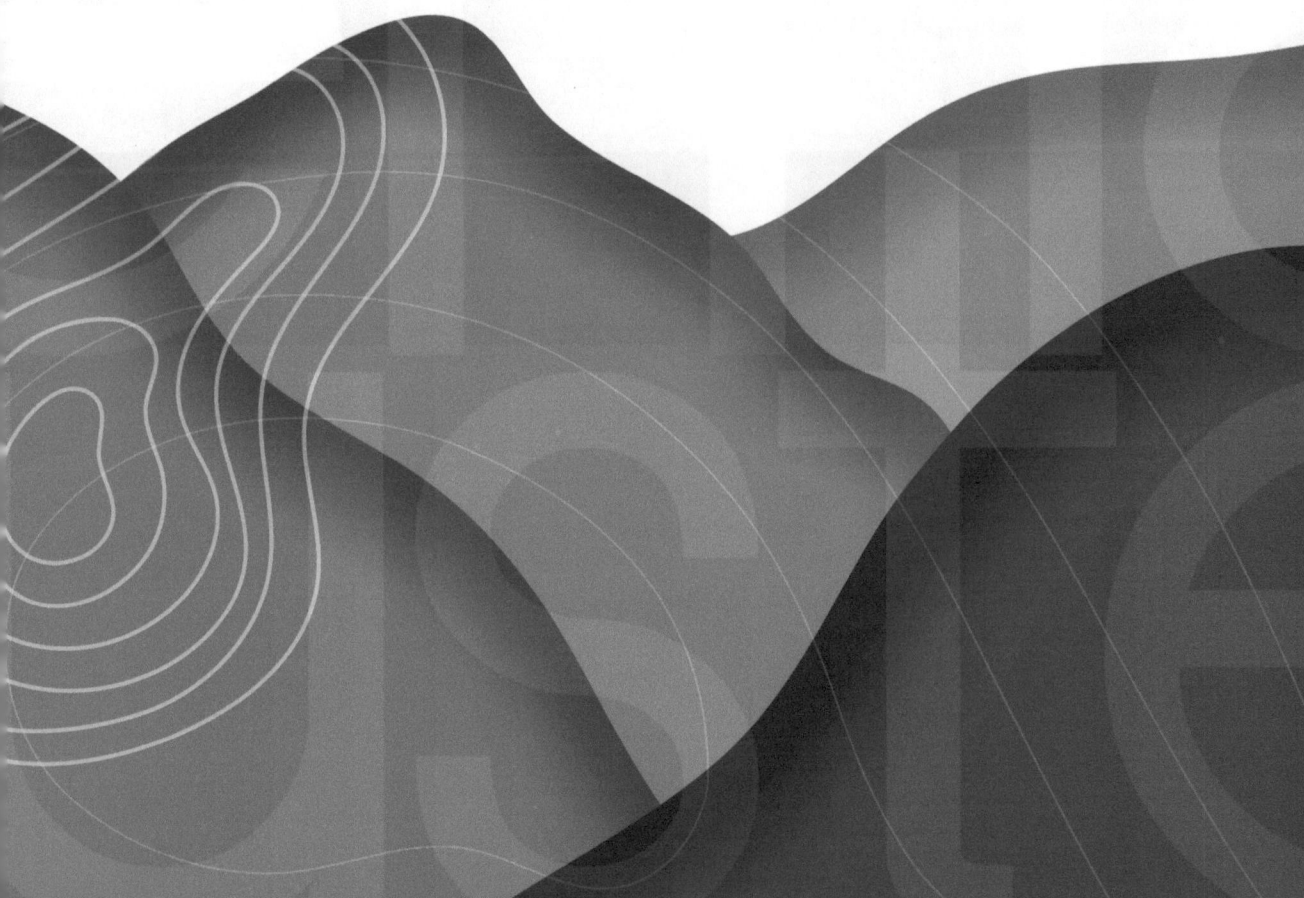

Chapter 7: Obsessive-Compulsive Personality Disorder

Chapter map	
7.1	Introduction
7.2	The Demanding Mode
7.3	Chairwork with the Demanding Mode
7.4	The Perfectionistic Overcontroller
7.5	Chairwork with the Perfectionistic Overcontroller
7.6	Chairwork variant – 'charging the chair'
7.7	Negotiating with the Perfectionistic Overcontroller during imagery rescripting
7.8	Child Modes in Obsessive-Compulsive Personality Disorder
7.9	Stimulating spontaneity and play in the Happy Child
7.10	Sticking points when working with Obsessive-Compulsive Personality Disorder
7.11	Chapter summary

7.1 Introduction

This chapter describes the objectives of treatment for Obsessive-Compulsive Personality Disorder. In short, the aim with these clients is to get them more in touch with their emotions and basic emotional needs, especially the suppressed needs for play, spontaneity, relaxation, autonomy and justice. That means they need to learn to let go more often of their familiar Perfectionistic Overcontroller mode, mainly in order to create space for emotions and basic needs. To achieve this, it will be necessary to fight the internalized demanding messages.

In practice, it can be very difficult to achieve these goals. Obsessive-compulsive clients do not view their Perfectionistic Overcontroller as a problem; instead, they say that they actually enjoy working and completing tasks. To them, it seems impossible not to work hard. This inability is fed by a belief that the messages from the Demanding Mode are actually true. It can be difficult to fight these demanding assumptions because, on the one hand, therapists sometimes have the *Unrelenting Standards* schema themselves, and on the other, clients with Obsessive-Compulsive Personality Disorder often resist to tasks that should lead to more relaxation, spontaneity and play. They tend to find activities that most people find relaxing to be a frustrating waste of time. This chapter describes how to handle these challenges and problems.

The box below describes the application of the different methods and techniques for clients with Obsessive-Compulsive Personality Disorder. In this chapter, we will focus on one specific therapeutic technique each for the Demanding Mode, the Perfectionist Overcontroller, the Disappointing/Underperforming Child and the Over-Diligent Child. These techniques may also be suitable for clients with Dependent or Avoidant Personality Disorder. Table 1.1 shows the chapters where you can find different methods and techniques for each mode.

> **Application of methods and techniques in clients with Obsessive-Compulsive Personality Disorder**
>
> *Experiential techniques:*
> - Imagery rescripting
>   *Trying to make direct contact with emotions and needs by closing one's eyes and focusing the attention on perceptions.*
> - Imagery rescripting
>   *Negotiating with the Perfectionistic Overcontroller is part of the visualization (for a detailed description of this variant of imagery rescripting, see later in this chapter).*
> - Historical roleplay
>   *Acting out significant past experiences provides greater access to the emotional experiences of the Vulnerable Child.*
> - Chairwork
>   *Negotiating with the Perfectionistic Overcontroller in another chair.*
>
> *Cognitive techniques:*
> - Discussing advantages and disadvantages
>   *In the short term, there mostly seem to be advantages, but are there any disadvantages in the long term?*
> - Probability calculation
>   *What are the realistic chances of something serious going wrong if you do not work as hard and with such perfectionism?*

Behavioural techniques:
- Behavioural experiments

  The client tests the adverse effects of working less hard and perfectionistically in practice.

Therapeutic relationship:
- Empathic confrontation

  You confront your client with the detrimental effects of the Perfectionistic Overcontroller on the therapist, the therapeutic relationship, and the therapy process.

- Using crises

  In moments of crisis, when the Perfectionistic Overcontroller has lost control, you offer care and support – making the client aware of the positive effects of being more in touch with their emotions and needs, and of connecting more with significant others.

7.2 The Demanding Mode

The aim of therapy is to reduce the influence of old, demanding assumptions. At the beginning of therapy, as the therapist, you have a leading role in fighting the Demanding Mode. However, this is often difficult, and both you and the client may find it difficult to come up with counterarguments. Unlike a Punitive Mode, the arguments of a Demanding Mode are not patently wrong or unrealistic; after all, people do have responsibilities and there are tasks and chores to be done. So, when the Demanding Mode stresses the need to take responsibility and to work hard, it can be difficult to argue against it.

Many therapists themselves have the *Self-Sacrifice* schema as well as the *Unrelenting Standards* schema (Simpson *et al*, 2019; Kaeding *et al*, 2017), which means they often have their own Demanding Mode and believe in the importance of working hard and taking responsibility. As a result, it can be difficult for them to think of something when they need to fight a client's Demanding Mode. However, the argument against this view is that by focusing on a single basic need – competence and the need to be productive – we miss the importance of fulfilling other essential basic needs.

Fighting the Demanding Mode, then, does not so much mean discussing whether work needs to be done as pointing out that paying attention to other basic needs – such as the need for spontaneity and play – is just as important.

Below are some general tips that can be helpful when working with the Demanding Mode in therapy.

7.2.1 Create distance

It is only possible to think critically about the assumptions of the Demanding Mode when you can put a little more emotional distance between you and that position. Writing down the assumptions on a whiteboard, applying chairwork (putting the Demanding Mode on a separate chair and contradicting it) or using imagery rescripting (addressing the people who were at the origin of the Demanding Mode) are all methods by which you can create more emotional distance from the Demanding Mode.

7.2.2 Prepare for cognitive restructuring

With that distance in place, you can prepare to fight the Demanding Mode. Before the session, with or without the help of colleagues, make a list of arguments as to why relaxation, play and spontaneity are not luxuries but essential basic needs. During the session, but before beginning the exercise, you and the client can also prepare for the cognitive restructuring that will take place during imagery rescripting or chairwork by talking through these arguments together.

7.2.3 Be alert to small emotional responses

When fighting the Demanding Mode, it is important to pay specific attention to the client's emotional responses, which will often be small. It is unrealistic to expect that fighting assumptions that are so ingrained in the client will suddenly trigger large, corrective emotional reactions. That can sometimes be the case when fighting a Punitive Mode, but because the Demanding Mode is often perceived as realistic and helpful, casting doubt on its assumptions will not immediately have a major emotional impact. Even so, standing up for basic emotional needs like play and spontaneity will trigger a more pleasant emotional response than the constant pressure of the Demanding Mode. Asking specifically for that emotional response, and paying attention to small differences in the emotional experience, can help the client to become more aware of the positive effects of fulfilling basic needs other than hard work and productivity.

There are various methods and techniques that can be used to apply this strategy, such as imagery rescripting, cognitive techniques such as multidimensional evaluation, and chairwork. Chairwork with the Demanding Mode is described in the next section.

7.3 Chairwork with the Demanding Mode

This section describes how chairwork can be used as an intervention in fighting the Demanding Mode. The essence of chairwork, as we have seen, is that chairs are used to represent something that has meaning for the client – such as a thought, a feeling, a person or, in the case of schema therapy, a mode. There are many different ways to perform chairwork, and following a step-by-step plan can be useful.

Step-by-step plan for chairwork with the Demanding Mode
Step 1: Become aware of the Demanding Mode.
Step 2: Rationale for chairwork.
Step 3: Have the client sit on another chair and interview the Demanding Mode.
Step 4: Have the client sit on the chair of the Vulnerable Child and offer compassion for the emotional response.
Step 5: Discuss arguments against the Demanding Mode from a standing position.
Step 6: The therapist fights the Demanding Mode while the client listens from the chair of the Vulnerable Child.
Step 7: Review and homework.

7.3.1 Step 1: Become aware of the Demanding Mode

The first step towards change is to recognize the Demanding Mode when it is active. The Demanding Mode is characterized by a critical appraisal of oneself and one's own performance. The client is in a state where they look critically at themselves, convinced that they could and should have been and done better. Unlike a Punitive Mode, the self-criticism here relates specifically to performance rather than the whole person. The tone in which a Demanding Mode speaks is critical and urging, but not as harshly condemning as with a Punitive Mode. For a further description of the differentiation between the Demanding Mode and other modes with obsessive-compulsive clients, see Chapter 3.

You can help your client to become aware of the Demanding Mode by explicitly naming it as a side of them and supporting this with gestures, as if you were pointing to another person in the room.

> **Example of becoming aware of the Demanding Mode**
>
> **>>Therapist:** "How have you felt over the past week?"
>
> **>>John:** "Well, I don't really know how I felt. But I was busy! I have a lot to do, and I should have organized it better. I have another deadline at work, and a lot depends on that, and now I'll have to work really long days. And, of course, I have to keep time free for exercise and cleaning as well."
>
> **>>Therapist:** "Okay, so I asked you how you've been feeling over the past week, but I didn't hear so much about what you felt (*points to client's belly*) as about how busy you were (*points to a spot on the ground to signify the Demanding Mode*). And it sounds like you aren't satisfied with how you managed all that. As if you look at yourself and that work pressure (*points to spot*), and then I hear you say things like: 'You should have done that differently, you just should have finished.' Is that true?"
>
> **>>John:** "Yes."
>
> **>>Therapist:** "I know you can feel differently too, but as you sit there now (*points again to spot*), you're completely in that critical state of not being satisfied with what you've done. Could it actually be that Demanding Side of you that I'm hearing then?"
>
> **>>John:** "Yes, maybe…"

7.3.2 Step 2: Rationale for chairwork

Now that the client is more aware of the Demanding Mode, the next step is to introduce chairwork. Qualitative research has shown that clients find chairwork to be valuable, but also somewhat strange and uncomfortable at first (Krans & Van der Wijngaart, 2022). Some clients will therefore have some inhibition in going along with the proposal to play this strange game of 'musical chairs.' Their willingness tends to increase, however, if the procedure and its benefits are clearly explained, and if they feel they can decide, in consultation with the therapist, whether or not to do it (Krans & Van der Wijngaart, 2022).

Example of the rationale for chairwork

>>Therapist: "So, I'd like to do an exercise. If that critical, demanding side of you is active now anyway, let's just give it a place in the room. Then we can take a closer look, and together we can try to understand why that conviction is so strong. And, of course, I'd like to help you, so you leave here feeling better than when you came in. How does that sound?"

>>John: "Yes, in itself it would be good to feel better... but how?"

>>Therapist: "I'll grab an extra chair, and in a moment I'll ask you to sit on that chair, and from there talk about what you think was wrong with everything you did last week. That shouldn't be too difficult, because you were already in that state of mind, but by expressing that perception while sitting on that chair and then looking at it together from here, we can get a better understanding of what is going on inside you and I can help you from there. I see you're not convinced – you have a look of... 'what now?!'"

>>John: "Well, it sounds a bit strange... surely I could just stay sitting here and tell you what I think?"

>>Therapist: "Sure, we can also just talk about it from the chairs we're sitting in now. But research has shown that it really helps to put that side of you in a separate chair, and that has been my experience too. As strange as it sounds, when you then stand up from that chair and look at it from a small physical distance, it actually gives you a little more emotional distance from those critical thoughts and feelings. And that distance can help you do something with it. Because when you can look at it from outside, you aren't stuck in that thought and feeling any more. I could say more about it, but I think it would be best just to experience it. Would you like to try it, and afterwards we can look back and see whether it had anything to offer?"

>>John: "Okay then, fine."

7.3.3 Step 3: Have the client sit on another chair and interview the Demanding Mode

As with its use in the treatment of other disorders, the objective of chairwork in schema therapy with the Demanding Mode is to generate a corrective emotional experience. The biggest pitfall here is talking in detail about the modes or sides of the client, which ultimately makes the exercise too cognitive. You can help the client with this by giving clear directions about what you want: in the chair of the Demanding Mode, you want them to relive that experience, to fully inhabit that part of themselves.

Example of having the client sit on another chair and interviewing the Demanding Mode

>>Therapist: "As you sit in that chair now, I actually want you to be that demanding, critical side of yourself. Now just be that critical voice, that Demanding Side. And I want you to look at John (*pointing to the original chair*) from that perspective. So now I'll actually address you as if you were that Demanding Side: What do you (*pointing to the client in the chair of the Demanding Mode*) have to say about him?" (*Points to the empty chair that now symbolizes the Vulnerable Child Mode.*)

>>John: (*starts listing all the to-do's*) "You just have to get on with it don't you – you're being paid for it, by the way! Other people manage, don't they!? If you'd just planned a bit better, and if you just work a little bit harder now, you should just get it done!"

>>Therapist: "Okay, okay, I'm going to pause you there for a moment. You're doing fine, but I'd like to ask you to come and sit on this chair here beside me."

7.3.4 Step 4: Have the client sit on the chair of the Vulnerable Child and offer compassion for the emotional response

There is no simple answer to the question of when to interrupt the client in the Demanding Mode to move to the next step of the technique. On the one hand, you need information about the demands the client is experiencing; on the other, the aim of the exercise is not to make them focus even more on those demands but instead to break free from them.

It is usually good to interrupt after a few arguments from the Demanding Mode, and to ask the client to sit in the chair of the Vulnerable Child. If the need arises, you can always let them articulate more demands from the Demanding Mode's chair later. The Vulnerable Child's chair could be the original chair, or could be a separate chair. Provided switching chairs is clearly understood as being a change of state of mind, and is supported by the therapist with clear instructions and a gentle pace, this is more a matter of personal preference and there is no strict 'right' or 'wrong' approach.

Example of having the client sit on the chair of the Vulnerable Child

>>**Therapist:** "When you get up from that chair, remember that it's the chair where you can be critical of everything you've done and not done in the past week. You can be critical about that there (*pointing to the chair of the Demanding Mode*), but only there (*pointing again to the chair of the Demanding Mode*). When you get up, leave all that criticism behind, as if it was glued to the chair. Come and sit next to me now."

(*John sits down in the chair of the Vulnerable Child.*)

>>**Therapist:** "Okay, so there (*pointing to the chair of the Demanding Mode*) I hear quite a critical voice. That's the one I hear saying, 'You just have to do it, you should have organized it better', and his voice also sounds harsh, a bit like… (*mimicking loud demanding talk*). How do you feel when you hear me use that critical voice like that?"

>>**John:** "Well… it's right, that's all true!"

>>**Therapist:** "I hear that you agree with him. But I didn't ask if you believe him, but how you feel when you hear those demands, and experience that kind of pressure? Does it make you feel good to hear what you didn't do right, or not so good?"

>>**John:** "No, it doesn't feel that great, no…"

>>**Therapist:** "And can you put words to that feeling, not as an analysis, but more to characterize it? Is it an unpleasant sad feeling, or an unpleasant tense feeling?"

>>**John:** "Well, both actually."

Clients with Obsessive-Compulsive Personality Disorder do not always find it easy to connect with their emotions, which can make it difficult or even impossible for them to answer questions above about emotional responses when they are in the Demanding Mode. If this happens, you can help verbalize and give more perspective to those emotions. For example, you can suggest how you would feel if something like that was said to you, and then ask the client if they are able to recognize that.

The next section describes how you can elaborate on this further (see also section 7.6 on 'charging the chair'). As before, chairwork aims to generate a corrective emotional experience, and to achieve that some emotional arousal through schema activation must occur. Because of this, it is important to focus on the client's emotional responses to the demanding messages.

Once the client is able to recognize and articulate the emotions evoked by activated schemas, your next step is to show compassion in the form of explicit acknowledgement. Compassion, acknowledging emotional pain, is first and foremost a way to connect with the client's experience. Additionally, compassion has a soothing, calming effect, which helps to facilitate the cognitive restructuring of demanding assumptions.

> **Example of offering compassion to the Vulnerable Child**
>
> **>>Therapist:** "I can understand that. Of course you feel sad and angry when you're told that, despite all your hard work, you didn't do well enough. Especially if you've had that criticism many times before – if it's not just this week, but the umpteenth time you've heard that you don't work hard enough. Of course that makes you feel sadness and perhaps some anger. Does that make sense, the way I describe it?"
>
> **>>John:** "Yes, that's true, yes…"
>
> **>>Therapist:** "How do you feel when you hear that I understand you? Does it feel nice to be understood, or not so nice?"
>
> **>>John:** "It feels nice, yes…"

7.3.5 Step 5: Discuss arguments against the Demanding Mode from a standing position

Although the client has already put some distance between themselves and the Demanding Mode by getting up from the chair, it may very well be that they are still convinced of the value of the critical, demanding assumptions that the Demanding Mode makes.

Thinking calmly and realistically about those assumptions requires more of their Healthy Adult. By getting up from the chair of the Vulnerable Child and looking at both chairs together from a standing position at some distance, it is easier for the client to get into a healthier state of mind, where realistic and critical thinking can take place.

> **Example of discussing arguments against the Demanding Mode from a standing position**
>
> **>>Therapist:** "So from here, you can feel the effect of the criticisms and demands that come from him (*points to the chair of the Demanding Mode*) very clearly. But that doesn't change the fact that you still feel that most of what he says is actually true – that you believe that his arguments are essentially correct. Is that right?"
>
> **>>John:** "Yes – after all, it is really true that all those to-do's have to be done…" →

>>**Therapist:** "Okay, let's step back a bit more, so we can take a moment just to think about everything that is being said from over there, and together we'll consider whether it really is all true. Come and stand next to me here."

(Therapist and client stand side by side looking at the chairs.)

There are several cognitive methods and techniques that can help to examine demanding assumptions critically. A few of these seem to work particularly well (see box below).

Useful techniques to test demanding assumptions

- Compare the emotional responses provoked by the Demanding Mode and the therapist's compassion – which gives the better feeling and the most energy?
- Is working hard and achieving things the only need that matters in life?
- When are you most productive, when you have energy or when you're tired?
- The Demanding Mode says that you can rest once the work is done. But is it ever completely done, or is there always something else to do?
- Does perfection exist? When is something good enough?
- Why might it be useful to stop and rest?
  (Variant: 'What happens if you don't charge your phone in time?')

Example of testing demanding assumptions

Reflecting on the effect of the Demanding Mode

>>**Therapist:** "So over the past week, this is what was going on inside you: your Demanding Side was constantly sending you messages about all the things you hadn't done yet and what you still needed to do. And you felt sad because of that, and perhaps also a little angry. And this didn't only happen last week; it's something that happens all the time: it's go-go-go-go, criticism-sadness-criticism-sadness, and so on. What do you think, when you look at it like that?"

>>**John:** "I think it's a bit wretched… a bit dark…"

Reflecting on whether hard work and achievement is the only need in life.

>>**Therapist:** "What does that sense of sadness actually need, do you think? What does that Sad and Vulnerable Child need? A hard kick up the backside?"

>>**John:** "No, of course not! Just some relaxation…"

>>**Therapist:** "Quite! What would you like to look back on in twenty years' time? More of the same cycle of criticism-sadness-criticism-sadness, or a bit more freedom away from all the tasks that need to be completed in life?"

>>**John:** "The last one…"

7.3.6 Step 6: The therapist fights the Demanding Mode while the client listens from the chair of the Vulnerable Child

The client should by now have a rational understanding of why the assumptions of the Demanding Mode are not realistic. However, these cognitive arguments may still need to be reinforced. To achieve this, ask the client to sit back in the Vulnerable Child's chair and listen to how you fight the Demanding Mode using the arguments you have discussed.

> ### Example of the therapist fighting the Demanding Mode
>
> **>>Therapist:** I don't agree with this Demanding Side of yours, for all the reasons we've just discussed. Would you like to feel what it's like when I tell him exactly why I disagree with him?"
>
> **>>John:** "Uh… yeah, sure…"
>
> **>>Therapist:** Then I'll go back to my chair for a moment, and I would ask you to sit back in the chair of that Vulnerable Side."
>
> (*John sits down.*)
>
> **>>Therapist:** "Good, now you're back in that place where you just felt how dispiriting it is when you keep getting criticized for everything you do. Do you remember all the criticism that he levelled at you?"
>
> **>>John:** "Yes, that I should have organized everything differently and just tried harder to do my best…"
>
> **>>Therapist:** "And does that give you a nice feeling?"
>
> (*John shakes his head.*)
>
> **>>Therapist:** "Then listen, and you'll feel what it's like when I go against him."
>
> (*The therapist turns towards the chair of the Demanding Mode.*)
>
> **>>Therapist:** "The problem I have with you is that you make John feel sad and angry. Not only that, but you don't seem to think this matters, because you're so work-focused. You're so concerned with tasks that John doesn't seem to be in the picture at all – he's just an afterthought. John does matter, and he's much more than just a production machine. There's a lot more to life than work, and it certainly isn't the only thing that John will want to look back on in twenty years' time."
>
> **>>Therapist:** (*turning to client*) "How does it feel when you hear those arguments? Do they feel right to you?"
>
> **>>John:** "Yes, well, yes… it's true what you say."

With these questions about feelings and emotional responses, you direct the client's attention to the corrective emotional experience that you are providing through the exercise. The client can now experience what it is like to stand up for needs that have been denied or suppressed for so long.

7.3.7 Step 7: Review and homework

The review of this exercise and the subsequent homework are designed to consolidate the corrective emotional experiences. On the one hand, the homework will consist of remembering that the emotional response to the compassion and cognitive restructuring offered was much more pleasant than the emotional responses to the Demanding Mode. On the other hand, it will also have to involve remembering the cognitive arguments against the Demanding Mode. To do this, you can either write the key arguments on a whiteboard and ask the client to take a photo of them, or you could record an audio flashcard summarising the major themes and arguments. Alternatively, you could ask the client to spend time writing down the main arguments at home.

7.4 The Perfectionistic Overcontroller

In the Perfectionistic Overcontroller mode, clients with Obsessive-Compulsive Personality Disorder try to protect themselves from making mistakes by working excessively hard and being very perfectionist. They seek to control themselves, as well as others, in a compulsive way, which may cause them to be perceived as overly critical. This is a state of mind in which clients with Obsessive-Compulsive Personality Disorder are detached from all their feelings and needs other than the sense of satisfaction they get from completing tasks or working efficiently. For more information on distinguishing the Perfectionistic Overcontroller from other modes, such as the Demanding Mode, see Chapter 3.

Working hard or trying to make as few mistakes as possible is not problematic behaviour in itself; such behaviour is also relevant to the Healthy Adult. However, in the Perfectionistic Overcontroller mode, the client focuses excessively on this aspect of their life and loses touch with other feelings and needs. The aim of therapy is to make these feelings and needs more accessible. To achieve that, the Perfectionistic Overcontroller will have to be made into a less dominating presence in the client's life. Unlike for the Demanding Mode, the strategy is not so much to fight the Perfectionistic Overcontroller as to engage in a form of negotiation with it, so as to encourage the client to want to let go of this side of themselves more often.

Schema therapy offers various ways to engage with, and lessen the influence of, the Perfectionistic Overcontroller (see Chapter 2). The first, and perhaps most important, step, is to explicitly name it as part of the client. Naming the familiar experience of task orientation as a mode creates a certain emotional distance between it and the client. This provides an opportunity for the client to think about alternatives to incessant perfectionism and hard work.

However, sometimes the Perfectionistic Overcontroller can be so strong that standard methods do not work well. For instance, the client might do a visualization but continue to talk rationally throughout the exercise. Or they may sit in the Vulnerable Child's chair but not seem to feel any emotions. In such situations, you will have to perform chairwork or imagery rescripting differently to achieve the desired result. Some options are described below.

7.5 Chairwork with the Perfectionistic Overcontroller

With chairwork, you can ask the client to voice the Perfectionistic Overcontroller on a separate chair, then make contact with the Vulnerable Child on another chair. Being physically distant from the Perfectionistic Overcontroller gives the client more space to connect with their underlying emotions and needs. The step-by-step plan described below can serve as a guide for this technique in the initial phase. The first part of chairwork with a strong Perfectionistic Overcontroller is no different to how chairwork is applied with other Coping Modes. The variation, which will be described in section 7.6, comes at Step 5, if it seems that the client is not yet experiencing feelings and emotions when sitting in the chair of the Vulnerable Child.

Step-by-step plan for chairwork with a Perfectionistic Overcontroller
Step 1: Recognize the Perfectionistic Overcontroller.
Step 2: Name the experience as a mode.
Step 3: Have the Perfectionistic Overcontroller sit on another chair.

Step 4: Negotiate with the Perfectionistic Overcontroller.   ■ Explore its advantages.   ■ Explore its disadvantages.   ■ Ask for permission to make contact with the Vulnerable Child, while offering reassurance, control and hope.
Step 5: Have the client sit in the chair of the Vulnerable Child.
Step 6: Validate the relevant basic needs.
Step 7: Review and homework.

7.5.1 Step 1: Recognize the Perfectionistic Overcontroller

Chapter 3 describes the characteristics of the Perfectionistic Overcontroller. We therefore only give a brief summary of how to recognize this mode here. It can be recognized by the fact that the client talks excessively about what they have done or are doing, without sharing any emotional experiences. The tone of voice is not emotional but functional, with little modulation or affect. As a therapist, you will find that do not feel emotionally connected to the client in this mode, and it can even trigger feelings of boredom or irritation.

> **Example of recognizing the Perfectionistic Overcontroller**
>
> **>>Therapist:** "Good to see you again. How have you felt over the past week?"
>
> **>>John:** "Well, I've been busy. Lots of projects on the go. One is a waterfront construction project, and there is a whole set of regulations for building next to water, and I've tried to make those people understand that, but it seems like they don't want to hear it."
>
> **>>Therapist:** "Okay, so I'm hearing what you did. But how did you feel about it?"
>
> **>>John:** "Well, it was sometimes quite frustrating, because I'd grab the handbook to show them the regulations, and, for example, there is a provision about the height of construction next to water, which was always 2.3 metres but that was in 2018… no, wait, it was 2017… no, actually 2018, yes, I remember, because…"
>
> *(The therapist is starting to have trouble concentrating on the story, and he is also becoming somewhat impatient because a clear answer is not being given to a simple question.)*

7.5.2 Step 2: Name the experience as a mode

The next step in working with the Perfectionistic Overcontroller is to name that state of mind as a side of the client – a mode. A mode model for the client has already been created in the case conceptualization, so here you can use the specific name for the Perfectionistic Overcontroller that you chose together. If, at this early stage of therapy, the client does not yet have much awareness of their different modes, it might be wise to start by explaining what state of mind you think you are currently observing.

> **Example of naming the experience as a mode**
>
> **>>Therapist:** "I'd like to take a moment to consider how we're talking now. Listening to you, it's clear that you find it easy to talk at length about what you did. But it seems like you find my questions about how you've been feeling much harder to answer. As you sit there now (*the therapist points to a spot next to John*), I mostly see the John who is busy with work, thinking about what needs to be done and how to handle it. The John I see then (*therapist points again to the spot next to John*) mostly seems to be absorbed in his hectic experience of work, tasks, chores and to-do lists. Does that sound right?"
>
> **>>John:** "Yes, that's true. But there really was a lot of work, and I'm very busy with it. That's okay, isn't it?"
>
> **>>Therapist:** "Of course, life can be busy sometimes. But I know that you're more than just a hard worker. You're also an emotional person, with humour, feelings and other needs besides work (*at this, the therapist points to John's belly*). So there seem to be two sides to your experience – sometimes there's more of that emotional part, and at other times there's more of that state where you're focused on working hard. We might say there are two parts of you, an Emotional John and a Hard Worker. How does that sound?"
>
> **>>John:** "Yes, that does make sense, I can acknowledge that, yes."

7.5.3 Step 3: Have the Perfectionistic Overcontroller sit on another chair

Now that the Perfectionistic Overcontroller has been identified as a mode, chairwork can be introduced. Earlier in this chapter, we mentioned that some explanation of the process and benefits of the technique is important to help clients overcome any resistance, as it may initially seem strange to them. Here, too, it is important to be clear in your instructions.

Example of having the Perfectionistic Overcontroller sit on another chair

>>Therapist: "Okay, so we've agreed that there are different sides of you, and the side you're predominantly in right now is the Hard Worker. And I think there's a reason for that. I'd like to do an exercise that will help us to understand why this Hard Worker is so active at the moment. It will also help you – by doing the exercise, I'll be able to find other ways for you to deal with work pressure. Ways you might even feel better about. Is that okay?"

(John nods.)

>>Therapist: "Good, then I'll pull up an extra chair."

(The therapist places an extra chair at the spot that was pointed to a few times in the previous conversation when discussing the Hard Worker. Note – this should be a different place and chair from the one where you put the Demanding Mode.)

>>Therapist: "And I want to ask you to go sit on that chair now."

(John goes and sits on the chair of the Hard Worker.)

>>Therapist: "On this chair, I want you to get fully into that feeling of working hard, doing your best, and finishing to-do lists. I don't think you'll find that difficult, because I think you were already in that state of mind when you came in. But now, on this chair, just be that Hard Worker. And all the while you're sat there, that's what I'll call you – the Hard Worker."

(John nods.)

7.5.4 Step 4: Negotiate with the Perfectionistic Overcontroller

Now start the negotiation with the Perfectionistic Overcontroller. To get the client to the point of being willing to let go of the Perfectionistic Overcontroller, it is important to start the negotiation with plenty of understanding and recognition of its benefits.

7.5.4.1 Explore the advantages of the Perfectionistic Overcontroller

Go into detail about the benefits of hard work and to-do lists. Many therapists are quick to talk about the disadvantages of this Protector, but it often works better to take some time to acknowledge its benefits. For example, you might say: 'Yes, I understand that. If you can get lots of tasks done with hard work, then of course that's great. Then there's less to worry about, and less sitting on the to-do list. To be honest, I think I do it myself:

sometimes I choose to get on with work rather than reflect on feelings I might have. Your hard work also used to serve an important function, because your father was always very critical and at the slightest mistake he would say that you were wrong or lazy.'

7.5.4.2 Explore the disadvantages of the Perfectionistic Overcontroller

The drawbacks can then be discussed quite easily by asking the client whether their fears, worries or frustrations are actually resolved by the Hard Worker.

> **Example of negotiating with the Perfectionistic Overcontroller**
>
> **>>Therapist:** "Okay, so you (*gesturing to John as the Perfectionistic Overcontroller*) protect him (*gesturing to the chair of the Vulnerable Child*) by keeping all those feelings away, by working hard and definitely not talking too much about feelings. I have a Hard Worker like that myself, and I recognize that sometimes it's more pleasant than dwelling on unpleasant feelings of sadness or worry. But what happens to those feelings of his then, when you work so hard? Does working hard help solve them?"
>
> **>>John:** "Yes, it does – then I feel good... well, yeah, I suppose it's not really solved, well at least in that moment it is, I mean, I might feel sort of bad again later."
>
> **>>Therapist:** "Okay... so you can do a good job of protecting him in the moment itself, by getting absorbed in work, but that doesn't resolve those feelings. So you aren't a real solution for him, no matter how well you manage to shield him from those feelings of fear and sadness in those particular moments...?"

7.5.4.3 Ask for permission to make contact with the Vulnerable Child, while offering reassurance, control and hope

Having recognized that the Perfectionistic Overcontroller is only an emergency measure and not a permanent solution, offer the client a better alternative by connecting them with their Vulnerable Child. Introduce this with hope and reassurance, because you're really asking the client to let go of a familiar way of surviving – and they'll need lots of encouragement to do it. Emphasize that they can really start to feel better, and offer reassurance and control by stressing that they stay in control, that they can stop the exercise at any time, and that you will help them to complete the exercise safely.

7.5.5 Step 5: Have the client sit in the chair of the Vulnerable Child

Once you have consent for the next step, ask the client to sit in the chair of the Vulnerable Child. Again, clear instructions will help the client to transition from one chair to another calmly – and to understand that changing chairs is more than just a physical act. In this instance, it represents a change from a closed state into a more open, emotional state.

> **Example of having the client sit in the chair of the Vulnerable Child**
>
> **>>Therapist:** "Good, then in a moment I'll ask you to stand up and come sit next to me here. Bear in mind that the chair you're in now is the Hard Worker's chair, and when you get up, you must leave him behind, stuck to the seat with superglue."
>
> (*John stands up and goes to sit on the chair next to the therapist.*)
>
> **>>Therapist:** "Okay, while you were sat there (*pointing to the chair of the Perfectionistic Overcontroller*) I heard the Hard Worker, who's all wrapped up in to-do lists and only sees the work that needs to be done. He's quite content with that, and he thinks it's better than sitting here (*the therapist turns to John next to him*), with feelings and emotions that aren't quite as easy to tick off or cross out. The Hard Worker (*the therapist points again at the empty chair where John was just sitting*) is afraid that all those feelings will only cause problems. But what feelings is he talking about? (*The therapist then turns to John next to him and asks that question in a slightly softer, more emotional tone.*) How do you feel?"
>
> **>>John:** (*in the same tone as before*) "Yeah, well, just busy, not much else or anything."

Here, you have hit a common problem when working with Perfectionistic Overcontrollers, which is that, in the Vulnerable Child's chair, the client remains unable to connect with their needs and emotions and is therefore still actually in Perfectionistic Overcontroller mode. Arriving at this point, you will have to adjust the technique and 'charge the chair' to achieve the desired result. The guidance for this can be found in the next section (7.6). Once the client has been helped to recognize and experience some emotions and needs as the Vulnerable Child, you can move on to the next step of the process – validating those needs.

7.5.6 Step 6: Validate the relevant basic needs

Schema activation is a necessary in order to generate a corrective emotional experience. This experience will be derived from listening to and positively reinforcing the message that acknowledging the need for spontaneity and play instead of retreating into work is essential. You can offer the necessary positive reinforcement by showing compassion. As described earlier in this chapter (7.2.2), compassion has a soothing, healing effect. On the one hand, you explicitly identify the negative consequences of the client's unmet need for spontaneity and play, while on the other you acknowledge any attempt to listen to that need. In both cases, check how it feels for your client when compassion is offered. Does it feel nice, or not?"

Example of validating the relevant basic needs

>>Therapist: "I understand – that you don't feel much of anything when all life seems to be nothing but work and deadlines. That seems like a perfectly normal reaction; no one thinks all work and no play is fun. And as you've said, this isn't a one-off experience for you – it's actually the pattern of your whole life. All your life, you've had to work hard. There was always something else to do, and you never quite got round to just relaxing and having fun. Does that sound accurate at all, as I describe it?"

>>John: "Yes, it really is, yes..."

>>Therapist: "So I've understood correctly then, how things are and have been for you. How does that feel, to be understood like that? Is it a nice feeling, or not so nice?"

>>John: "It's nice..."

>>Therapist: "And again, I think it's only natural, with all that unavoidable work, to feel a bit sad an d angry. Because what might you be doing otherwise? What would you like to be doing right now, instead of work, if you had a free choice?"

>>John: "Now? I don't know, just to sit in the garden for a while, I guess. I did regret it a bit when the weather was nice and I didn't get to go out and enjoy it."

>>Therapist: "Nice idea! What does sitting in the garden look like? With a drink, a book?"

>>John: "Yes, with a good book..."

>>Therapist: "I really enjoy hearing what you feel like doing. I also think it's great, and insightful, that now you seem to be paying attention to what you (*pointing to John*) really need instead of listening to him over there (*pointing to the place of the Perfectionistic Overcontroller*) and still just thinking that a lot still needs to be done. How does it feel to hear this, to be complimented for listening to other needs besides work?"

>>John: "It's nice, yes..."

7.6 Chairwork variant – 'charging the chair'

If the Perfectionistic Overcontroller is particularly strong, and as a result the client needs a bit more encouragement and support to make contact with the Vulnerable Child, you can verbalize those underlying emotions and needs by 'charging' the Vulnerable Child's chair with emotions before the client sits in it. Step-by-step guidance for this is shown below.

'Charging' the chair of the Vulnerable Child step-by-step
Step 1: Identify the client's difficulty in making contact with the Vulnerable Child.
Step 2: Ask the client to observe from a distance, for example from the therapist's chair.
Step 3: Sit in the Vulnerable Child's chair and 'charge' it with emotions.
Step 4: Ask the client to express these emotions and needs from the Vulnerable Child's chair.
Step 5: Raise emotional awareness by paying attention to the emotional, physical and cognitive components of those emotions.

7.6.1 Step 1: Identify the client's difficulty in making contact with the Vulnerable Child

The fact that the client is finding it difficult to connect with their feelings should be clearly apparent by this point in the exercise. Referring back to the case conceptualization, explain to them they that have never learned to maintain a connection with their own feelings and needs. In this way, the client's inability to connect with their Vulnerable Child can be reformulated in a positive way, from an apparent problem into a central objective of therapy.

> **Example of identifying the client's difficulty in making contact with the Vulnerable Child**
>
> **>>Therapist:** "I notice how difficult it is for you to put your feelings into words when the Hard Worker is so active. There (*pointing to the Hard Worker's chair*), it's clear what you're experiencing – it's all about to-do lists and tasks. But here (*pointing to the chair where the client is sitting now*), it's still a question mark. It's perfectly understandable that you don't yet really know what you feel. →

How would you? In your childhood, you mostly trained the Hard Worker and didn't learn to recognize your own feelings and needs. You don't have to be able to do it all at once, and you don't have to do it all by yourself. I'll help you get some perspective on what you're feeling and what you need when the Hard Worker is so busy."

7.6.2 Step 2: Ask your client to observe from a distance, for example from the therapist's chair

Ask the client to sit in your chair. Explain that you will now sit in the Vulnerable Child's chair yourself. You can then help to verbalize the client's underlying emotions and needs by exploring what they might potentially experience when they are in the chair of the Vulnerable Child. In this way, the Vulnerable Child's chair becomes more strongly associated with those feelings and needs. At first, the client just observes from a distance, in order to understand cognitively, and as realistically as possible, what feelings and needs might be at play.

> **Example of switching chairs**
>
> **>>Therapist:** "Then I'd like to suggest that we switch chairs: you come and sit on my chair here, and I'll sit on your chair. Once I'm there, I'll try to articulate the feelings you might have with all that hard work and not having time to relax. And you can just watch and listen from here, from my chair. Just try to absorb some of what you hear me say."
>
> (*The therapist and client switch chairs.*)

7.6.3 Step 3: Sit in the Vulnerable Child's chair and 'charge' it with emotions

Sit in the Vulnerable Child's chair and try to verbalize what you assume to be the client's underlying emotions and needs. Do this as authentically as possible in order that this component of chairwork can be an emotional experience, not just an unemotional conversation about emotions.

Ways in which you can access the emotions and needs that the client might be expected to experience as the Vulnerable Child include:

- Describing the client as a child as you have seen them in photos or visualizations.
- Describing the emotional reactions of children in general in such situations.
- Describing how you would feel in that context yourself.
- Describing the emotions in the present tense, and as authentically as possible.
- Describing the underlying basic needs.

> **Example of the therapist 'charging' the Vulnerable Child's chair**
>
> **>>Therapist:** "So I'm sitting here now, and I've just heard all about how hard I've been working. And we were talking about the past week, but I recognize that experience of hard work: I've done it for much longer than that. It brings up images of the past for me – times when I always had jobs to do as a child, when there were always tasks to be completed. Then I'm reminded of that image we were talking about last week, of having to tell my friends at the door that I couldn't come to play because I still had to help with all kinds of chores. Then I do feel some sadness. I didn't want to just work, I wanted to play too… to be free and play, just a bit. Constantly having to do things, it doesn't feel great. I feel that here again (*points to chest*). All that work (*points to the Hard Worker's chair*) makes me (*points to own chest*) feel sad, angry and like I just really want some time off to relax. Okay, now let's switch chairs again."

7.6.4: Step 4: Ask the client to express these emotions and needs from the Vulnerable Child's chair

Immediately after expressing the emotions as authentically as possible, ask the client to sit in the Vulnerable Child's chair. Do not reflect or think about what you expressed while sitting there – just ask the client to repeat those feelings and needs as literally and as directly as possible. By expressing those experiences out loud, they are able to take more 'ownership' of them. Your job as a therapist is to coach them in expressing these feelings and needs.

> **Example of the client expressing feelings and needs from the Vulnerable Child's chair**
>
> (*The therapist and client switch chairs again – the client now sits in the Vulnerable Child's chair and the therapist sits in his own chair again.*)
>
> **>>Therapist:** "Now you're sitting in the chair where I was just talking about what I would feel in your position, with all that hard work and everything that happened in the past. Do you remember what I said, the words I spoke?"

> **John:** "Yes…"
>
> **Therapist:** "And what did I say about how it felt to be in that chair?"
>
> **John:** "Not great… sad…"
>
> **Therapist:** "And what did you hear me say about what I would really want?"
>
> **John:** "Playing, just being free…"
>
> **Therapist:** "Can you repeat that: 'I don't want to work all the time, I want some freedom'?"
>
> **John:** "I don't want to work all the time, I want some freedom…"

7.6.5 Step 5: Increase emotional awareness by paying attention to the emotional, physical and cognitive components of those emotions

Repeating the feelings and needs expressed by the therapist is an attempt to achieve some schema activation in the client, along with some awareness of the emotions associated with this. However, the client is not used to experiencing emotions, and because of this unfamiliarity and possible discomfort, the experience may not be consolidated sufficiently. That is why the final step of this technique is to increase the client's emotional awareness by explicitly directing their attention to different aspects of these emotional experiences.

> **Example of increasing the client's emotional awareness**
>
> **Therapist:** "But all that Hard Worker (*points to the Hard Worker's chair*) wants to do is work, harder and more. He's completely focused on his lists of tasks and chores. How does that feel for you, pleasant or unpleasant?"
>
> **John:** "Not great…"
>
> **Therapist:** "Not-great sad? Not-great angry?"
>
> **John:** "Both, really…"
>
> **Therapist:** "Can you say that out loud, that you feel sad and angry when you hear that there's only room for work, and that you always have to work even harder?"
>
> **John:** "It makes me sad, that I'll just have to work harder, that it's never enough…"
>
> **Therapist:** "And where do you feel that sadness in your body?"
>
> **John:** "About here, I think." (*Points to chest and stomach area.*)

7.7 Negotiation with the Perfectionistic Overcontroller during imagery rescripting

A strong Perfectionistic Overcontroller can make it difficult for a client to visualize meaningful emotional images. One way forward in such cases is to instead ask the client to visualize this Perfectionistic Overcontroller and take on that role, and for you to then negotiate with them in their role as the Protector within the visualization.

The box below describes what this variant of imagery rescripting might look like.

Step-by-step plan for negotiating with a visualized Protector
Step 1: Try to visualize the Vulnerable Child.
Step 2: Identify and explore the resistance experienced.
Step 3: Ask the client to visualize the resistance experienced.
Step 4: The therapist steps into the picture and the client observes what is happening.
Step 5: The therapist negotiates with the Protector to connect with the Vulnerable Child.
Step 6: Show compassion for the Vulnerable Child and make the client aware of the healing effects of that compassion.
Step 7: Review and homework

7.7.1 Step 1: Try to visualize the Vulnerable Child

Ask the client to recall an image of a significant emotional experience from their past. That might follow the discussion and visualization of a recent trigger situation, but you could also begin the exercise by visualizing an image from the client's past. If a client with Obsessive-Compulsive Personality Disorder indicates that they don't see any images, you can ask them to think of one of the photos from the case conceptualization. Ask them to describe that photo, and prompt them with questions like: 'What kind of light do you see?', 'How does the child in that photo look?', 'How do they feel?' After your client has described the child in the photo, ask them if they can put themselves in that child's place: 'Just be that little child in the photo now…'

In many cases, perseverance – the photo, paying attention to the sensory information and taking time for the exercise – are enough to get past the resistance from the Perfectionistic Overcontroller and to get more in touch with the client's Vulnerable Mode. However, for some clients this still is not enough; indeed, it may even seem that resistance has increased.

7.7.2 Step 2: Identify and explore the resistance experienced

Of course, if the previous attempts have not worked, you might choose to pause the exercise and try to overcome the Perfectionistic Overcontroller another way – with chairwork, for example. However, you could equally stay in the visualization and ask the client to expand on their resistance: 'Where do you feel that resistance?', 'What do you not want to do?', 'What would you like to do now?' Also, be sure to ask if this resistance is familiar. Such questions help to build awareness that this is an old, familiar experience – a side of the client, in other words.

7.7.3 Step 3: Ask the client to visualize the resistance experienced

The next step is to ask the client to attach an image to the resistance they are experiencing. This can be any image that best represents the resistance for them: a wall, a barbed wire fence, or anything else. For the remainder of the exercise, it is a little easier if the client visualizes themselves surrounded by that image of resistance.

> **Example of the client visualizing the resistance experienced**
>
> **>>Therapist:** "Now can you form an image of that feeling of resistance? What do you look like when you don't feel like paying attention to feelings? What do you look like when you'd rather get to work and take care of chores?"
>
> **>>John:** "Well, just like myself!"
>
> **>>Therapist:** "Okay, so you see yourself as you are now? Can you describe to me what you look like now? Just literally say what you see."
>
> **>>John:** "Well, just as I am now..."
>
> **>>Therapist:** "So do you see yourself sitting there?"
>
> **>>John:** "No, somehow I actually see myself standing now."
>
> **>>Therapist:** "Okay, and do you see anything that shows that this John doesn't want to talk about feelings? From the look on his face? His posture?"
>
> **>>John:** "Well... it's clear, he really has that look of: 'No come on, we're not going to talk about this now, don't you know how much work I still have to do!'"

By describing this image, the client is already putting some distance between themselves and the resistance experienced. Instead of feeling that there is still so much work to be done and that they don't feel like having emotions, the client is talking objectively about their resistance, looking at it instead of completely identifying with it.

7.7.4 Step 4: The therapist steps into the picture and the client observes what is happening

In the preceding steps, a situation has been visualized of the child from the photo and the Perfectionistic Overcontroller. Next, ask if you can step into the picture. Your goal is to negotiate with that visualized Perfectionistic Overcontroller just as you might in a chairwork exercise. By asking the client to keep watching during that negotiation, you prevent them from immediately identifying with the perceived resistance again.

> ### Example of the therapist stepping into the picture
>
> **>>Therapist:** "Good, so now you see the little boy from the photo sitting there. And you still see the Hard Worker – that adult who doesn't feel like it and just wants to get on with something? Where do you see him? To your left or right, or right in front of you?"
>
> **>>John:** "Well, a little to the right…"
>
> **>>Therapist:** "Can you point the Hard Worker out, so I know where you see him?"
>
> (*John gestures to a spot to the right in front of him.*)
>
> **>>Therapist:** "And that little boy, the little boy from the photo, where do you see him?"
>
> **>>John:** "A little bit behind the other one, the Hard Worker."
>
> **>>Therapist:** "Okay, so now I'd like to come into that picture. Can you add me?"
>
> **>>John:** "…"
>
> **>>Therapist:** "When you listen to my voice now, and you think of me, do you perhaps see me in your mind's eye, a little way in front of you?"
>
> (*John nods.*)
>
> **>>Therapist:** "Great, so can you put me in the picture then? Put me close to the Hard Worker, just between him and the little boy. Can you see me?"
>
> **>>John:** "Yes, a little bit, I think."
>
> **>>Therapist:** "Excellent, you're doing well!"

7.7.5 Step 5: The therapist negotiates with the Protector to connect with the Vulnerable Child

Now you negotiate with the Perfectionistic Overcontroller in the way described as part of the chairwork section (7.5.4). You offer plenty of recognition and understanding for all the benefits of hard work, and as you speak to the Hard Worker you turn your head toward the place where the client has visualized it. Keep asking the client to indicate how the Perfectionistic Overcontroller responds, and each time you ask for that feedback, turn back to the client. Your voice should be different when you talk to the Perfectionistic Overcontroller than when you talk to the Vulnerable Child. The tone in which you talk to the Perfectionistic Overcontroller should be level and neutral; when you talk to the Vulnerable Child, use a friendly, supportive tone. This increases the vividness and reality of the visualized situation.

After the advantages, the disadvantages of the Hard Worker are also discussed. In your negotiation, emphasize that you can actually make the child in the photo feel a little better.

7.7.6 Step 6: Show compassion for the Vulnerable Child and make the client aware of the healing effects of that compassion

A detailed description of showing compassion can be found in the section earlier in this chapter on chairwork with the Demanding Mode (7.3.4). In summary, address the visualized child and identify explicitly what he or she lacked: play and spontaneity. Identify the resulting emotions of sadness, loneliness and agitation, and explicitly acknowledge these feelings. Ask the client if what you just described seems accurate. Then check the primary emotional responses to this recognition. Does it feel good or bad to be understood? Without becoming aware of these positive effects of compassion, the client could easily overlook this positive experience.

7.7.7 Step 7: Review and homework

The corrective emotional experience produced by this exercise must be remembered and consolidated. A review of the exercise contributes to this consolidation. During this review, reflect on the experience in detail, what the client learned from it, and what they want to take away and remember.

Finally, give the client some homework so that these learning experiences are contemplated and repeated between sessions.

7.8 Child Modes in Obsessive-Compulsive Personality Disorder

Clients with Obsessive-Compulsive Personality Disorder lacked in their childhood fulfilment of the basic needs for spontaneity and play, autonomy and justice (see Table 3.10). Child modes frequently seen in obsessive-compulsive clients include the Disappointing/Underperforming Child and the Over-diligent Child, both related to the schema of *Unrelenting Standards* and their focus on hard work.

As a role model of the good-enough parent these clients should have had in their childhood, you therefore need to be a 'parent' in therapy who encourages and validates their needs for spontaneity and play, autonomy and justice. For this reason, provide space for relaxation during the sessions, so that the whole session does not have to be productive. If you leave space in the therapy to chat a bit about everyday things, share a joke, show a video on the internet that you liked, or share something personal that wasn't just productive or efficient or clever, this can be a corrective experience for the client.

You may be pursuing more spontaneity and play in your client's life, but don't make it a requirement – leave sufficient room for autonomy. Validating the need for autonomy is especially relevant in the middle and final stages of treatment. For example, validating autonomy means leaving room for choices made by the client that do not match your own expectations for the therapy. That is the client's right. However, at such moments you do need to emphasize that you would like it to be the Healthy Adult making the choice, and not the Perfectionistic Overcontroller or the Demanding Mode.

7.9 Stimulating spontaneity and play in the Happy Child

The learning history of clients with Obsessive-Compulsive Personality Disorder is characterized by constant reinforcement of the value of hard work and high performance. By contrast, doing nothing, relaxing, or having fun has never been validated, and may even have been punished or criticized. As a result, obsessive-compulsive clients do not enjoy letting go of the schema of *Unrelenting Standards* or following spontaneous impulses such watching television, playing games or simply doing nothing. Their unhealthy patterns are maintained by the constant validation of hard work on the one hand, and by feeling uncomfortable with spontaneity and play on the other.

These clients must learn to tolerate, and even appreciate, the feeling of 'idleness'. Explain to the client that it will take time for them to get used to the unfamiliar feeling of doing nothing, but given time, they will learn to enjoy it. So, encouraging spontaneity and play is a kind of learning – learning to gain, or to regain, an appreciation for activities that these clients perceive, with their compulsiveness, as useless and even tedious. It is important that the client understands this rationale, and realizes that tolerating discomfort in playful, spontaneous activities is part of that positive learning.

It is best to do the first playful exercises in this domain together, during the session. That way, you can maintain some control over how they are performed and be alert to the client's slight emotional responses when doing them. The client can easily miss these responses because of the strong Perfectionistic Overcontroller. As a therapist, you retain the ability to coach the client to process the learning experiences from these exercises in a realistic way, so they actually become corrective emotional experiences and not just forced assignments that the client will abandon as soon as possible.

Examples of exercises to stimulate the Happy Child in a session
- Watch funny videos on the Internet.
- Tell the client your funniest joke.
- Play non-intellectual games.

Examples of homework assignments to stimulate the Happy Child
- Take a wrong turn three times in a row on the way home, so you end up in a new area.
- Tell the therapist's funniest joke to at least three other people.
- Play with children.
- Play with cats or dogs.

7.10 Sticking points when working with Obsessive-Compulsive Personality Disorder

Some clients with Obsessive-Compulsive Personality Disorder seem to have lost touch with their emotional life completely. In cases where the exercises described above have little effect because the client cannot recognize their feelings at all, it may be necessary to introduce a phase in which they can practice emotional awareness in a broad sense. These exercises focus on becoming sensitive to the emotional and physical responses that these experiences can evoke. With them you try to answer questions such as 'When do I feel angry, scared, sad, relaxed, happy, and how do I notice these feelings?'

Exercises to stimulate emotional awareness during the session
- Mindfulness exercise.
- Task concentration training (taken from the protocol for Social Anxiety Disorder).

Homework exercises to stimulate emotional awareness
- Choosing appropriate music for different emotions (happy, angry, sad, scared).
- Choosing appropriate films for different emotions.

7.11 Chapter summary

This chapter has described how fighting the client's Demanding Mode is different from fighting a Punitive or Blaming Mode. The Demanding Mode focuses solely on competence, and a key strategy in fighting it is to pay attention to other basic needs and to argue that fulfilling these other basic needs is not a luxury, but a necessity.

You will sometimes have to help an obsessive-compulsive client to connect with their emotions and needs by sitting in the Vulnerable Child's chair yourself, as the therapist, and imagining your client's emotional responses. In this way, you can 'charge' the Vulnerable Child's chair with emotions, which you can then use to help the client connect with those feelings in that same chair.

The Perfectionistic Overcontroller – a common part of obsessive-compulsive clients – can be addressed using visualization and imagery rescripting. This enables you to do an experiential exercise while at the same time working on the client's blocked feelings through a visualized negotiation with the Perfectionistic Overcontroller.

Encouraging play and spontaneity involves targeted exercises to elicit emotional responses such as joy and relaxation from the client. This might involve playing games in the session, watching funny clips, or something similar. Obsessive-compulsive clients need to learn to appreciate the feeling of relaxation and playfulness, and, as the therapist, you can help them achieve this by being alert to small positive emotional responses during the exercises and making the client aware of them.

Chapter 8: The middle phase of therapy

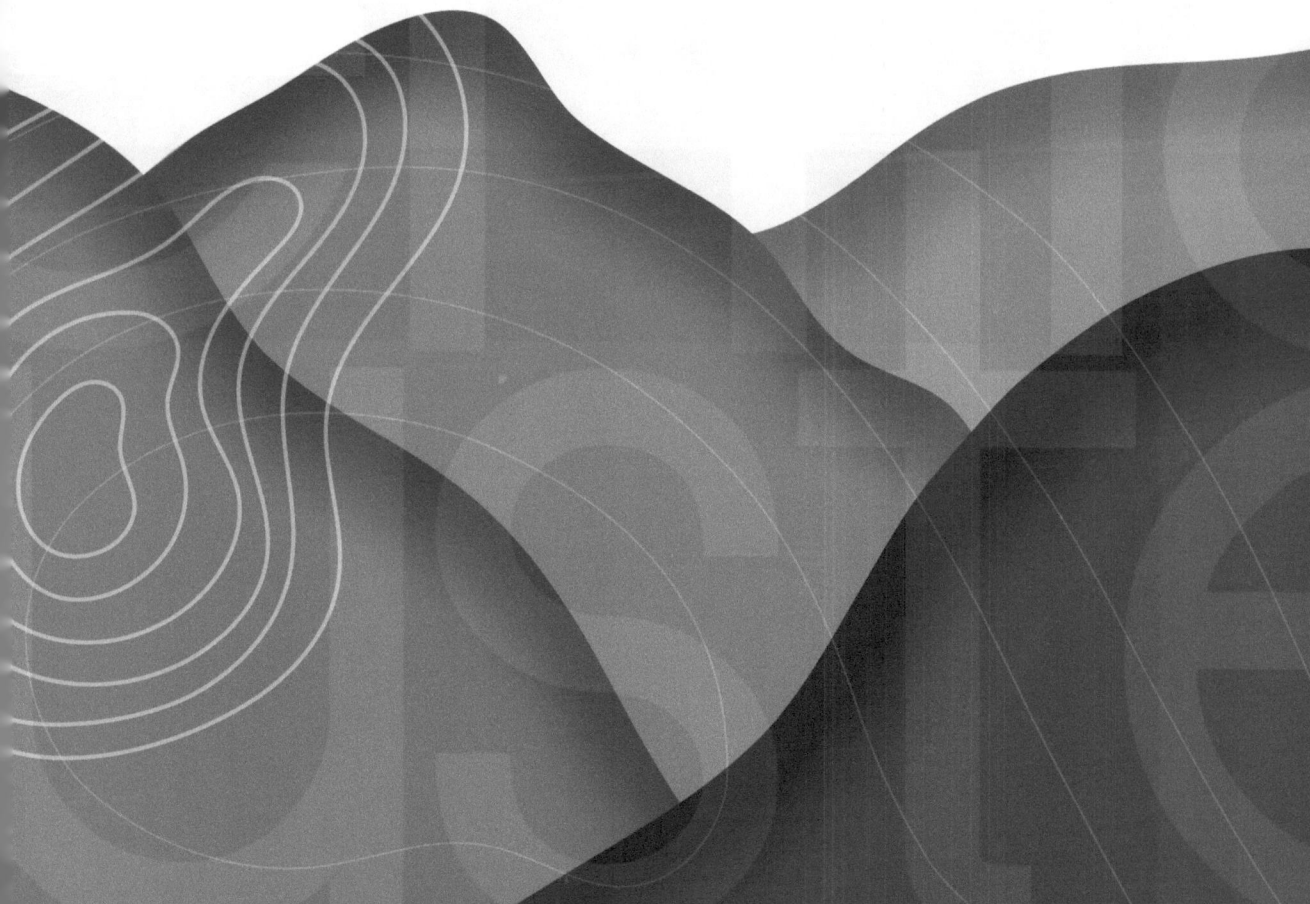

Chapter 8: The middle phase of therapy

Chapter map	
8.1	Introduction
8.2	Visualizing the Healthy Adult
8.3	The three steps of the Healthy Adult
8.4	Chairwork with the three steps of the Healthy Adult
8.5	Imagery rescripting in the middle phase
8.6	Chairwork in the middle phase
8.7	Chapter summary

8.1 Introduction

The initial phase of therapy focused on increasing awareness and generating corrective emotional experiences. Your primary function in this phase was to act as a guide, helping to articulate the client's modes and needs. To achieve that, you took the role of a good-enough parent. In that role, you stepped into visualizations and rescripted meaningful events, you negotiated with Avoidant and Inverted Coping Modes, and you challenged and changed Critical Modes. The healthy experiences your client gained in this way can now serve as a basis for his own Healthy Adult to grow.

In the middle phase of therapy, the Healthy Adult will take on a more central role. In this phase, the client will learn to validate his own basic needs independently. In the safety of therapy, he can practice the skills that you have demonstrated. Building on these exercises, behavioural patterns in daily life can increasingly be broken in the final phase.

This chapter describes how to work with the Healthy Adult in the middle phase of therapy. It does not focus specifically on any one of the cluster C personality disorders because the processes, methods and techniques it describes apply equally to all three of them.

8.2 Visualizing the Healthy Adult

In the middle phase of therapy, your objective is for the client's Healthy Adult Mode to take over and start doing the things you demonstrated in the initial phase. First and foremost, the client must learn to become aware of his own different modes. Further, as a Healthy Adult, he must also learn to validate his own basic needs independently.

Before the client can use the Healthy Adult to validate his basic needs, he must learn what his own Healthy Adult looks like. Like all the other modes, the Healthy Adult is a side of your client, and he will have to get to know this side of himself well. He will also have to learn to connect with the Healthy Adult even when schemas are activated. The box below gives step-by-step instructions for teaching the client to visualize and gain a better understanding of his own Healthy Adult. It is intended only as a guide, not as an objective in itself, and there are many other ways to achieve this.

Step-by-step plan for learning to visualize the Healthy Adult
Step 1: Provide psychoeducation regarding the Healthy Adult.
Step 2: Share a personal memory of your own Healthy Adult
Step 3: Use this memory as a tool to connect with the Healthy Adult
Step 4: Ask the client to visualize their own Healthy Adult
Step 5: Review and homework

8.2.1 Step 1: Provide psychoeducation regarding the Healthy Adult

Clients may have distorted ideas about what a 'Healthy Adult' looks like. A client with Dependent Personality Disorder is likely to think it is 'healthy' if everyone is happy, even if that comes at the expense of their own needs and feelings – but what they are really seeing is the image of the Compliant

Surrenderer. And a client with Obsessive-Compulsive Personality Disorder is likely to think it is 'healthy' to deliver the best possible standard of work at all times – but this is really just the image of their own Demanding Mode.

You will have to explain to your client that there are two characteristics of a true Healthy Adult. On the one hand, a Healthy Adult is in touch with his feelings and needs. This is how the client feels what touches him, what makes him insecure or sad. On the other hand, a characteristic of a Healthy Adult is that he can manage these feelings, as well as the context in which they are triggered, by also paying attention to rational thoughts and logic, thereby forming healthier interpretations of events and the world around him.

8.2.2 Step 2: Share a personal memory of your own Healthy Adult

There are a few advantages to providing the client with personal examples of your own Healthy Adult. First of all, this can give him a realistic idea of what a Healthy Adult looks like, providing you with an opportunity to adjust any unrealistic expectations.

Secondly, sharing experiences in which you felt insecure, tense or stressed has the added effect that the interaction between you and your client can become somewhat more equal. In this middle phase of the treatment, more space is needed for the client to develop autonomy, and he will not develop that autonomy properly if you continue to represent an unattainable ideal of serene perfection as a therapist.

> ### Example of sharing a memory of your own Healthy Adult
>
> **>>Therapist:** "Sometimes, I have to be really proactive in mobilizing that Healthy Side of myself. If I find myself in a difficult situation, I really need to pay attention to it. When that happens, I find it helpful to recall situations where I was that Healthy Adult. By thinking of an appropriate memory, I can feel that Healthy Side of myself, and try to become that Healthy Adult again. For example, if I know I have to do something difficult, I might close my eyes (*here, the therapist closes his eyes for a moment*) and think back to a challenging situation I experienced recently."

Here, you could choose an example that might also be relevant for your client. For example, for an avoidant client like Jenny, you might choose a situation in which you faced a difficult social situation. For a dependent client like Claire, you might choose a time you stood up for your opinion despite someone else not liking it. And for an obsessive-compulsive client like John, who we will focus on, you might choose a situation in which you felt under pressure from a high workload, but still chose a relaxing activity.

> **Example of sharing a memory of your own Healthy Adult – continued**
>
> **>>Therapist:** "I recently had a couple of very long, busy days. There were several deadlines on top of my normal work. And I can remember lying on the sofa at the end of the day and being quite tired. And for the first half hour, it was just nice. Just relaxing after working hard. Can you imagine yourself there?"
>
> (*John nods emphatically.*)
>
> **>>Therapist:** "But after half an hour, I suddenly remembered that I still had something left to do. That made me feel grumpy, because I really just wanted to rest, so at first, I tried to ignore it. But the thought kept coming back: 'It won't take care of itself – if you just do it now, you won't have to worry about it and then you can really relax.'"
>
> **>>John:** "Yes, exactly, I have that a lot, too. In that kind of situation, it's good just to do it because then you know it's done. Otherwise, you're kind of fooling yourself."
>
> **>>Therapist:** (*smiling*) "I thought this would be familiar to you. And it really seemed at the time that it was best to take action, just as you say. But that isn't the Healthy Adult I want to talk about. That's the Old Me, the way I'm used to seeing things, based on my background. That's the Demanding Side of me. It's the old message not to put off until tomorrow what you can do today and so on. So no, that isn't my Healthy Adult. He did arrive shortly afterwards though. It was at the moment I was just about to get up from the sofa, when I thought: 'Yeah, but wait a minute, I'm saying that this is just one more task before I can really rest. But the reality is, there will always be more tasks to do. So you could just keep working, which would be great for the to-do list, but what do you actually need right now? Yet more work? Or a bit of overdue downtime? Something else in your life?' Try to find a good balance between work and relaxation."

8.2.3 Step 3: Use this memory as a tool to connect with the Healthy Adult

Hopefully, the example you provide will help your client to learn that life is full of difficult moments – times when they will have to make choices and try to take healthy courses of action. You also show your client that we all need to try to recognize old patterns and sides of ourselves, because recognizing them is the first step toward handling challenging situations in a healthier way. Using your own memories like this, you can demonstrate to the client how you connect with your Healthy Adult and what tools you use to do it.

Example of sharing a memory of your own Healthy Adult – continued

>>Therapist: "When I think back to that, I feel the same way I felt in that moment… a kind of peace, a calmness within me. I feel that here (*points to his abdomen*), and I notice again that I sit up a bit straighter - not leaning forward like when I was thinking about all the things I still had to do, but more upright, balanced. Do you notice that?"

>>John: "Yes, yes, of course… you're sitting straighter, and yes, you do sound a bit calmer or something…"

>>Therapist: "Really, I sound different? Nice! How do I sound compared to just now?"

>>John: "Well, you're speaking more calmly now, more slowly. When you were just talking about needing to do tasks, you talked faster or something."

>>Therapist: "I'm glad you noticed that. And it's good to hear, because although I knew about other characteristics of my Healthy Adult, I didn't know that one. It's helpful to know what my Healthy Adult looks like, feels like and sounds like. The more I know about him, the better I can connect with that side of myself. Characteristics, like sitting up straight, speaking calmly and the actual memory itself are sort of like keys that unlock my Healthy Adult. For example, I know that the words 'The reality is…' really help me to connect with my Healthy Adult. So, by saying those words, 'The reality is…', I automatically make some contact with that healthy side of myself."

8.2.4 Step 4: Ask the client to visualize their own Healthy Adult

Now comes the step at which the client must learn to form a mental picture of their own Healthy Adult. With your example, the client has been given an idea of what kind of memories are involved – memories in which schema activation was managed well.

As such, there are different elements to visualizing the Healthy Adult. First, ask your client to recall an image in which schema activation occurred.

Example of recalling a situation in which schema activation occurred

>>**Therapist:** "I want to ask you to keep your eyes closed for the next ten minutes. You can just focus on a point ahead of you if you're more comfortable with that. The idea is to focus your attention inward, and not to get distracted by your surroundings. In this exercise, you'll form a picture of the Healthy Adult, of you as the captain of your ship."

Concentrating on the breath:

>>**Therapist:** "So just take a deep breath… and close your eyes. It starts with just becoming aware of yourself in this moment. After all the hustle and bustle of the day, with travelling and people, now there's only time for you. Be aware of your feet on the floor, of those places where you're in contact with the chair beneath you. Notice your breathing. You don't have to change anything about it… just notice that it seems to have its own rhythm… sometimes a little faster, sometimes slower. A bit like standing on the shore and watching the waves come and go. Sometimes they come a little faster, sometimes slower, but they keep going without you having to change anything."

Recalling the picture of the Healthy Adult:

>>**Therapist:** "And now, from this position, I want to ask you to let an image, a memory, of your Healthy Adult come to mind. What kind of image might it be? These are often memories of moments when you had a tricky situation or a difficult time, but you handled it well. They're memories where you have a satisfied, or maybe even proud, feeling. What images or memory comes to mind? Something challenging – not an easy situation, but one that you handled well?"

(John keeps his eyes closed and seems focused on his thoughts)

>>**Therapist:** "Once you have an image, I want you to try to relive it, as if you were there again now. So just take a moment to have a good look around. Where are you? Just calmly turn your head from left to right, and take a good look around where you are. What can you see? Who's there? What kind of light do you see? Is it day or night? Do any sounds that come to you? Smells? And what is happening?"

Next, ask the client to become aware of that schema activation by asking about its cognitive, emotional and physiological aspects. The step from *experiencing to becoming aware* is the first step in working on the Healthy Adult. With this, you ask your client to take the position of an observer from the experience of the activated Child Part.

Example of becoming aware of schema activation

>>**Therapist:** "How do you feel now? What is that unpleasant feeling? Is it like fear, or insecurity? Or a form of anger? Sadness, or something else? And where do you feel it in your body? Just put a hand on the area where the feeling is strongest. It isn't nice, I understand that, but I want to ask you to keep in touch with it anyway. And ask yourself: is this feeling new, or do I recognize it? Is there something familiar about it? And if the answer to that question is yes, realize that the feeling you have now is really an old pain from the past. What you feel now is the same feeling you had when you were a young, vulnerable child. You're encountering that child again now."

After becoming aware of the Vulnerable Child, ask your client to visualize how they handled that challenging situation and the schema activation in a healthy way.

Example of experiencing the Healthy Adult

>>**Therapist:** "But there's more to this picture than just pain. It's also a good image. Now, think about what it is that makes this a good memory for you, something you can look at with satisfaction, or even pride. Fast forward to the moment when it became a positive experience for you. And once you're there, what are you doing that you feel so good about? Or maybe what are you not doing? And what's the good feeling you are experiencing? Is it something like pride? Power? Balance? Don't analyse it; just try to sense it a bit. What is that pleasant feeling? And where do you experience it in your body? Put a hand on the place where you feel it most strongly, make contact with it."

The client has now made contact with the Healthy Adult by focusing their attention on this healthy memory. Ask the client to become immersed in this experience as much as possible, and, in the process of that, to converge and become one with the Healthy Adult. Ask them to form an image of themselves in this state. This teaches the client to visualize the Healthy Adult in a way that, with practice, can be replicated in everyday life.

Example of visualizing the Healthy Adult

>>**Therapist:** "Now let that feeling grow, and grow… let it fill you up, so it flows all the way through you. And also find a posture that fits with the feeling that's going through you right now. Check for yourself if this posture matches the feeling. Remember, this feeling is your Healthy Adult, this is the captain of your ship. Zoom out a little so you can look at yourself now, in this state of mind. You don't need to be in exactly the same posture – you might see yourself standing, for example. But just look at the person in front of you. That's your Healthy Adult – that's the captain of your ship."

At this stage, ask the client to become aware of the different facets and modalities of this state – explore the emotional, physiological and cognitive aspects of this side of them.

> **Example of becoming aware of the emotional, physiological and cognitive aspects of the Healthy Adult**
>
> **>>Therapist:** "And how can you tell that this is your Healthy Adult? Is it something in their posture? The look on their face? What does the caption for this image say? What words does this person speak? This is you… maybe the best you. Climb back into the skin of that Healthy Adult you're looking at, and just be that captain again. Feel how good it is. Where is that pleasant feeling in your body again? Enjoy it, that great feeling."

Aside from visualizing the Healthy Adult, you also want your client to learn to connect with it when schemas are activated. Some practice with switching from a Child Mode back to the Healthy Adult can already be done during this visualization; however, it isn't yet necessary, and adding this element does make the exercise a little more complex. For this reason, you might want to keep things as simple as possible for the client.

If you do want to practice switching at this stage, you can ask the client to direct their attention to the schema activation that they experienced – their Vulnerable Child Side. Then ask to them bring their attention back to the Healthy Adult. This teaches the client to switch back to the Healthy Adult whenever they notice that schemas are activated.

> **Example of switching between the Child Mode and the Healthy Adult**
>
> **>>Therapist:** "But of course, it isn't only nice – that little child you just encountered is still there. Where are they now? To your left, or your right? Or are they sitting on your lap? Take a look at where the little one is. And now turn your head towards them, as if you're looking at them. Just look at that little child… do you see any of their pain? How do you see that this little one is uncomfortable, scared, sad, or maybe angry? And I think you do understand where that feeling comes from, right? Of course, this little child feels that way because… can you finish that sentence within yourself? What makes it so understandable that this little one feels that way?"
>
> *(The therapist pauses to let the client experience these emotions.)*
>
> **>>Therapist:** "When you focus your attention on the little child that way, on that pain, maybe you can feel something of that pain too? Realize that you

> feel the child's pain, and understand it well, but realize also that this pain is not you. You are not the child, you are looking at them. It might be good to avert your eyes, for now. Just turn your head away a little. Not to ignore the little one, who is still there, close to you, but so that you can fully become that Healthy Adult again, right now. Just be that captain. Feel that pleasant feeling that comes with it. And, yes, the little one's pain is still there too, right there beside you, but for now it's just you, as the captain of your ship."

At this point, you can keep practicing this 'switching', or you can conclude the exercise. It is important to pay attention to the consolidation of the Healthy Adult, so ask your client to focus their attention on all aspects of that side of themselves.

> **Example of switching between the Child Mode and the Healthy Adult – continued**
>
> **>>Therapist:** "Just enjoy the good feeling. Where do you feel it in your body again? Put a hand on the place where you encounter the feeling... stay in contact with it. Even when we end the exercise in a moment, I want you to keep in touch with it. Now let the images fade, but keep hold of the feeling. Even as you let this therapy room come back to your mind, stay in contact with it. Now move your hands and feet to anchor you back to the here and now again a little more. And then, as you open your eyes, in your own time, maybe you can bring that feeling back with you into the here and now."

8.2.5 Step 5: Review and homework

Reviewing this exercise is an important part of the process. Through this review, which includes paying explicit attention to all aspects of the Healthy Adult, you help the client become aware of this side of themselves. You also help them become aware of the ways they can learn to connect with their Healthy Adult. However, the skill of 'switching' to the Healthy Adult requires a lot of practice. That's why you should give the client homework to regularly visualize their Healthy Adult. Ask them to choose music that best conveys the feeling and experience of the Healthy Adult, or an image or object that symbolizes it.

You may have to repeat this exercise several times in the therapy sessions before some clients get to know this side of themselves better.

8.3 The three steps of the Healthy Adult

Now that your client has a picture of their own Healthy Adult, the next step is for them to learn to generate self-correcting healthy experiences and to validate their own basic needs. To achieve this, you must explicitly communicate the healthy strategy you demonstrated in the initial phase. You can summarize that strategy in three steps:

1. Compassion
2. Cognitive restructuring
3. Behaviour modification

For clients, these three somewhat technical steps can be translated into:

1. Be kind to yourself
2. Think calmly and realistically
3. What do you need and how can you act on it in this situation?

These three steps of the Healthy Adult are described in more detail below.

8.3.1 Step1: Compassion – be kind to yourself

When schemas are activated and old emotional wounds flare up, clients tend to react quickly to do something to diminish these feelings and emotions. For example, as soon as Claire becomes afraid that another person might be dissatisfied or angry, she will try hard to please them. Jenny immediately decided not to go to her friend's house when she heard that another person would be present. And at the end of a working day, John went straight back to work when he found that a job had not been completed by others.

Coping Modes are reflexive survival strategies that these clients developed long ago in response to real situations and challenges, and which have become firmly ingrained over the years. However, when schemas are activated in the present, immediate action is no longer necessary – instead, clients need to learn to pause and find compassion for themselves. Compassion, in the form of an explicit understanding of the unpleasant feelings associated with schema activation, has a soothing effect. This is a necessary prerequisite for calm and realistic thinking, as well as to make other healthy behavioural choices. However, many clients may not have learned to have compassion for the emotional pain they feel with schema activation. Indeed, the initial phase of therapy may have been the first time in your client's life that they have ever experienced compassion.

Begin by explaining that compassion is a form of explicit understanding. Ask your client to finish the sentence: 'Of course you feel so anxious/insecure/frustrated, because…' Then ask them to say something about the circumstances of the situation that justifies their feelings, and to pay attention to the fact that old emotional pain is at play in these experiences: 'I've had experiences in the past, which is why I feel this way now.'

8.3.2 Step 2: Cognitive restructuring – think calmly and realistically

After healthy regulation, and calming the emotions evoked, your client will now need to look critically at the assumptions associated with schema activation. In other words, your client will have to actively counteract the Coping Modes and Critical Modes that have been activated. In the initial phase, as a therapist, you offered arguments for why those sides of the client do not provide healthy ways to look at difficult situations. Now your client will have to practice this sort of realistic thinking independently.

Incidentally, we often talk about the different phases of therapy as though they are distinct blocks, in which you have completely different expectations of the client. In practice, it is more of a continuum or an organic process of growth. This means that, at the beginning of the middle phase, it is likely that you will still need to actively support your client when they try to argue against the Coping and Critical Modes.

8.3.3 Step 3: Behaviour modification – what do you need and how can you act on it in this situation?

To complete the three steps, your client will have to learn to handle situations, and the context in which schemas are activated, in healthy ways. However, you want their behavioural choices to be based on needs, and not just on reflexive repetitions of old Coping Modes. This third step therefore begins with the question: 'What do I need in this situation?' Again, we want to stress that this question can easily be confused with: 'What do I *want*?' While 'wants' and 'needs' may overlap, desires are not always the same as needs. This step is about what the Vulnerable Child needs now. For example, Jenny *wants* to get away from unpleasant situations as soon as possible, or not to get into them at all. But what Little Jenny *needs* is connection – more ability to speak up about those needs.

The next section describes how to use chairwork to practice these three steps.

8.4 Chairwork with the three steps of the Healthy Adult

Chairwork can be used to practice the three steps of the Healthy Adult. However, this is a different form of chairwork to the one previously described. Instead of representing the different parts of your client, this time the chairs represent the three steps of the Healthy Adult. The step-by-step plan below can serve as a guide to practice these steps.

Step-by-step plan for chairwork with the three steps of the Healthy Adult
Step 1: Explore the problem situation.
Step 2: Place three chairs facing the client and explain the exercise.
Step 3: The client sits in the first chair: Compassion.
Step 4: The client sits in the second chair: Cognitive restructuring.
Step 5: The client sits in the third chair: Behaviour modification.
Step 6: The client returns to the original chair and repeats the messages from the three chairs.

8.4.1 Step 1: Explore the problem situation

Introduce this technique by exploring a problem situation that recently occurred for the client, or one that is due to take place in the near future and is causing them concern. This might for instance be an appointment or a social arrangement.

When exploring the difficult situation, explicitly distinguish between the context (the discriminative stimulus), the primary emotional responses (the Child Modes that are activated), and the Coping and/or Critical Modes that are activated in response. Give each of these three components a distinct physical location in the room, by gesturing to different spots. Their positioning can be used during the exercise to bring the three steps of the Healthy Adult into better focus. The first step, to show self-compassion, focuses on the activated Child Modes. The second step, of cognitive restructuring, focuses on the activated Coping and Critical Modes. And the third step, of behaviour modification, relates to Coping Modes and the context and the situation in which this all took place.

Example of exploring the problem situation

>>**Therapist:** "How have you felt over the past week?"

>>**Jenny:** "Well, not great. There was a situation with this colleague at work, who I share an office with."

>>**Therapist:** "Oh? Could you share with me what happened?"

>>**Jenny:** "Well, she'd arranged to go for a drink with some colleagues, and then she asked me if I wanted to join them after work too."

>>**Therapist:** "Ah, great! How nice that they invited you. I know it's stressful for you to interact with colleagues, but I'm glad that they gave you the opportunity to join in."

>>**Jenny:** "Yeah, maybe… but it was mostly stressful for me. I really didn't know what to say and all I could think of was how to get out of it."

>>**Therapist:** "So, what made you want to get out of it so badly?"

>>**Jenny:** "Well, just again, that I won't know what to say… that they'll think I'm stupid, and I'll spoil the mood." I'd feel bad for them… I'd rather not have to go through all that."

>>**Therapist:** "Okay, so what I hear is that your colleague asked you to go for a drink with them. (*When naming the context, the situation, the therapist gestures to a spot on the floor, in front of Jenny and the therapist.*) And in that situation, all sorts of things happened. I hear that you felt very stressed. Anxious, I think?"

(*Jenny nods in agreement.*)

>>**Therapist:** "So in that situation, you mostly felt fear and tension. (*The therapist gestures at Jenny's belly.*) And if I've heard correctly, there were mostly all sorts of thoughts about how you'd spoil the mood. (*Here, he gestures to a spot diagonally behind Jenny.*) That others wouldn't have a good time because you were there?"

(*Jenny nods again.*)

>>**Therapist:** "It sounds like part of you was seeing that situation, but already internally picturing how others would be disappointed afterwards. How others would be disappointed by something you might have done?" (*At this, the therapist gestures again to a spot diagonally above Jenny.*)

>>**Jenny:** "Yes, exactly… that I've spoiled everything for them, when the idea was to enjoy some time together for a while."

>>**Therapist:** "Exactly, I hear that. (*Gestures again to the spot diagonally above Jenny.*) And what I also hear you saying is that, with all that bad feeling, you were mostly preoccupied with the idea of how you could get out of the situation as quickly as possible?'" (*Now gesturing to a spot next to the chair where Jenny is sitting.*)

(*Jenny nods.*)

>>**Therapist:** "So, a lot happens in that kind of situation. It's good that you've brought this up. It sounds like a situation in which you could well use your Healthy Adult, the captain of your ship. What do you think?"

>>**Jenny:** "Yes, I think so too… But I have no idea how else I could deal with it… I mean, things like that really are very stressful for me."

>>**Therapist:** "I get that. I think this is a bit of an Everest for you – a vast mountain that you look up at and can't imagine ever getting to the top of?"

(*Jenny nods.*)

8.4.2 Step 2: Place three chairs facing the client and explain the exercise

Place three chairs opposite your client. These three chairs represent the three different steps of the Healthy Adult. If you don't have three different chairs in your room, you can use just one extra chair and go through the three steps while your client remains seated on that. If you do this, consider moving the chair slightly for each step to emphasize that your client now has a different task. Alternatively, you could put three sheets of paper on the floor that say 'compassion', 'think calmly' and 'what are you going to do now?' and ask your client to walk past the sheets, stopping at each one.

Example of chairs representing the three steps of the Healthy Adult

>>**Therapist:** "So now I'd like to do an exercise to strengthen the captain of your ship, your Healthy Adult. Let's use this situation for that, even if it's already behind us, because it's a good opportunity to practise with the Healthy Adult. Okay?"

>>**Jenny:** "Okay…"

>>**Therapist:** "Great! Then I'll grab three chairs and just put them opposite you…" (*The therapist stands up, takes three chairs and puts them in a row opposite Jenny.*)

>>**Therapist:** "Why three chairs, do you think?"

>>**Jenny:** "Well… they're for the Prosecutor, the Silent One… and Lonely, Shy Jenny?"

>>**Therapist:** "Well done – that's how we used those chairs before, right? To pick apart those different sides of you. And you've seen that achieving that is a realistic possibility. But now I want to use the chairs a bit differently…"

>>**Jenny:** "Oh…?"

>>**Therapist:** "Yes, my idea now is that the three chairs I'm putting here stand for your Healthy Adult. So, the three chairs together represent the Healthy Adult. But why three chairs for the Healthy Adult, do you think?"

>>**Jenny:** "I don't know…"

>>**Therapist:** "That's okay. Just because I'm asking doesn't mean you have to know the answer. I'm always just curious about your ideas and thoughts on things. That's why I ask. Anyway, the three chairs stand for the three steps you need to learn to take in life as a Healthy Adult. Do you remember the three steps I'm referring to?"

>>**Jenny:** "Like being kind to myself?"

>>**Therapist:** "Exactly! Very good! Yes, being kind to yourself, and compassionate, is the first step to take as a Healthy Adult. Because that compassion has a calming effect and makes it possible for you to think more steadily and realistically. And that's the second step. So that second chair represents steady, realistic thinking. For you, that means you can certainly take a moment to check whether the Prosecutor and the Silent One are present. And if they are, it means that you also think for a moment about why they aren't right, why it isn't wise to go along with those sides of yourself. And then the third chair… that represents the action that is needed. You're in a situation, and yes, you do have to say something, do something. But what's the best, the healthiest choice? In taking that third step, then, it's important that you pause for a moment to consider what your needs are in the situation."

(*Jenny looks at the three chairs rather uncertainly.*)

>>**Therapist:** "Is it clear when I go through it like that? So, we have a situation (*points to the spot on the floor in front of them*) and in that situation, you feel all kinds of things, think all kinds of things, and tend to fall back into that avoidance. (*The therapist gestures to the places where the Prosecutor, the Silent One and the Vulnerable Child were indicated earlier.*) Okay, on that first chair, you just need to be kind to yourself. Why is it actually quite understandable that you feel so tense, stressed and guilty? In the second chair, you'll practice being a Healthy Adult and giving some resistance to that Prosecutor who accuses you of ruining an evening before it even happens. But in that second chair, as a Healthy Adult, you can also take a moment to think about why the Silent One doesn't represent the best

course of action. And then, in the third chair, as a Healthy Adult, you can practice thinking about healthy ways to deal with this kind of situation. What are your needs that you need to be especially aware of? And what's the best way to listen to those needs in this kind of situation? Let's practice, shall we?"

(Jenny looks a little unhappy, but nods.)

>>Therapist: "I know you don't like this. These exercises I'm suggesting aren't exactly your favourite, right?"

>>Jenny: (laughs uncomfortably with some resignation) "No, I do find it quite hard."

>>Therapist: "I get it! But you don't have to be able to do it all right away. You don't have to do anything with it right after the session either. But I do want to suggest using the safety of our session to practice making your captain a bit more competent, okay?"

(Jenny nods.)

8.4.3 Step 3: The client sits in the first chair: Compassion

From this point on, ask the client to sit in turn in each of the three different chairs. In the first chair, their task is to practice self-compassion. Give coaching where necessary. This will still be needed quite often at the beginning of the middle phase. Your treatment plan can help make sure you don't take the lead in this exercise for too long.

> ### Example of the first chair – self-compassion
>
> **>>Therapist:** "So just sit down on that first chair now."
>
> (Jenny sits on the first chair.)
>
> **>>Therapist:** "This is the first chair of the Healthy Adult. That means you have to make contact with the Healthy Adult first. Just put on that captain's hat... how do you do that? Can you take me through how you connect with the Healthy Adult?"
>
> **>>Jenny:** "Well, I always just close my eyes for a moment..."
>
> **>>Therapist:** "Go ahead, just do what you'd do at home to activate her."
>
> **>>Jenny:** (closes her eyes) "And then I think again of that situation during the team meeting where I felt anxious about voicing my opinion... but I did it anyway because I felt strong enough at the time."
>
> **>>Therapist:** "And do you have a specific posture you can assume now to help you really become that Healthy Adult?
>
> (Jenny sits up a little straighter.)   →

>>**Jenny:** "Then I see myself as more mature or something… calmer."

>>**Therapist:** "And what words?"

>>**Jenny:** "'I'm okay'… that above all. 'I'm okay, I'm not different to anyone else.'"

>>**Therapist:** "Very good. I see and feel that something has changed. Is that true?"

>>**Jenny:** (*opens her eyes*) "Yes, I feel a bit calmer…"

>>**Therapist:** "Good, then let's look back at that situation where your colleagues asked you to join them for a drink. (*The therapist points to the spot on the floor in front of the chairs.*) Jenny didn't feel comfortable in that situation. (*The therapist gestures to the original chair where Jenny was just sitting*). How does she feel in that situation?"

>>**Jenny:** "Anxious… tense… and guilty, that she's spoiling it for the others."

>>**Therapist:** "Exactly… But I think you and I can understand why she feels so anxious and tense, right? And so guilty?"

(*Jenny nods.*)

>>**Therapist:** "Can you say that to her, as if you're speaking to her, that anxious, tense Jenny who feels so guilty. (*The therapist gestures again to the original chair.*) 'Of course you feel so anxious and tense and guilty because…' Can you finish that sentence?"

>>**Jenny:** (*towards the chair where she was sitting first*) "Well, I do understand why you feel so anxious and tense… because this situation isn't very familiar to you yet. You don't know these people well, so you don't really know how it will go."

>>**Therapist:** (*gently prompting*) "Anyone would feel a bit tense about a situation they're not familiar with yet."

>>**Jenny:** "It would be stressful for anyone if they don't know the others very well."

>>**Therapist:** "Very good! But I think we can also understand that this is especially an awkward situation for Jenny, right? With what she's been through in the past? Why is it so understandable that she feels tense and anxious about this kind of situation?"

>>**Jenny:** "Well, because she never actually learned to speak up… because there was always some criticism of whatever she said."

>>**Therapist:** "Can you say that directly to her?"

>>**Jenny:** (*turning toward the original chair*) "Well, I do understand why you feel so anxious, because this has always been difficult for you. You never got compliments or felt that what you had to say was okay."

>>**Therapist:** "So it's natural…"

>>**Jenny:** "So it's natural for you to feel so tense and anxious in this situation."

>>**Therapist:** "Exactly, because it's an old emotional pain from the past…"

(*Jenny nods.*)

Practicing self-compassion is often an unfamiliar experience for clients. In the initial phase, they experienced that it was nice to receive compassion from you, but now they must say those words and provide that compassion themselves. This won't come easily, and it takes attention and repetition to master that language and self-compassion. For this reason, ask in depth about the experience, and consolidate the positive aspects of it.

Example of reviewing self-compassion

>>**Therapist:** "How does it feel to say this?"

>>**Jenny:** "Odd… uncomfortable."

>>**Therapist:** "Nasty uncomfortable? Or is there something nice in that discomfort?"

>>**Jenny:** "It is pleasantly uncomfortable… that's true."

>>**Therapist:** "Great! Where do you feel it, that pleasant feeling?"

>>**Jenny:** (*thinking for a moment then pointing to her chest*) "Here, I'd say… like it's getting a bit softer…"

>>**Therapist:** "Great. Well, then you can move to the second chair."

8.4.4 Step 4: The client sits in the second chair – Cognitive restructuring

In the second chair, the client can practice making their own counterarguments against the Coping and Critical Modes that have been activated. You have already presented these arguments on multiple occasions in the initial phase of therapy. In this middle phase, the client will have to contribute more themselves to combat the assumptions that can often still seem so credible during periods of schema activation.

Example of cognitive restructuring

>>Therapist: "Okay, so now you're in the second chair. You're still that Healthy Adult, but in this second chair, you have a different task. Just now (*therapist points to the first chair*), your job as a Healthy Adult was to be compassionate with all the fear and stress you felt in that situation. Now, in this second chair, I want to draw your attention to the critical voice of the Prosecutor who says you're bound to ruin things for others. But I also want to pay attention to the Silent One who immediately starts thinking very hard about how you can get out of the appointment."

>>Jenny: "Okay… so what should I do then?"

>>Therapist: "Good question. Well, first I'd like to reflect for a moment on what exactly the Prosecutor is saying. But before you answer that, a question. I keep pointing to a spot there diagonally above your original chair when it comes to the Prosecutor, but do you feel that's the right place?"

>>Jenny: "Yes, I'd say so, because it feels like all kinds of judgements are being made from on high…"

>>Therapist: "Okay, so that place makes sense. There's a lamp near it, so let's think of that lamp as the Prosecutor for a moment. What does the Prosecutor actually say?"

>>Jenny: "Well… that I still won't know what to say and then the whole atmosphere will be ruined because of me. And I would really hate that."

>>Therapist: "Keep being the Healthy Adult for a while and, as two Healthy Adults, let's reflect for a moment on what the Prosecutor is saying. Is that actually true? Are you sure the others really won't like it if you join in?"

>>Jenny: "No, of course, I'm not sure about that… I'm afraid of that…"

>>Therapist: "Okay, so the Prosecutor is making claims that aren't at all certain yet. What do you think of that?' How would you feel if someone told Linda, your good friend, that something really bad was going to happen, when it wasn't certain at all?"

>>Jenny: "Yeah, kind of stupid actually…"

Cognitive challenge techniques help to encourage the client to contradict the Critical Mode in this middle phase of therapy. Commonly used techniques include role reversal ('What would you advise your best friend?') and thinking of advantages and disadvantages. However, do try to include the already internalized arguments against the Critical Mode that you gave as the therapist in the initial phase.

Example of cognitive restructuring – continued

>>**Therapist:** "Do you remember what I used to say to the Prosecutor?"

>>**Jenny:** "What you said?"

>>**Therapist:** "Yes, you often heard me contradict the Prosecutor, in exercises like this with chairs. But even in visualization exercises, you've often heard my voice, my words. Do you remember what I said?"

>>**Jenny:** "Yes, you always said that the Critical Side is not at all about what you really need, those basic needs…"

>>**Therapist:** "Exactly! It's great that you remember that! Can you say something about that to the Prosecutor?"

>>**Jenny:** (*to the place of the Prosecutor, now represented by a lamp*) "You aren't helping me at all. I don't need you making me always feel bad and guilty. I need you to help me out sometimes, just a little bit of appreciation."

>>**Therapist:** "Nice, you did that really well!"

Aside from giving substantive counterarguments, your client will also have to learn to resist the Critical Mode more actively, and to send the Critical Mode away themselves.

Example of cognitive restructuring – continued

>>**Therapist:** "So, could you say something like that to the Prosecutor? Because it does exactly that to you…"

>>**Jenny:** (*turning slightly towards the lamp*) "Well… you really have no idea if they're all going to think it's annoying…"

>>**Therapist:** "And I think it…"

>>**Jenny:** "I think it's stupid that you say that…"

>>**Therapist:** "Great! Say it again, but this time twenty percent louder."

>>**Jenny:** (*slightly louder*) "I think it's stupid that you say that…"

>>**Therapist:** "Nice, well done! And what do you want the Prosecutor to do? To keep doing that?"

>>**Jenny:** "No, it needs to stop doing that…"

>>**Therapist:** "Say it differently then, that you think the Prosecutor needs to stop."

>>**Jenny:** "Stop that."

>>**Therapist:** "Say it again, but twenty percent louder…"

>>**Jenny:** "Stop that!"

>>**Therapist:** "Great! Once more, but like you really mean it."

>>**Jenny:** "You have to stop it! It just isn't true! You don't know that at all!"

>>**Therapist:** "Good. How does it feel to say that?"

>>**Jenny:** "Yes, pretty good, I think…"

>>**Therapist:** "Yes? What is that good feeling?"

>>**Jenny:** "A bit lighter, or something? Yes, a bit lighter…"

>>**Therapist:** "And where do you feel that light feeling in your body?"

>>**Jenny:** (*pointing to her chest*) "Here, I think…"

>>**Therapist:** "Good, you did that really nicely. But there is also the Silent One…"

From this point on, your job is to coach the client first to think critically about the Silent One and their strategy of using avoidance as a way of dealing with the invitation from colleagues. When completed successfully, the client should come independently to the conclusion that avoidance is not the outcome they really want at all. You can then coach the client – just as with the Blaming Mode – to address the Silent One.

8.4.5 Step 5: The client sits in the third chair – Behaviour modification

In the third chair, coach the client to find practical ways to keep listening to their own needs, even in difficult situations. Now that the client has shown compassion for the Vulnerable Child and contradicted the Critical Mode, space is created to think about different behaviours. This does not need to be complicated, and often involves behavioural instructions that are almost obvious. For example, your client needs to learn not to make immediate decisions when it comes to difficult choices, but to allow some time for reflection. Or they need to learn that they can draw on support figures or do something kind for themselves when they have been in a difficult situation. Behaviour modification means that you work with your client to find ways to break through old Coping Modes. For Jenny, that means she gets to do something other than avoidance.

Example of behaviour modification

>>**Therapist:** "Now I'd like to ask you to go to the last chair, the third chair."

(*Jenny sits on the third chair.*)

>>**Therapist:** "Okay, you've already done a lot. In that first chair, you had compassion for all the feelings that were evoked in that situation. And after you calmed down a bit, in the second chair, you quietly thought about it and gave some resistance to the Prosecutor and the Silent One. Anyway, it's obviously a very practical situation where you've been invited, so you have to respond in some way. So, in this third chair, I'd like you to think about what advice you'd like to give, as a Healthy Adult, to Jenny, on how best to deal with this situation."

>>**Jenny:** "And that isn't trying to get out of it?"

>>**Therapist:** "Well, in theory, your advice could be anything, but before you give it, first I'd like to ask you: 'What does Jenny need most of all in life? What did she lack in her childhood, and what does she need most of all now?'"

>>**Jenny:** "Connection… and that she feels good about herself… appreciation?"

>>**Therapist:** "Exactly! So, if that's the direction we're trying to follow, what advice would you give her? What do we think Jenny needs most of all, then? Avoiding it?"

>>**Jenny:** "No, I don't think so… That's what I always do."

>>**Therapist:** "Exactly, then she'd be following the Silent One. And you just told the Silent One why it shouldn't try to be in charge here. So."

>>**Jenny:** "Then she should actually accept the invitation…?"

>>**Therapist:** "Is that what she needs?"

>>**Jenny:** "Yes, I think so…"

>>**Therapist:** "Can you say that to her? 'Jenny, what you have to do now is…'"

>>**Jenny:** (*turns back toward the original chair*) "Jenny, what you need to do is go with them. You're afraid, and I get that, but if you don't go, you'll be alone again."

>>**Therapist:** "It's good that you include those considerations from just now. And what's your practical advice for her? What should she actually do now? Or not do?"

>>**Jenny:** "Okay… tomorrow you have to tell your colleague that you've thought about it a bit more and that, if you can, you'd like to come along after all."

Here, you can discuss more concrete tips and advice for handling the situation in a healthier way. This could range from taking a deep breath, looking away for a moment to order your thoughts, or whatever action is needed to handle both the needs and the specific situation as best as possible. Don't forget to ask the client how it feels to give this kind of practical advice to themselves. By creating this awareness, you consolidate the corrective experiences that these three steps represent for your client.

8.4.6 Step 6: The client returns to the original chair and repeats the messages from the three chairs

As an optional final step, ask the client to return to the original chair. In that chair, ask them to recall the challenging situation again. Putting themselves back into that difficult moment activates schemas again. At this point, as the therapist, repeat the messages from the three chairs of the Healthy Adult. Your client should now be in a position to receive those healthy messages and feel their full effect. Repeating these steps combined with your client's changed perspective can deepen the positive impact of this exercise.

As homework, ask your client to write down all the messages that have been practiced. You might also ask them to write down the spoken message that you, as the therapist, can then record as an audio flashcard. Such a recording is then the result of a collaborative partnership between you and your client's Healthy Adult Mode.

8.5 Imagery rescripting in the middle phase

In the initial phase of therapy, you stepped into the picture as the therapist during an imagery rescripting session. This exercise was not technically complicated. Your client visualized a significant situation from the past and experienced, from the child's perspective, how you came into the picture as the role model of a good-enough parent who does what is necessary to validate their basic needs.

In the middle phase, the client must learn to do the rescripting themselves. This is a bit more technically complex because the client must visualize themselves both as a child and as a Healthy Adult. The step-by-step plan below can help make this process easier.

Step-by-step plan for imagery rescripting by the client in the middle phase
Step 1: Visualize the Healthy Adult instead of the Good Place.
Step 2: Visualize a traumatic event from the child's perspective.
Step 3: Rescript this traumatic image from the perspective of the Healthy Adult.
Step 4: Repeat this rescripting, but now from the child's perspective.
Step 5: Review and homework.

Before the actual exercise begins, the first step is to explain the purpose of the exercise to the client. Although you have done imagery rescripting as an exercise before, it is important to explain to your client how the exercise will be different this time.

Example of explaining the purpose and process of the exercise

>>Therapist: "It's session 26 today. I'm not sure if that means anything to you."

>>Claire: "No, what do you mean exactly?"

>>Therapist: "Well, we made a plan at the beginning of your treatment where we agreed that the therapy would consist of a total of fifty sessions. That means that today we're right in the middle – and we're now in the middle phase of your treatment. And what's the most important thing about therapy again? And maybe about life?"

>>Claire: "Basic needs?" (*Has to chuckle a little at that.*)

>>Therapist: (*also chuckling*) "Exactly! You've learned well. And which basic need is especially important for you to keep in mind? What in particular did you miss out on in your childhood?"

>>Claire: "Do you mean autonomy?"

>>Therapist: (*nodding*) "Exactly. During your childhood, you weren't given sufficient opportunities to learn that you can do things yourself, that the world contains more than just dangers, and that you're competent and skilled enough to face the challenges of life. So that means that in this middle phase of therapy, we need to start coaching your Healthy Adult, the captain of your ship, to handle things more independently."

>>Claire: "Alright…"

>>Therapist: "That's why today I'd like to do another one of our visualization exercises. But now I want to start using more of the Healthy Adult you've worked on so much in the past few weeks. I want that Healthy Side to step into the picture now and do what Little Claire needs. But don't worry, I'm still going to help you. I do have confidence that you'll be able to do everything perfectly well on your own soon enough, but you don't have to be able to do it all independently right away."

8.5.1 Step 1: Visualize the Healthy Adult instead of the Good Place

Instead of starting imagery rescripting by visualizing a Good Place, it's better in the middle phase to start visualizing the Healthy Adult instead. In the exercise, the client must rescript the image as the Healthy Adult themselves. Starting the exercise by visualizing the Healthy Adult makes it easier to switch to that mode during the exercise.

Since you have now practiced visualizing the Healthy Adult regularly, you might want to leave more room for autonomy and competence by letting your client take the lead in this. If so, you can skip this step and begin the exercise at step 2. At the same time, you can ask supportive questions as appropriate in order to provide ongoing coaching.

> **Example of visualizing the Healthy Adult instead of the Good Place**
>
> **>>Therapist:** "So I'd like to ask you to close your eyes now and keep them closed for about the next ten minutes."
>
> (*Claire closes her eyes.*)
>
> **>>Therapist:** "And then I want you to evoke the image of that Healthy Side of you, the captain of your ship. Do you see her?"
>
> **>>Claire:** (*nodding*) "Yes, I see that image again…"
>
> **>>Therapist:** "Can you tell me what you see now?"
>
> **>>Claire:** "I see myself, but more self-assured."
>
> **>>Therapist:** "What shows you that this Claire feels more self-confident?"
>
> **>>Claire:** "She stands there, firm, with both feet on the ground… A kind of peace or calm in her eyes."
>
> **>>Therapist:** "What does the caption under this image say, what state of mind does this Claire project?"
>
> **>>Claire:** "I can handle it… confidence… self-confidence."

8.5.2 Step 2: Visualize a traumatic event from the child's perspective

The beginning of the exercise is identical to the imagery rescripting exercise in the initial phase. Ask the client to put themselves in a significant event from the past. Because you want them to practice rescripting for themselves for the first time, you might choose to use an image or memory that you have already rescripted for them. This will increase the chances of a successful experience. Ask the client to insert themselves into the image and, by asking questions about sensory information, try to activate the relevant schemas.

> **Example of visualizing a traumatic event from the child's perspective**
>
> **>>Therapist:** "So I'd like to ask you to let this image fade away now. We'll get back to her, to your Healthy Adult, in a moment. But now I want to ask you to bring up the image that we've worked on before; the situation when you were six and you wanted to play at your friend's house, but your mother didn't let you. Can you picture that situation?"
>
> (*Claire nods.*)
>
> **>>Therapist:** "Can you tell me what you see now?"
>
> **>>Claire:** "I see my mother and she's telling me that playing at Miriam's house is out of the question because it's in another neighbourhood. She says she wouldn't be able to reach me very quickly if something was wrong."
>
> **>>Therapist:** "Looking at yourself then, do you see yourself as a child there with your mother, from outside? Or are you actually that little girl now?"

This last question helps to define the image. It doesn't matter especially how your client answers, but it is a question that stimulates them to become aware of what they're actually seeing in that moment. If the client has more of an observer's position, they are watching the event from a distance and seeing themselves as a child as well as the other person. This observer perspective allows you to ask informative questions about the context, such as the age of the child being observed. Ultimately, however, you want the client to put themselves into the role of the visualized child and take a first-person perspective. This will increase the emotional experience of the visualized events.

Example of visualizing a traumatic event from the child's perspective – continued

>>**Claire:** "A bit of both. Maybe more that I'm looking at it, like a picture."

>>**Therapist:** "Fine, then can you tell me what the girl, Little Claire, looks like?"

>>**Claire:** "Quite cute… she's wearing a dress, with braids."

>>**Therapist:** "And where do you see your mother? Can you point to her?"

(*Claire points to a spot diagonally in front of her.*)

>>**Therapist:** "Just be that little girl now, be six-year-old Claire in your dress and braids."

(*The therapist now speaks slightly more softly, as if speaking to a small child.*)

>>**Therapist:** "Hey Claire, what's happening? What's going on?"

>>**Claire:** "I want to play at Miriam's house, but Mummy doesn't think I should."

>>**Therapist:** "No, uh, Mummy seems a bit worried about everything that could go wrong, is that right?"

(*Claire nods.*)

>>**Therapist:** "And how is that for you? How do you feel now, hearing that it's not allowed because Mummy is so worried?"

>>**Claire:** "I don't like it… it makes me sad."

>>**Therapist:** "And maybe also a tiny bit angry?"

(*Claire nods hesitantly.*)

>>**Therapist:** "Where do you feel that sadness, and maybe that anger, in your body?"

(*Claire points to her belly.*)

>>**Therapist:** "Just put a hand on that spot."

(*Claire puts a hand on her belly.*)

>>**Therapist:** "And if you connect with that sadness now, and that little bit of anger attached to it, what are you so sad about, Claire? What's going through your mind?"

>>**Claire:** (*in a slightly sadder voice*) "I just don't like it, I never get to play anywhere, while my friends all get to meet up with each other."

>>**Therapist:** "A bit lonely?"

(*Claire nods.*)

Again, try to gauge the level of emotional arousal. You want schemas to be activated so you can provide a corrective emotional experience. However, at the same time, you don't want your client to be overwhelmed by their emotional responses. In the example, Claire talks vividly about emotional experiences of fear and anger that she also experiences physically. Her voice sounds a bit more emotional. Even though she doesn't seem to be at the limit of her Window of Tolerance, it still seems a good moment to start rescripting.

8.5.3 Step 3: Rescript this traumatic image from the perspective of the Healthy Adult

Bringing in the Healthy Adult actually means a mode switch for the client, a transition from the Vulnerable Child to the Healthy Adult. You will have to guide that transition. You can help the client by being clear: 'I want you to be that Healthy Adult now', 'Be that Healthy Adult now'. However, you can start by visualizing the Healthy Adult before asking the client to put themselves into that state of mind.

> **Example of rescripting the traumatic image from the perspective of the Healthy Adult**
>
> **>>Therapist:** "So I think you could use some help and support right now… I'd like Grown-Up Claire to join us. Bring her in, where do you see her now?"
>
> **>>Claire:** "Over there, a bit farther along, by the door."
>
> **>>Therapist:** "Just point to her (*Claire points diagonally in front of her*) and turn towards her for a moment." (*Claire turns in the direction where she sees her Healthy Adult, Grown-Up Claire.*)
>
> **>>Therapist:** "Just look at Grown-Up Claire. What does she look like?"
>
> **>>Claire:** "Big… self-assured."
>
> **>>Therapist:** "Now I'd like you to be that Grown-Up Claire. Just be her… (*The therapist's voice changes to a more mature tone.*) So now you're there, Grown-Up Claire, and you see what's going on. There's the little girl, six years old, with her braids, and you also see your mother. And your mother has just told the girl that she isn't allowed to go and play at her friend's house. And the girl is sad about that. Do you see that too?"
>
> (*Claire nods.*)
>
> **>>Therapist:** "What do you think of that? What do you think about the little girl not being allowed to go and play with her friend?"

>>**Claire:** "Well, it's not right… of course she should be able to play at a friend's house. Isn't that very normal?"

>>**Therapist:** "So you understand that the little girl is sad, maybe even a little angry?"

(*Claire nods.*)

When coaching the Healthy Adult, follow the three steps of the Healthy Adult again: 1) compassion, 2) cognitive restructuring, and 3) behaviour modification.

Example of rescripting the traumatic image from the perspective of the Healthy Adult with compassion

>>**Therapist:** "Can you say that to her, that you understand how she feels? That you understand that it makes her sad?"

>>**Claire:** (*turning slightly towards the visualized Little Claire*) "I understand that you feel this way. Of course you feel sad. It really isn't nice when you want to go and play with Miriam but you aren't allowed to."

>>**Therapist:** (*prompting*) "And of course you feel quite sad, because this isn't the first time you've been told you aren't allowed to do something…"

>>**Claire:** "Yes… yes, of course you feel sad, and a bit angry, because this isn't the first time. Mummy never likes it if you do something and she can't be there herself."

Now that you have coached your client in expressing self-compassion, that corrective experience needs to be consolidated. Consolidation begins by fostering an explicit awareness of the healing effects of compassion.

Example of rescripting the traumatic image from the perspective of the Healthy Adult with compassion – continued

>>**Therapist:** "Just look at that little girl. How does she seem to feel about what you're telling her now?"

>>**Claire:** "It's good… she's calmer."

>>**Therapist:** "Very good! She feels a bit calmer?"

Coach the client to articulate counterarguments against their Critical or Coping Modes. In imagery rescripting, those counterarguments are directed against the origin of the schemas, which for Claire is her mother. Here, the therapist wants Claire to understand better and also believe that her mother's internalized ideas of independence are wrong.

Example of rescripting the traumatic image from the perspective of the Healthy Adult directed at the origin of the schema

>>Therapist: "So perhaps you could say something to your mother now. I think it's important for Little Claire to hear why what her Mummy is saying is wrong. Can you tell your mother why she's wrong? Just turn to her and say that you think Little Claire should be allowed to go and play with her friend."

(*Claire turns in the direction where she sees her mother.*)

>>Claire: "She should be allowed to play at her friend's house. It's a very normal thing. It isn't right that you're stopping her when she wants to."

>>Therapist: (*talking softly, prompting*) "Children need to be able to explore the world a bit…"

>>Claire: "It's very good that she wants to do things, and children actually need that."

>>Therapist: (*prompting*) "This will give her more self-confidence and make the world a bit safer…"

>>Claire: "She also needs to be able to do things to gain more self-confidence. This way, she'll only get anxious and worried about everything that could go wrong."

>>Therapist: "Very good! How does your mother react?"

>>Claire: "It's hard for her to hear… she's completely focused on all kinds of things that could go wrong."

Here, you need to decide whether or not to go further into the reactions of the visualized mother. It is important to state that the intention is not to change the visualized antagonist. This is often not even possible because clients have no real-life experience of the antagonists ever showing different, healthier behaviours.

Whether or not you continue the conversation with the visualized mother, eventually you need to ask the client to turn their eyes away from the antagonist. Ask your client to start focusing more on the corrective experience of that moment and their own needs.

Example of rescripting this traumatic image from the perspective of the Healthy Adult directed at the Vulnerable Child

>>Therapist: "And take a look at Little Claire. How does she feel about everything you've just told her?"

>>Claire: (*turns slightly towards the visualized Little Claire*) "She likes it. She feels supported."

→

>>**Therapist:** "Very good! And what do you want to do now? Do you want to say something to her? Or do you want to hold her? Or maybe both?"

>>**Claire:** "I would like to give her a cuddle for a moment."

>>**Therapist:** "Do that then… hold her nice and tight. Do you feel her against you?"

(*Claire nods.*)

>>**Therapist:** "Do you feel any of that relaxation you just saw? Or is that small body still a bit tense?"

>>**Claire:** "No, she is much more relaxed now… she's leaning against me."

Finally, the behavioural change is that your client learns to act more in accordance with her own needs. In Claire's example, this is the need for autonomy and competence.

Example of rescripting the traumatic image from the perspective of the Healthy Adult directed at behavioural change

>>**Therapist:** "And what do you want to tell her she can do now? Do you think she should be allowed to play with her friend?"

(*Claire nods.*)

>>**Therapist:** "Tell her then. Just find your own words, you can do that just fine."

>>**Claire:** "You know… (*Her voice sounds soft, like she is talking to that little girl.*) It's fine that you want to play with Miriam. I like the fact that you want that kind of thing, and that's allowed. There's nothing wrong with doing things like that, and Mummy is just a bit overprotective. Just listen to what you want, there's nothing wrong with that."

>>**Therapist:** (*prompting*) "The world is full of fun and interesting and sometimes exciting things, and it's good to discover some of that…"

>>**Claire:** "Yes, of course there are dangers in life, but there are also a lot of great things, and it really is very good to discover them!"

>>**Therapist:** "How does it feel to say this?"

>>**Claire:** (*nods*) "Yeah, good…"

>>**Therapist:** "Come, I'll take you to your friend's place now. Are you coming?"

>>**Claire:** (*hesitantly*) "Really?"

>>**Therapist:** "Yes, for sure, she's already waiting for you."

>>**Claire:** "I like that…"

8.5.4 Step 4: Repeat this rescripting, but now from the child's perspective

After the rescripting by the client as a Healthy Adult is complete, ask them to rewind the image to the point when the rescripting started. Ask them to visualize the rescripting again, but this time from the perspective of the Vulnerable Child. With this, you repeat the healing, corrective side of the exercise, which helps to consolidate the experience. By having your client repeat the schema-forming event and visualize it from the child's perspective, you help them to address other basic needs as well. Rescripting from the Healthy Adult perspective aligns with and validates basic needs such as competence and independence. In turn, rescripting from the child's perspective aligns with other basic needs, such as safe connection and appreciation. By incorporating other needs in this way, you deepen the corrective experience.

> **Example of repeating the rescripting, but now from the child's perspective**
>
> **>>Therapist:** "Great. Then I want you to rewind the picture now. Just rewind the film – go back in time until you get to that point where your Mum has just said that you can't go play. Are you there again?"
>
> (*Claire nods.*)
>
> **>>Therapist:** "And now I want you to be that little girl again. Just be that six-year-old. (*Here, the therapist talks softly again, as if talking to a child*). There you are. You want to play at Miriam's, but your mother, diagonally across from you, won't let you, right?"
>
> (*Claire shakes her head.*)
>
> **>>Therapist:** "But if you turn your head a little now, you can also see that Grown-Up Claire is here. Take a look at her…"
>
> (*Claire turns her head.*)
>
> **>>Therapist:** "Grown-Up Claire is standing there and comes closer. Do you see her?"
>
> (*Claire nods.*)
>
> **>>Therapist:** "And what does Grown-Up Claire say to you?"
>
> **>>Claire:** "That she understands that I feel bad… that it makes sense that I'm sad and a bit angry."
>
> **>>Therapist:** "How does it feel to hear those words?"
>
> **>>Claire:** "Yes, it does feel nice…"   →

>>**Therapist:** "Where do you feel that in your body?"

(*Claire points to her belly.*)

>>**Therapist:** "Just put a hand on that side of your belly where you feel that pleasant sensation most strongly."

(*Claire puts her hands on her belly.*)

>>**Therapist:** "Just feel that sensation. What is its temperature? Is it warm or cool?"

>>**Claire:** "Warm… relaxed…"

>>**Therapist:** "Very nice, enjoy it!"

Again, ask the client to become aware of the healing, corrective experiences generated by the intervention. By focusing on this, you make the client aware of experiences they might otherwise easily overlook. Focusing on the corrective experiences is also a way to consolidate them. You can then turn your attention to the cognitive arguments against the internalized schema beliefs.

Example of repeating the rescripting, but now from the child's perspective – continued

>>**Therapist:** "And what do you see Grown-Up Claire doing now? Does she say anything else to your mother?"

(*Claire nods.*)

>>**Therapist:** "What does she say?"

>>**Claire:** "She says: 'It's not unusual at all that Claire wants to play at her friend's house, and that's fine. It isn't all that dangerous, and if you only talk about what could go wrong, you only make her anxious about it.'"

>>**Therapist:** "And how does your mother react to that?"

>>**Claire:** "Mummy actually has a hard time hearing it, it seems. As if in her head she's mostly occupied with all the dangers."

>>**Therapist:** "Then I want you to take your eyes off your mother for a moment and focus on Grown-Up Claire. What is she doing now?"

>>**Claire:** "She's holding me…"

>>**Therapist:** "And how does that feel?"

>>**Claire:** "… Yes, very good…"

>>**Therapist:** "Just feel that big body, lie against it for a bit. Is it nice?"

(*Claire nods.*)

>>**Therapist:** "And what else does Grown-Up Claire say to you?"

>>**Claire:** "That I will get to play at my friend's house now. That it's actually great to do new things, to discover things."

>>**Therapist:** "How does it feel?"

>>**Claire:** (*nodding*) "Yes, nice… warm."

>>**Therapist:** "Is there anything else that Grown-Up Claire says?"

>>**Claire:** (*smiling*) "Yes, she also says that she'll take me to Miriam's house."

>>**Therapist:** "And what's it like to hear that?"

>>**Claire:** "Yeah, nice… very nice."

Finally, to further strengthen healthy schemas about competence and autonomy, ask the client to practice using a new, more competent self-image.

Example of repeating the rescripting, but now from the child's perspective – continued

>>**Therapist:** "Very good. Just enjoy that nice feeling, the realization that it's good to feel you want to try things, that it's okay to go out into the world and have new experiences. You're perfectly capable of that. You can handle it just fine; you really are strong enough for it. Just say that: 'I can handle it, I'm strong enough for that.'"

>>**Claire:** "'I can handle it… I can handle it, because I'm strong enough for that…'"

>>**Therapist:** "How does that feel?"

>>**Claire:** "Yeah, nice… good."

>>**Therapist:** "And then Grown-Up Claire also says you can play at your friend's house. Can you hear her say that?"

>>*Claire:* "Yes, she says it's fine that I want to play at Miriam's house… that there is nothing wrong with exploring the world like that. And she also says my mother is overprotective…"

>>**Therapist:** "And how does it feel to hear that?"

>>**Claire:** "Yes, very good. It feels really nice: solid, supportive."

>>**Therapist:** "Could you say that? Something like: 'It's good to listen to what I want; my needs matter.'"

>>**Claire:** "It's good to feel what I want, there's nothing wrong with that. My needs matter."

8.5.5 Step 5: Review and homework

In the review of this exercise, reiterate the most important lessons and experiences that can be taken forward into the future. In an atmosphere of positive reinforcement, discuss the client's successes and compliment their independent action. Also, make agreements about homework. Again, your client should take more control of the process at this point by thinking more actively about the best form of homework themselves.

8.6 Chairwork in the middle phase

As well as imagery rescripting, chairwork was also used in the initial phase of therapy. In the middle phase, too, you will continue to use both techniques frequently. Chairwork is used in the middle phase to negotiate with the client's Coping Modes and to contradict their Critical Parts in order to validate the needs of the Child Modes. However, in the middle phase, your client will take a more active role in the exercises.

From this point forward, you add a chair for the Healthy Adult during the exercises, and your client works with you from this chair when working on the unhealthy modes. Your role as a therapist is now more that of a coach than a leader. It is important to recognize this shift of role, otherwise there is a chance that you will continue to lead the client just as you have done up to now. So far, you have always taken the initiative in recognizing and working on the different modes. Be aware that you are now in a different phase, and make sure you do not get 'stuck' in the same active role you had in the initial phase of therapy.

> #### Example of chairwork in the middle phase
>
> **>>Claire:** "And when I filled in that form, I made a mistake, and I was so upset about that! I could have kicked myself!"
>
> **>>Therapist:** "Well, that sounds a bit strong, Claire! I understand that it wasn't great that you made a mistake, but it happens to everyone once in a while."
>
> **>>Claire:** "Yes, but I always make stupid mistakes like that. I'm just so stupid! I actually just need to be more aware of that. I always make a mess of things like this."
>
> **>>Therapist:** "I find myself wondering who I'm listening to now when you say this. I hear you saying you're stupid. That you always mess everything up. Who says things like that? Not your Healthy Adult, that's for sure."

> **Claire:** "No… you mean this is the Strict One?"
>
> **Therapist:** "I can well imagine it being the Strict One, yes. So, what do you see that makes you think of the Strict One?"

In the middle phase of therapy, it is appropriate to call a little more on the insights your client has gained up to this point. Ask more open-ended questions, for instance when it comes to recognizing their different modes. If your client is able to recognize these modes well, you might ask how they were able to do so. In this way you encourage self-expression and autonomy, which are very important for Claire in the example.

> ### Example of chairwork in the middle phase – continued
>
> **Claire:** "Well, that I'm feeling stupid, mostly. Also, because that's what Dad always said."
>
> **Therapist:** "Yeah, right? I immediately thought of him too, because you said that seemed to be his standard comment, that you're stupid. If the Strict One is so active anyway, I'd like to give her a chair here in the room."
>
> (Here, the therapist stands up and puts a chair diagonally opposite Claire.)
>
> **Therapist:** "So the Strict One is sitting there. And what does the Strict One say?"

It is no longer essential for the client to sit in the specific chair for the Critical Mode. You have done chairwork so many times now, with the same chair in the same place in the room each time, that it is likely that the empty chair already sufficiently represents the Critical Mode. If it is still difficult for your client to detach from that mode, you can always ask them to articulate those critical perceptions from the chair of the Critical Mode first.

> ### Example of chairwork in the middle phase – continued
>
> **Claire:** "She says that I can't do anything anyway, that I'm stupid…"
> (Here she bows her head, and her voice sounds sad.)
>
> **Therapist:** "And how do you feel now, hearing that criticism from the Strict One?"
>
> **Claire:** "Small… sad."
>
> **Therapist:** (*in a soft voice*): "I can well imagine that, Claire. That's quite a thing to hear, that you're stupid. That would make anyone sad. But then again, this is the Strict One that rants about that sort of thing all the time, right?"
>
> (Claire nods.)

> **Therapist:** "And when that has been said to you so often, and when it is still being said all the time, yes, of course you get sad. You're only human after all. This seems to me like a good time to bring in your Healthy Adult."
>
> *(At this, the therapist stands, pulls up an extra chair and places it next to Claire.)*

The ultimate goal of therapy is for your client to be able to connect with their Healthy Adult independently whenever schemas are activated. In the middle phase, it is still necessary to provide them with some aids for that transition. The extra chair for the Healthy Adult allows the client to distance themselves not only physically but also emotionally from the feelings that are triggered by the schema activation.

Example of chairwork in the middle phase – continued

> **Therapist:** "Please get up from the chair where you're sitting now. But you know, when you get up, leave all the emotions and pain behind, in the chair. Leave that pain stuck there with superglue, and then take a seat on the chair there next to you."
>
> *(Claire gets up and sits down in the extra chair.)*
>
> **Therapist:** "And in this chair, I'd like to ask you to take a moment to put on your captain's hat. Just make contact with your Healthy Adult. Can you take me through how you do that by saying out loud what that Healthy Adult looks like?"

Here, ask the client to use the image of the Healthy Adult that you practiced in the previous sessions, and then coach the Healthy Adult first to show compassion for the emotions they were feeling. Then coach the client to contradict the Critical Mode.

Example of coaching the client to contradict the Critical Mode

> **Therapist:** "So the Strict One says that Claire is stupid, and, quite understandably, she is sad about that. What do we think about that, that the Strict One just does that? Would you wish that on a friend, that kind of criticism?"
>
> **Claire:** "No, definitely not!"
>
> **Therapist:** "No, right? But why not?"
>
> **Claire:** "Well, you just don't say that! It makes no sense just to call someone stupid."
>
> **Therapist:** "I agree completely. But can you tell the Strict One that as well?"
>
> **Claire:** *(to the empty chair of the Strict One)* "You don't say that…"

>>**Therapist:** "Fantastic! But it could be more powerful. Say it again, but this time twenty percent louder."

>>**Claire:** (*slightly louder*) "You don't say that."

>>**Therapist:** "Again, and throw yourself into it, stand up for Little Claire."

>>**Claire:** "You don't say that! Behave yourself!"

>>**Therapist:** "Very good! It's great to hear your anger too, I love hearing that from you!"

This is just one example of what coaching the Healthy Adult can entail in chairwork. There are many different conceivable variations, depending on the type of mode being worked on, and also on your individual client's mood and feelings. Sometimes your client will feel a bit more vulnerable and there might seem to be a slight setback, which hinders the connection with the Healthy Adult or their ability to speak from that mode. In such cases, you may temporarily have to give them a bit more support.

8.7 Chapter summary

This chapter has described how to help the client form a picture of their own Healthy Adult. We explained how you can make the client aware of all aspects of this mode, and how you can then explain the strategy that springs from that Healthy Adult state of mind – the three steps of self-compassion, cognitive restructuring and behaviour modification. We also described how the client can practice these steps using chairwork, where, instead of representing different parts, the chairs represent the three steps of the Healthy Adult.

Your role as a therapist shifts in the middle phase of therapy, from being a guide to being more of a coach. For imagery rescripting, this means that the client starts to act from their own Healthy Adult to rescript images themselves. As a result, your client now has two positions and perspectives in any visualizations that you explore – the perspective of the Vulnerable Child, and the perspective of the Healthy Adult, who provides good care for that child. Your role is to teach the client to experience the rescripting from both perspectives, so that different basic needs can be addressed and validated from each one.

Chapter 9: The final phase of therapy

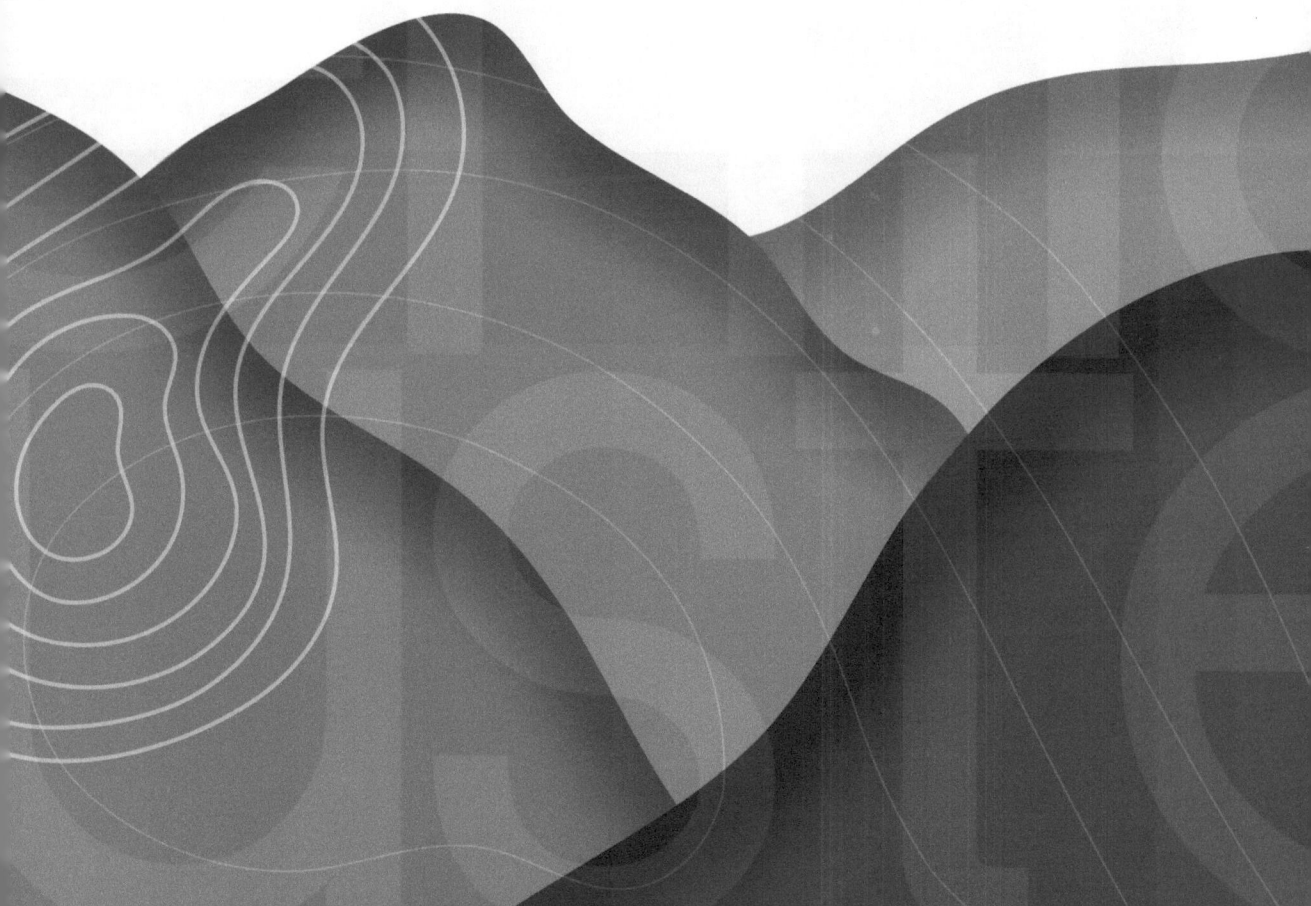

Chapter 9: The final phase of therapy

Chapter map	
9.1	Introduction
9.2	Historical roleplay in the final phase
9.3	Future-oriented imagery
9.4	Chairwork with the therapist as the Coping Mode
9.5	Roleplay with role reversal
9.6	Empathic confrontation in the final phase
9.7	Ending the therapy
9.8	Chapter summary

9.1 Introduction

In the middle phase of therapy, you spent some time working on behavioural change. However, in the final phase of treatment, the goal is for that behavioural change to increasingly carry over into their daily life. A dependent client will need to do things independently and stand up for their own needs. An avoidant client will need to get out among people and speak up more when they do. And an obsessive-compulsive client will need to work less and take more time for relaxation and playfulness. If the ingrained patterns of behaviour are not actually broken, your client will slip back into them.

The sessions are scheduled with lower frequency in the final phase, about once per month. Due to this low frequency, you will naturally have a different role as a therapist. In the sessions, you will spend more time listening to your client's news, rather than guiding the client through your plan. Try to be aware that your role in this final phase really is qualitatively different. In the middle phase, you were an active coach who still sometimes participated in the exercises. In this final phase, you continue to coach – but from the sidelines. Of course, you are still involved in what is going on in your client's life, but you do so from a distance and give the client space to live their own life.

After many months of therapy, you may actually have less insight into your client's behavioural patterns. That might sound strange, because you've just worked on change so intensively together. However, you primarily focused on your client's perceptions, schemas and modes – their origins, and how to work on them. With so much focus on thoughts and feelings, you may have asked less about the client's behaviour.

It is therefore wise to take a fresh look at your client's behavioural patterns at the start of the final phase. What do they do differently now, and what hasn't changed that much on a behavioural level? To answer these questions, you can refer back to the case conceptualization, but now with these behavioural patterns in mind. You can also ask partners, parents or children to come along again, as you did after the case conceptualization.

This kind of evaluation of behavioural change can occasionally be somewhat confrontational. For example, you may have thought the therapy was progressing successfully, but your client's partner doesn't mention anything to you about an actual change in their behaviour. Fortunately, it is not too late to find this out, and you still have enough time to work on that behavioural change in the final phase.

Example of re-evaluating the client's behavioural patterns at the start of the final phase

You have discussed with Jenny that her therapy is entering its final phase and that the goal of these last ten sessions is to put what she has learned into practice. You not only referred back to the case conceptualization, but you also asked Jenny to bring her friend Linda to therapy. Linda came along once at the beginning of therapy; as Jenny's best friend, and actually as Jenny's only real social network, you have explained the modes and purpose of Jenny's therapy to her. Linda liked hearing that the therapy aims to get Jenny to listen to her basic needs more. This is exactly what Linda herself has often said to Jenny. Although Linda is not a co-therapist during treatment, it was nice that Linda was aligned with you as the therapist on this. Now that Linda has come again, you ask her specifically what she has noticed in terms of changes in Jenny. Linda says that →

Jenny shares more with her and that she likes that. However, she says that Jenny still cancels or reschedules arrangements quite often, both with her and at work. During the conversation, Jenny sits looking rather defeated. You recognize the same shame she often felt with you at the beginning of therapy.

\>\>**Therapist:** "Jenny, would you share what is happening for you now, when you hear Linda talking like this?"

\>\>**Jenny:** (*with bowed head*): "I don't feel great…"

(*The therapist does have an idea of what Jenny means by this, but in this final phase he thinks she can express more of what she is experiencing.*)

\>\>**Therapist:** "And that is a feeling of…?"

\>\>**Jenny:** "Shame…"

\>\>**Therapist:** "That you feel bad about what Linda says about you?"

\>\>**Jenny:** "Yes…"

\>\>**Therapist:** "And who is it, then, that makes you feel so bad about yourself? I don't mean Linda of course, because she isn't doing anything wrong – she's just saying what she's seen. But what side of you is making you feel so bad when she says that?"

\>\>**Jenny:** "The Prosecutor?"

\>\>**Therapist:** "It does sound a lot like the Prosecutor, yes. And when Linda says that you still avoid things, what does the Prosecutor translate that to mean?"

\>\>**Jenny:** "That I make it so difficult for everyone, that it's my fault that she has trouble with that…"

\>\>**Therapist:** "And you? I'm reaching out to you as the captain now, as the Healthy Adult. What do you think about that? Do you agree?"

\>\>**Jenny:** "It does feel that way, yes…"

\>\>**Therapist:** "Yes, I can imagine that does it still feel that way, because the Prosecutor can still be quite dominant and give you that wretched feeling. But I didn't ask if it felt that way; I asked if you, as the captain, agree with the Prosecutor that you've done something wrong and that it's your fault if Linda feels bad?"

\>\>**Jenny:** "No…"

\>\>**Therapist:** "Because…?"

\>\>**Jenny:** "Because… Linda didn't say she feels bad or that she thinks I'm annoying."

\>\>**Therapist:** "And so…"

> *The therapist continues to use Socratic questioning into the counterarguments Jenny now has against the Blaming Mode. With this, he encourages the Healthy Adult to speak up more and stand up for Jenny. You decide to make the focus of the next session the issue of joining colleagues when they go for drinks on the last Friday of the month.*

Now that you know what behavioural patterns are still active in the client's life, you can use the remaining sessions to break them as much as possible. Your role as therapist is not only as a coach on the sidelines, but also as someone who helps the client to remember what they were trying to achieve. If the client does not do what has been agreed, a somewhat firmer empathic confrontation is called for.

In this final phase, you actually use the same methods and techniques as you used in the initial and middle phases, but these now have the objective of changing behaviour. As a result, some of the techniques, such as imagery rescripting and chairwork, are done slightly differently. In addition to the techniques already applied, in this final phase you can also use any other methods and techniques that help to facilitate behavioural change. Behavioural therapy offers a variety of options for this, ranging from skills training to self-control procedures, and from exposure to communication training. The application of several methods and techniques from the final phase is described below.

9.2 Historical roleplay in the final phase

Historical roleplay is another way to strengthen the Healthy Adult. You have already used this technique in treatment in the initial phase (see Chapter 5), but at that time you were a role model for the good-enough parent, so that your client could experience sufficiently good care. Now, this technique allows the client to practice standing up for their own needs independently in the last step of the roleplay.

In the box below, we repeat the step-by-step plan for historical roleplay in the initial phase from section 5.5, with a difference at step 7.

Step-by-step plan for historical roleplay in the final phase
Step 1: Explore current symptom patterns.
Step 2: Identify a meaningful related event from the past.
Step 3: Re-enact event: client as child; therapist as antagonist.
Step 4: Review first roleplay and identify schemas formed.
Step 5: Re-enact event: client as antagonist; therapist as child.
Step 6: Review second roleplay and identify any schema-refuting information.
Step 7: Re-enact event: client as child, but with Healthy Adult insights and the capacity to stand up for their own needs.
Step 8: Review exercise and formation of healthy schemas.

These steps are explained in more detail below using John as an example. Because historical roleplay has already been explained in Chapter 5, we will touch only briefly on the replicated steps and spend more time on the new elements (particularly Step 7).

9.2.1 Step 1: Explore current symptom patterns

By this phase of therapy, you will already know a good deal about the patterns in your client's life and the modes associated with them. This will enable you, together with your client, to quickly identify those patterns in the everyday situations they talk about.

> **Example of exploring current symptom patterns**
>
> **>>Therapist:** "So, if I understand you correctly, you'd had a long day at work and you were lying on the couch exhausted, but then you remembered a little job you still had to do. So you got up from the sofa and went back to work. Is that true?"
>
> **>>John:** "Yes, that's true."
>
> **>>Therapist:** "Well, it's a familiar example, I must say. Basically, it's another situation in which there doesn't seem to be room for any leisure or relaxation, but where work and your responsibilities take priority."
>
> **>>John:** "Yes, I know we've talked about it a lot, but at times like that I think it's really hard not to do that work… I mean, the job won't take care of itself or anything…"

>>**Therapist:** "I understand that. I understand that it's very hard for you to see things differently at times like that. There's a reason you have this recurring pattern in your life, that you work so hard and work often comes before relaxation or rest. Perhaps we could do an exercise today to reflect on that again. It will help us to gain more understanding of how work could have become such a major theme in your life. But in it, I'll also help you deal with this issue in a different way. What do you think of that?"

9.2.2 Step 2: Identify a meaningful related event from the past

By this stage, you have a good deal of insight into the origins of your client's patterns and modes. You have done imagery rescripting many times, in which you linked recent problem situations to past events. At this point in treatment, you can therefore assume that your client knows which past events can be linked to current patterns.

Example of identifying a meaningful related event from the past

>>**Therapist:** "So, this week you had one of those situations where you got up from the couch because there were still tasks to be done. And by now I think we have a pretty good idea where that sense of responsibility, that pressure, comes from, right?"

>>**John:** "Yes, I think so, yes…"

>>**Therapist:** "Can you recall a memory from your childhood when something like that also seemed to happen? It should be a situation from your past where you might have felt like you really wanted to relax, but you also felt pressure to get to work."

>>**John:** "I'm reminded of that situation with my father which I mentioned earlier. I'm standing at the piano and my father is standing in front of me. A friend has just rung at the door to see if I'm coming out to play, and I want to. But my father says I'm not allowed because I haven't practiced the piano. The situation from the past week reminds me of that, because it's another task that has to be done before I can relax."

9.2.3 Step 3: Re-enact historical event: client as child, therapist as antagonist

In Chapter 5, we explained that historical roleplay consists of three rounds. The first of these is acting out the historical event as it actually happened in the past.

Example of introducing the first round of roleplay

>>**Therapist:** "Let's revisit this situation in a roleplay, like we've done before. This past event is apparently connected to what happened last week when you got up from the couch because you still had a job to do. Shall we act out this situation so we can take a closer look at exactly what happened?"

(*John nods.*)

>>**Therapist:** "We'll literally act out that situation here in this room, as if we're bringing the past into the present. First, let's just re-enact exactly what happened. Afterwards, I want to look at that situation with you, so we can understand together what the boy from that time learned from the situation."

Don't keep talking about the event for too long; get up from your chair fairly quickly to set up the roleplay area, together with the client.

Example of setting up the first round of roleplay

>>**Therapist:** "Good, so first I'd like to come and stand next to me for a moment."

(*The therapist stands up and John follows so they are standing next to each other in the room. The therapist gestures to a side of the room that will be the roleplay area.*)

>>**Therapist:** "Let's re-enact the past situation with you and your father here. Take me with you for a moment: where did it happen, in the living room at home?"

>>**John:** "Yes, in the living room, where the grand piano was."

>>**Therapist:** "And the grand piano is… where?"

>>**John:** "Well, if this is the living room… the grand piano would be here. (*Gestures to a spot in the room.*) So there's the sitting area…"

>>**Therapist:** "And where is your father?"

>>**John:** "He's standing there (*pointing to a spot near the piano*). So I'm standing here (*points to a spot near the father*). Because I've just come in through the front door."

>>**Therapist:** "Because you'd just been talking to your friend at the door who asked if you were coming out to play, right?"

(*John nods.*)

You already know the antagonist well at this stage, from the many stories you have explored during therapy, and you will therefore be able to play the role fairly easily. Of course, you can still briefly ask for any specific instructions for this roleplay.

Example of preparing to play the antagonist

>>**Therapist:** "Okay, so you've just come in through the door there and you're standing here, and you tell your father about the plan to go play outside. Now I'm about to play your father, so can you tell me how he acts? How exactly does he tell you that you can't go play and that you need to practice the piano?"

>>**John:** "Well, he doesn't say it angrily or anything, but more as if it's self-evident… as if it's the most normal thing in the world, and there is no question of doing otherwise."

>>**Therapist:** "So, a little bit strict? But not angry?"

>>**John:** "Yes, exactly, just like: 'This is how it is, and this is how we're going to do it,' and there is no argument possible."

>>**Therapist:** "And I guess he's talking like a history teacher again, with that very official language."

>>**John:** "Yes, using words like 'irrelevant', 'obviously', 'punctual', that kind of thing."

>>**Therapist:** "Good, I'm getting a bit of a picture. Now you'll be playing yourself as a child in the roleplay. How old are you in this situation?"

>>**John:** (*having to think about it*) "Well, I think I started playing piano when I was eight. So I guess this happened when I was about ten?"

Before you start the roleplay, take a moment for the client to get into the perspective of the child they are about to play, even if by now you and they are very familiar with what life was like for them as a little boy back then.

Example of re-enacting event: client as child, therapist as antagonist

>>**Therapist:** "Okay, so you're back from school, and a friend, or friends, have just rung at the door to ask if you want to come out and play football. So you go and ask your father if you can go play outside. Okay?"

(*John nods.*)

>>**Therapist:** "Then just start when you're ready…"

>>**John:** "Dad, that was Tom just now, and they're going to play football. I want to go with them. Can I go outside?"

>>**Therapist:** (*tries to look at him like the father he has come to know from John's stories; a bit flat, functional and not really like a warm parent*): "No, John, you can't because you haven't practiced your piano yet. You need to do that first."

>>**John:** "Yeah, but Dad…"

>>**Therapist:** "No, John, piano first and then play. That's how it is, and you won't change it. But the sooner you start, the sooner you'll be done, and the sooner you can go out and play." (*At this point, the therapist turns away as if on his way to a new task.*)

>>**John:** "..."

9.2.4 Step 4: Review first roleplay and identify schemas formed

Return to your seats and discuss how the first roleplay went. Pinpoint the conclusions that the client has drawn about themselves and the other person from this interaction. These are the more cognitive aspects of the schemas that formed in the circumstances you have just acted out. Remember to check the credibility of those assumptions, so you can explore whether anything changes in them during the exercise.

Example of reviewing first roleplay and identifying schemas formed

>>**Therapist:** "Okay, let's stop here. First, a question: did that look like the situation? Is that at all how you remember it?"

>>**John:** "Yes, it was like that. My Dad might have said even less – maybe just 'practice first, lad' before going back to his work, but it really did feel like the way it was then."

>>**Therapist:** "Stay in this experience for just a little while longer. Keep being the ten-year-old boy. How do you feel now?"

>>**John:** "I don't know – sad maybe? Well, maybe mostly a bit irritated..."

>>**Therapist:** "Okay, sad but mostly irritated. So let's step out of this situation for a moment and look at what happened from a distance."

(*The therapist walks to the place where they discussed the exercise beforehand and, with the client beside him, they look back over to where the roleplay was performed.*)

>>**Therapist:** "Okay, now if we just look back at what happened over there from the stillness and space we have here, what do you think that ten-year-old boy learned?"

>>**John:** "Well... that he should just do as he's told?"

>>**Therapist:** "Yes, that sounds right. And what proved more important in that situation, that the boy wanted to play, or that there was still work to be done?"

>>**John:** "That there was still work to be done."

>>**Therapist:** "Right. So, what did the boy learn about his need for play and relaxation?"

>>**John:** "That it didn't matter as much…"

>>**Therapist:** "Exactly. So the little boy actually learned that 'what I feel, my need for play and relaxation, is not important'?"

>>**John:** "Yes, something like that…"

>>**Therapist:** "Just see if that fits with how you experienced it. 'What I need, my feeling that I want some relaxation and free time to play, that's not important.' Does that kind of fit with how you experienced the situation?"

>>**John:** "Yes, that's just how it is."

>>**Therapist:** "And from your perspective as a ten-year-old boy, how true is that thought? How credible is it?"

>>**John:** "As a ten-year-old?"

>>**Therapist:** "Yes, how did that little boy you just played experience that? Was it a hundred percent true that it didn't really matter what he needed? Or less?"

>>**John:** "Well… no-one ever said that it was completely unimportant. But in practice it very often seemed to be, and it still does now. So ninety-five percent, maybe?"

>>**Therapist:** "Okay… and what did the little boy learn about others? How does that little boy look at the father he sees before him in that past situation?"

>>**John:** "That's a difficult question. Look, for me, that's just the way it was."

>>**Therapist:** "What your father said were kind of just the rules in life, I think?"

>>**John:** "Yes, exactly – work first and only relax afterwards."

>>**Therapist:** "So it's not so much about your father himself in that situation, but the norms and rules he imposed. And the rule is: 'Work first and relax after'?"

>>**John:** "Yes, exactly!"

>>**Therapist:** "And how strongly does the ten-year-old boy believe that rule?"

>>**John:** "One hundred percent."

Write down your client's statements, and note the credibility of their self-image, which you have just identified, and the image they have of others and the world around them.

9.2.5 Step 5: Re-enact event: client as antagonist, therapist as child

In the second round of roleplay, the original event is played out again, but this time you are the child and the client is the antagonist. With this change of perspective, even more information can be gained about the circumstances in which the schemas were formed.

> **Example of re-enacting event: client as antagonist, therapist as child**
>
> **>>Therapist:** "Now let's re-enact the same situation again, but this time we'll switch roles. Now you'll be your father, and I'll play you as a ten-year-old boy. Your father is about forty years old then, right?"
>
> (*John nods.*)
>
> **>>Therapist:** "And what does his life look like?"
>
> **>>John:** "Well, he's a history teacher at the same school as my mother. He works hard – he's always preparing lessons or marking homework or tests. And he's also busy with activities around the school."
>
> **>>Therapist:** "Now let's step back into the past again." (*The therapist walks over to the roleplay area, but now stands in the place of the ten-year-old boy.*)
>
> **>>Therapist:** "I want you to be the father now. So you're back from work, you have a lot of work to do and now there's your ten-year-old son, John. Okay, let's start."
>
> **>>Therapist:** (*playing the role of the ten-year-old boy as well as he can based on what he has observed, and speaking in a somewhat childlike voice*) "Dad, that was Tom at the door, and they're going to play football. I'd like to go and play with them, can I?"
>
> **>>John:** (*playing his father and speaking in a decisive voice*) "No, it's out of the question because you haven't done your piano practice yet. Go and start on that."
>
> (*John turns and starts moving to walk away.*)
>
> **>>Therapist:** "Okay, okay! Let's stop here… phew! Now I understand a bit better what you meant when you described your father. He's really quite firm, isn't he?"
>
> **>>John:** "Yes, not angry or anything. But that's how it went."
>
> **>>Therapist:** "Well, I notice that I feel all kinds of things about what just happened. I still feel that it's very annoying to be spoken to like that when actually I do have a right to go out and play – I can feel some of the irritation you just mentioned. And I can also feel some of that sadness that what I say or feel doesn't seem to matter at all."

>>**John:** (*looking at the therapist inquiringly*) "Do you really mean that?"

>>**Therapist:** "Yes, definitely! I can easily understand that this isn't nice for a ten-year-old boy. How is that for you to hear?"

>>**John:** "Well, good actually… It's nice that you see and experience it the same way, that it's not completely my fault."

>>**Therapist:** "No, of course it isn't your fault! But can you stay in the role of your father for a bit longer? Just stand here a moment, and I'll speak to you as him, okay?"

(*John nods.*)

>>**Therapist:** "John's father, I heard that you won't let John go and play outside. Can you tell me again why you think it's so important for him to practice the piano first?"

>>**John:** "He'll still need to practice anyway. That's just the deal, and a deal is a deal."

>>**Therapist:** "Yes, I do understand that sometimes certain things need to be done in life. But John is only ten, and playing is important for children, too, don't you think?"

>>**John:** "Well, I'm not so concerned with that. He just needs to practice his piano, and I still have a lot of work to do, and that's the end of it for me."

>>**Therapist:** "So you aren't concerned so much with John and what he needs as with all the tasks that are still to be done – piano practice, schoolwork and so on?"

>>**John:** "Yes, absolutely!"

>>**Therapist:** "Okay, we'll stop here. Let's step away for a moment, and go back over there where we can think about everything that happened."

(*The therapist and John walk back to the original position to talk about the roleplay.*)

As shown in this example, after the second roleplay, you can give feedback on what you experienced in your role as the child. By talking about the impact of the antagonist's behaviour, you acknowledge the feelings your client might also have had as a child.

9.2.6 Step 6: Review second roleplay and identify any schema-refuting information

In Chapter 5, we explained that switching roles does not necessarily lead to different conclusions. Sometimes, the role reversal simply confirms the conclusion that your client's needs didn't matter much to the antagonist. However, role reversal may affect the client's self-image and the image they have of others. For example, a common effect of role reversal is that your client comes to realize that the antagonist in the re-enacted situation did not have the presence of mind or capacities to address the child's needs. When the client comes to realize this, it can result in them seeing the source of the problem less as themselves, and more as the antagonist. It wasn't the client as a child who was the problem in the example, but the antagonist, who fell short as a parent.

Example of reviewing second roleplay and identifying any schema-refuting information

>>Therapist: "Okay, well let's take a quick look at what we just learned. What do you take away from this roleplay?"

>>John: "Yeah, I don't really know… well, maybe it's that my father wasn't actually that concerned about me at all."

>>Therapist: "Yes, I noticed that too, when I was talking to him. Does it still matter to you that he said he wasn't concerned with your needs, but mostly with his own tasks?"

>>John: "Yes, a little bit… it's still aggravating that he didn't pay any attention at all to what I needed, but it wasn't so much because he begrudged me having what I wanted, it's just not where his attention was."

>>Therapist: "So how do you view now that idea: 'What I feel and need don't matter'?"

>>John: "Now? How do I look at it now?"

>>Therapist: "Yes, having just been in your father's position, and looking back on the whole situation. How do you see the idea that your feelings and needs don't matter?"

>>John: "Well, for my father, it didn't matter that much. But he was just occupied with other things. Talking about it like that now, it does feel different, that my needs and feelings are important, but he just wasn't concerned with them."

>>Therapist: "So how credible does that thought feel to you now: the thought that your feelings and needs don't matter?"

>>John: "Yes, a bit less… fifty percent or so?"

>>Therapist: "Great. And then the thought that work must be done before you can relax. How do you see that after this second roleplay, with the knowledge you have now? And can you now begin to look at something like this as your Healthy Adult?"

>>**John:** (*looking thoughtful, in silence*) "Well, somewhere it still feels like it's true. But it is fair to say that now I'm more aware that this is just how my father saw it, and that doesn't mean it's automatically true forever and for everyone."

>>**Therapist:** "So with that realization, that this is how your father might have seen it but it doesn't have to be right for everyone and forever, how true does that idea feel that there's always work to be done before you can relax?"

>>**John:** "Yeah, less… also something like fifty percent?"

>>**Therapist:** "That's great. It's not about right or wrong, it's just about taking a measurement of how it is for you now, with all the information we've discussed."

9.2.7 Step 7: Re-enact event: client as child, but with Healthy Adult insights and the capacity to stand up for their own needs

This round differs from the historical roleplay in the initial phase of treatment, as presented in Chapter 5, because now it is the client who stands up for their own needs. In the final round of historical roleplay, your client will have the opportunity to do this. Emphasize to them that, as a child, in the situation as it was then, they could not stand up for themselves. But now, with all the insights and learning experiences from therapy, they can. First, discuss what they would like to say to the antagonist in the roleplay. Then act out the original situation again, with the client playing the role of the child. They use that role to speak out against the antagonist with the insights of the Healthy Adult Mode.

Example of preparation for third roleplay: client as child, but with Healthy Adult insights and the capacity to stand up for their own needs

>>**Therapist:** "Good, then there's one last round. We've now re-enacted the situation as it really occurred, with you as the child. Then we reversed the roles, and that gave us extra information. But of course, you're not that ten-year-old anymore. You're a grown man and, in therapy, you've also learned about what children need, their basic needs. With everything you've learned, and with all you now know, when you look back on that situation, what do you think that little boy really needed in that situation?"

>>**John:** "To go and play football, of course!"

>>**Therapist:** "That seems to be very clear to you, right?"

>>**John:** "Yes. It also makes me a bit angry that it wasn't allowed… partly because that's always how it was. There was always some task or chore that had to come first. I mean, he would say, 'Just get to work quickly, because then

you can relax sooner', but that moment never actually came. There was always something else I had to do."

>>Therapist: "The way you look at it now, as the Healthy Adult, the captain of your ship, you get angry about everything that happened here, is that right?"

>>John: "Yes I do!"

>>Therapist: "Then I'd like to suggest that we act out that situation again, but now you include everything you just told me. So you're about to play ten-year-old John again, but this time bring your Healthy Adult into that role. So in a moment you'll be standing there, not as a ten-year-old, but as the Healthy Adult, using the role of the little boy to express what you'd actually like to say to your father now. Does that make sense?"

>>John: "Yes, but it wouldn't really have been possible to say something like that to my father…"

You have already indicated that John, as a child, could never have spoken out against his father in the way you're preparing to do now. Even so, it's important to emphasize that message a few more times. Clients with strong Critical Modes can easily interpret this discussion as an expectation, a demand for how they should have reacted as children.

> ### Example of re-enacting event: client as child, but with Healthy Adult insights and the capacity to stand up for their own needs
>
> **>>Therapist:** "Yes, I understand that. And it's good that you say it again, because I'm certainly not trying to give you the idea that you should have said all this to your father at the time. You couldn't have! Ten-year-old John did what he could, and that was fine! As a ten-year-old, you can't stand up for yourself against a father who is so strict and firm. But now, as a Healthy Adult, you can. And I'd like us to act that out, to give you the experience of what it's like to stand up for your needs. Shall we give it a try?"
>
> **>>John:** "So I'll play the ten-year-old then, but as I see it now?"
>
> **>>Therapist:** "Exactly!"
>
> (*The therapist and John walk back to the roleplay area, with the therapist in the father's spot and John in the ten-year-old boy's spot.*)
>
> **>>Therapist:** "Very good, let's start then."
>
> **>>John:** "Dad, that was Tom. He asked if I want to come out and play football. I'd really like to do that, can I?"

>>**Therapist:** (*now as the father*) "No, out of the question. Go and practice your piano first, you still have to do that."

(*The therapist begins to turn away as John had just acted that out.*)

>>**John:** "Dad, you can't say that. What do you mean I can't go and play? I'm a child! You always say there's time to relax once the work is done, but that moment never seems to come. I don't want to just work; I want to enjoy myself sometimes. I've been to school, I do all kinds of chores here at home, now I just want to play for a while!"

Arriving at this point, you must decide how to react as the antagonist now that the client is standing up for their own needs so well. You could give a healthy response – compliment the client for speaking up, for example. However, the question is whether the antagonist as your client knows them would have done that. You can also interrupt the roleplay here and indicate that you don't know how the antagonist would have reacted. However, you know how you would react if you had been the antagonist and your child had stood up for himself like that. By expressing, or playing out, that natural response, you can offer the client another corrective experience, just as you did in the initial phase.

Example of giving a personal reaction in the role of the antagonist

>>**Therapist:** (*makes a stop gesture to interrupt the roleplay*): "Wow! You did that so well! Really powerful!"

(*John beams.*)

>>**Therapist:** "Really very good! I could feel that you really meant it. That makes it a bit tricky for me now, because I'm not sure how your father would react if you had said that to him. I have serious doubts about whether he would have been able to let go of his rigid way of thinking. What do you think?"

>>**John:** "No, there's no way he would have changed his mind. He never did."

>>**Therapist:** "Exactly. I sensed that. I can tell you how I would react if I was a father in that kind of situation, and my child came to me and said he really just wanted to play, and that he'd already worked so hard and didn't feel like any more jobs right now. I would say: 'I understand, son! Of course you can! You've had a long day, and now I'm trying to give you even more to do. Sorry, lad, I wasn't paying enough attention there. Of course you should go enjoy yourself, go have fun playing football. The piano isn't going anywhere, you can do that later. Now just enjoy yourself for a bit! Have fun! Now that I think of it, I was tempted to go straight to work myself but it suddenly strikes me that what I'm saying applies equally to me. So I'd like to come with you and play football too, if that's okay – what do you think of that?'"

>>**John:** (*laughing*) "Yes, alright. I think you really could use some relaxation too! But my father would never do that in real life."

The client has practiced standing up for their needs. You have already reinforced this healthy behaviour with compliments and your reaction as the antagonist in the roleplay. Now this positive experience needs to be consolidated as much as possible. To do this, reflect on the experience at length, paying attention to all aspects of it.

> **Example of consolidating the positive experience**
>
> **>>Therapist:** "How does this feel to you? A reaction like that?"
>
> **>>John:** "Yes, it feels fun. And nice that you said you were wrong for a moment."
>
> **>>Therapist:** "Well, you helped with that too, because the way you stood up for your needs was great! How does it actually feel to you when you say it like that, with so much force, that you've had enough of all the and you just want to play for a while?"
>
> **>>John:** "Yeah… it's good…"
>
> **>>Therapist:** "Where do you feel that good feeling, in your body, I mean?"
>
> **>>John:** (*points to his chest*) "Here, maybe?"
>
> **>>Therapist:** "Okay, then just put a hand on that spot on your chest, and try to reconnect with that feeling for a while. Where in particular did you feel this pleasant feeling in your chest? When you said you'd had enough of all that work?"
>
> **>>John:** "Yes, I think it was at that moment when I said I was done with it for a while."
>
> **>>Therapist:** "Just say that again: 'I've had enough of just working for a while, I just want to enjoy myself!'"
>
> **>>John:** "I've had enough for now, I've done enough, I want to take it easy for a bit."
>
> **>>Therapist:** "What does it feel like? Is that the pleasant feeling in your chest?"
>
> **>>John:** "Yes, that is the feeling, yes."

9.2.8 Step 8: Review exercise and formation of healthy schemas

The final step of the exercise is to reflect with the client on the credibility of their core thoughts. Remember to look back at the reason for doing the historical roleplay in this session, namely that the client has recently fallen back into old patterns and has now been able to practice new, more healthy behaviour. You encourage your client to take that experience into everyday life and to stand up more for their needs.

Example of reviewing the exercise

>>Therapist: "Now, with this experience, let's step out of the past again and take a moment to look back at everything that happened."

(The therapist and John walk to the place where they look back at the roleplay area.)

>>Therapist: "Right, you had a very different experience there, when you stood up for your need to relax. When you bring that experience to mind again, how credible is the thought for you, now, that 'My feelings and my need for relaxation don't matter'?"

>>John: "Yeah, it's really much less now."

>>Therapist: "How much less? It was fifty percent just now."

>>John: "Well, it hasn't completely gone, but it's a lot less, maybe twenty percent."

>>Therapist: "That's a substantial change. And as far as I'm concerned, this says most of all that this experience was very meaningful for you. Is that right?"

>>John: "Yes, it was."

>>Therapist: "So how do you feel now about the idea that you must 'Work first and only relax afterwards'? That was fifty percent credible for you too."

>>John: "Yes, that's also much less, maybe about the same? Ten percent?"

>>Therapist: "Okay, so in that respect too, this experience really did change things. Now let's take a look back at how we started this. At the start of the conversation, you talked about a situation in the past week where you were lying on the sofa at the end of a long day, and then got up anyway because there were still jobs to do. With all that we've done, discussed and experienced now, how do you see that situation?"

>>John: "Yes, it's the same as the one we just did really. It's kind of sad that I just keep working and don't relax. And I didn't even have my father telling me I had to do it."

>>Therapist: "I get that, and you don't really need your father to think these things anymore, do you? You've actually internalized his messages, it's that Demanding Side of you that drives you to do work, tasks and chores instead of listening to your need for relaxation. But here, looking at the situation and with the awareness you have now, as a Healthy Adult, as the captain of your ship, what do you think you should do next time you're in a situation like that and lying on the sofa after a long day at work?"

>>John: "Stay on the sofa, I think."

>>Therapist: "That seems like a significant conclusion to me. But I also understand that while you can draw that conclusion now, it will be difficult to

> get back to that yourself when you're in a situation like that in real life. So let's take a look at how you can help yourself actually remember the conclusions we've reached today. Then you'll be able to use that knowledge in situations like the one you had this week."

9.3 Future-oriented imagery work

Up to this point, you have been using imagery rescripting to work with images from the past, in order to generate new and healthier experiences. In the final phase of therapy, you must also begin to prepare the client for schema-activating situations that will arise in the future. It is precisely these sorts of situations in which they will tend to fall back into their old coping modes and patterns of behaviour.

There are therefore several reasons to use future-oriented visualizations to help break avoidant, dependent and obsessive-compulsive patterns. In future-oriented imagery, events seem to be 'pre-lived', just as memories can be 're-lived' in the imagination (Schacter & Addis, 2007; Schacter et al, 2008). Furthermore, future-oriented imagery seems to have a motivating effect for behavioural change (Libby et al, 2007). There is evidence that watching yourself from an observer's perspective as you perform new behaviour is more effective for behavioural change than taking a first-person perspective in which you visualize the new behaviour as if you are actually doing it. The expression 'I can see myself doing it' seems to have relevance here (Krans, 2022).

Furthermore, future-oriented imagery is not restricted to observable behaviour. It is possible to practice every aspect of healthy schema activation: being aware of that activation, healthy handling of the emotional and cognitive components of the activated schemas, and, of course, behavioural change. In the example described below, the exercise focuses on recognizing schema activation and handling the emotional and cognitive components of those activated schemas in a healthy way.

There are no strict scripts for future-oriented imagery work, but the step-by-step plan below will help guide you through the options and choices offered by this kind of exercise. The steps are then explained in more detail, with Jenny as the example.

Chapter 9: The final phase of therapy

Step-by-step plan for future-oriented imagery work
N.B. The individual steps can be spread over several sessions if desired.
Step 1: Preliminary discussion.
Step 2: Visualize the Healthy Adult.
Step 3: Visualize the feared disaster scenario.
Step 4: Connect with the Healthy Adult.
Step 5: Follow the three steps of the Healthy Adult.
Step 6: Review and homework.

9.3.1 Step 1: Preliminary discussion

With future-oriented imagery, several choices have to be made in advance. First, it is necessary to choose a scenario for the exercise. What problem situations are likely to arise in the future? What schemas will then potentially be activated, and what patterns of behaviour is your client likely to fall back into? Second, you must also choose which new skills you will have your client practice during the exercise. Will they practice becoming aware of those old behavioural patterns? Will they practice self-compassion, realistic thinking, or a new behaviour? Or will it be a combination of all three?

With all these options, the preliminary discussion of the exercise is somewhat more detailed than you may be used to.

> **Example of preliminary discussion of future-oriented imagery work**
>
> *You agreed in the previous session that Jenny would work purposefully on going out with colleagues for drinks on the last Friday of every month. Jenny is not necessarily enthusiastic about this idea, but she does acknowledge that one of the treatment goals you have agreed on is to engage more socially. In discussing this situation, it first seems important for Jenny to practice becoming aware of the Silent One. Sometimes she feels so bad she is convinced she is sick, only to realize later that she was probably suffering from stress. You also discuss that Jenny should actively use the counterarguments you have explored against the Silent One. Finally, it is important to focus the exercise on actually going for drinks. Together, you very carefully take stock again of the signals that identify the Silent One, and what counterarguments Jenny now has. Beyond that, you concretely discuss how she will attend the get-together.*

9.3.2 Step 2: Visualize the Healthy Adult

The exercise begins with visualizing the Healthy Adult. Using this as the start of the exercise increases the chance that your client will be able to connect with the Healthy Adult when you introduce the feared scenario later on. By now, the client has practiced visualizing the Healthy Adult many times, so this part of the exercise does not need to take a lot of time or can be skipped. Be sure to give the client more space for autonomy. Instead of leading the visualization yourself, ask the client to connect with the Healthy Adult in their own way for a moment, and have them do it out loud so you can listen in.

9.3.3 Step 3: Visualize the feared disaster scenario

As agreed in the preliminary discussion, ask the client to visualize the situation in which they fall back into old behavioural patterns. Direct the focus onto those aspects of the situation that the client finds particularly difficult. This makes the exercise challenging. In the final phase, this is recommended because it will help your client to prepare for difficult moments that will occur after therapy ends. Of course, you do also want and need your client to stay within their Window of Tolerance, so don't make it so difficult that your client is consumed by fear and cannot do the exercise.

> ### Example of visualizing the feared disaster scenario
>
> **>>Jenny:** "And just as I'm finishing work, this colleague comes by the office and asks if we're coming along for drinks today. The colleague who shares my office always goes, but now he says he's skipping today."
>
> **>>Therapist:** "And how do you feel now?"
>
> **>>Jenny:** "Tense... anxious... I never know what to say, and I'm afraid it's going to be very awkward."
>
> **>>Therapist:** "And now the colleague who shares your office isn't going. Maybe you could say you're not feeling well so you're not going either?"
>
> **>>Jenny:** "Yes..."
>
> **>>Therapist:** "Maybe next time then, and just go home today?"
>
> *(Jenny looks a little confused, as if she is thinking but not quite sure what to do next.)*

9.3.4 Step 4: Connect with the Healthy Adult

The purpose of the exercise is to practice handling schema activation in a healthy way. The first step is for the client to become aware of old patterns being activated. In that awareness, they gain a little more distance from the perception they were in danger of falling into. Unlike in the initial phase, the client must now learn to take this step alone. You can help with encouragement and questions, but it is important that you do not take over, as this will not strengthen the autonomy that the client needs at this time.

> ### Example of connecting with the Healthy Adult
>
> **>>Therapist:** "It's your choice, no one is forcing you into anything. Do you recognize the feeling that you could maybe go next time? And today take it easy, and go home?"
>
> **>>Jenny:** "Yes..."
>
> **>>Therapist:** "Where do you recognize that feeling from?"
>
> **>>Jenny:** "I always have that feeling."
>
> **>>Therapist:** "And who is it that always makes you feel you could just go next time?"
>
> **>>Jenny:** "That's the Silent One..."
>
> **>>Therapist:** "Do you want to follow the Silent One now, or let the captain take over?"
>
> **>>Jenny:** "The captain."
>
> **>>Therapist:** "Okay, then make contact with the captain – put on the captain's hat."
>
> (Jenny sits up a bit straighter.)

9.3.5 Step 5: Follow the three steps of the Healthy Adult

Once your client is in their Healthy Adult mode, they can practice the skills you have discussed. This might be a specific element, such as practicing self-compassion or behaviour change. Or it could be a combination of the three different elements, as is the case with Jenny. In chairwork with the three steps of the Healthy Adult in the middle phase (see section 8.4), we described in detail how self-compassion, cognitive restructuring and behaviour modification can be practiced. In the final phase of treatment, as the therapist, you are more reserved in guiding your client. Encourage the client to practice those steps themselves. Sometimes this requires you to push a bit harder, but that pushing is a necessary step as you approach the end of therapy, after which you will no longer be there to help the client when they face similar situations.

> **Example of drawing on the three steps of the Healthy Adult**
>
> *Jenny has just spoken words of understanding and compassion from her Healthy Adult, and she is now about to contradict the Silent One.*
>
> **>>Therapist:** "And as a Healthy Adult, what do you want to say to the Silent One who mostly just thinks it makes sense not to go this time, and says you can always go next time? Why isn't it good for Jenny to think like that?"
>
> **>>Jenny:** "I don't know…"
>
> **>>Therapist:** "No problem, take your time. What's wrong with the Silent One's logic? What argument could you make against it?"
>
> **>>Jenny:** "I really don't know…"
>
> **>>Therapist:** "Well, to be honest, I don't believe that. I don't mean to be critical, but you've heard me talk to the Silent One many times. I think you must have some of my words stored in your mind. What would I say to the Silent One?"
>
> **>>Jenny:** "That avoidance does help me to relax in the short term, but doesn't really help me in the longer term, because it doesn't change anything about the anxiety?"
>
> **>>Therapist:** "Yes, that's something I might say. But now you're here, so you say it."
>
> **>>Jenny:** "I do want to avoid it, but that doesn't help me progress. It'll just make it more difficult to go next time."
>
> **>>Therapist:** "Great! Again, but this time twenty percent louder, as if you mean it!"

For a more detailed discussion of future-oriented imagery work, see *Imagery Rescripting: Theory and Practice* (Van der Wijngaart, 2020, Chapter 5).

9.3.6 Step 6: Review and homework

Reviewing this exercise is a way to consolidate the experience gained. Extensive discussion of the skills practiced and paying attention to experiential aspects helps internalize these experiences. Review in the form of homework leads to further consolidation. Homework tasks might include listening to a self-recorded audio flashcard or writing down and re-reading the main conclusions from an exercise. Of course, the client will also have to try to put what they learned in the exercise into practice. The homework is discussed concretely and specifically in advance to prevent misunderstandings and to minimize the chances of your client avoiding it.

9.4 Chairwork with the therapist as the Coping Mode

Chairwork has already been used extensively during therapy. In the initial phase, you were the one trying to reduce Coping Modes and contradict Critical Modes. In the final phase, chairwork can be used to strengthen your client's Healthy Adult. One way to strengthen the Healthy Adult is to give it more challenges. To do this, as the therapist, you can use chairwork to take on the role of a Coping Mode or to represent a Critical Mode. The client can then make counterarguments from their chair as the Healthy Adult.

> **Example of preparing for chairwork with the therapist as the Coping Mode**
>
> *Claire and her boyfriend, Jonas, were making plans for the coming weekend and Jonas wanted to visit his family. Claire didn't feel like it and needed some quiet time to herself, or with just the two of them. At first she did say that, but she soon noticed that Jonas really wanted to visit his family and for her to go with him. So she agreed. In the therapy, she starts out by explaining that it was actually a good plan, because they haven't visited for a long time. Jonas also has a lot on his mind, and she likes being there for him. After all, he is very important to her too. When the therapist asks whether she would have chosen to do this if Jonas did not have such a clear preference for a family visit, Claire hesitantly confesses that she had really wanted to stay at home.*

In this example, we can hear Claire's Coping Mode again. The Coping Modes of clients with cluster C personality disorders are particularly intractable. It is thus unsurprising if the client is still prone to fall back into these modes, even towards the end of therapy. In this final phase of treatment, however, it is important that they actively recognize these modes themselves, and that you do not have to help with this awareness as often.

> **Example of recognizing the Coping Mode**
>
> **>>Therapist:** "So you really wanted something else, but you went along with Jonas?"
>
> **>>Claire:** "Yes, but I didn't mind or anything."
>
> **>>Therapist:** "No, and I believe you. But who are we hearing when you do what someone else wants, even if that isn't what you really need yourself?"
>
> **>>Claire:** "Well, that is what I actually think." →

> **Therapist:** (*sighs briefly*) "Yes, of course it feels that way, but who are we hearing when you do something that someone else wants?"
>
> **Claire:** "Are you angry?"
>
> **Therapist:** "No, not angry… maybe a bit impatient. We've often discussed this, that you tend to do what others need instead of what you need… so who is doing that?"
>
> **Claire:** "The Pleaser?"
>
> **Therapist:** "You say it like a question, but do you really recognize the Pleaser?"
>
> **Claire:** "Yes, maybe I do…"

If, at this stage of treatment, a client still seems unable to recognize for themselves which Coping Mode is active, an empathic confrontation like the one described above may prove necessary (see also 9.6). After all, you can assume that the client does have this knowledge by now, and that are therefore evading the issue somewhat.

Now that the Coping Mode has been recognized, explain that it will come up again and it is important that the Healthy Adult knows how to handle it. Emphasize that the client now has all the knowledge and skills needed to do this. However, you want to use these final sessions for the client to practice these skills. At this point, you can introduce chairwork as a way to strengthen the Healthy Adult. Explain that you want to put the Coping Mode back on a separate chair. However you, the therapist, will now represent the Coping Mode, while the client has the role of the Healthy Adult who must resist what the Coping Mode says.

Example of chairwork with the therapist as the Coping Mode

> **Therapist:** (*in the chair of the Pleaser*) "It's fine, Jonas really wants to do that, and I like seeing his family too. We haven't seen them for a while, so it's good to do that."
>
> **Claire:** "…"
>
> **Therapist:** (*leans sideways slightly, in the role of therapist, to encourage the client*) "Your job now is to give some resistance to me, to the Pleaser. What's wrong with what I just said? What's still missing?"
>
> **Claire:** "I don't know… it's actually fine. I really do like his family, I mean, I don't have any problems with them or anything."
>
> **Therapist:** (*again stepping out of the role to encourage*) "Yes, that's just the sort of thing I want to say from this chair, as the Pleaser. But your role is different now. →

> You have to try to think as your Healthy Adult, not as the Pleaser. So be the Healthy Adult. And as Claire's Healthy Adult, what can you say when the Pleaser says it's fine if everyone is happy? Or what did I always ask you when we talked about this before?"
>
> **>>Claire:** "What my needs are…?"
>
> **>>Therapist:** "Exactly! Can you say something about that now as the Healthy Adult?"
>
> **>>Claire:** "Well, Jonas might think it's important, but I would actually much rather stay home and do something cosy together."

In this final phase, as the therapist you can slowly increase the pressure by making things a little harder for your client, and you don't have to be too quick to be happy with every healthy step the client takes. When the therapy is over, it's likely that the client will often find themselves stuck in old patterns. It is therefore better to practice hard for those difficult moments now, than to be satisfied too easily.

> ### Example of chairwork with the therapist as the Coping Mode – continued
>
> **>>Therapist:** (*in the role of the Pleaser again*) "Yes, but it's nice to visit his family, isn't it? And he said he really needs to do that, so it wouldn't be that cosy anyway if we just stayed home and did what I wanted…"
>
> (*Claire looks doubtful.*)
>
> **>>Therapist:** (*gently prompting*) "Maybe you could say something about your needs being just as important as his?"
>
> **>>Claire:** "Oh yes… well… Yes, it's true that he'd really like to visit his family, but actually I need something else, and we'll have to work that out together."
>
> **>>Therapist:** "Very good! Keep going…"
>
> **>>Claire:** "And if we have to compromise, we shouldn't just do whatever he wants."
>
> **>>Therapist:** (*gently prompting*) "After all, who is primarily responsible for your needs?"
>
> **>>Claire:** "I have to do that myself… Yeah, I shouldn't immediately give in to what he wants, because I'm the one who has to stand up for my own needs first of all."

9.5 Roleplay with role reversal

Clients sometimes do not realize the effect that their behaviour has on others. Avoidant clients, for example, tend to think that *not* doing something or avoiding unpleasant situations is harmless. Dependent clients do not realize that their dependent behaviour can irritate others at times. And obsessive-compulsive clients do not realize that they can often come across as quite critical. Roleplay with role reversal is a way to explore this, giving the client a chance to experience the kinds of responses that they arouse in others, and to learn to handle situations differently as a result.

> ### Example of roleplay with role reversal
>
> *John does not understand why his wife Laura stormed out angrily last night after he once again put his work ahead of doing something relaxing and fun with her.*
>
> **>>Therapist:** "Let's see how the conversation with your wife went before she walked out. So, I'll play your wife, and you play yourself. What was the trigger?"
>
> **>>John:** "We were supposed to go to the cinema, but I came home late and still needed to make a couple of phone calls. My wife said I should just do it tomorrow."
>
> *(The therapist takes two chairs and suggests replaying the conversation on them.)*
>
> **>>Therapist:** *(now in the role of John's wife)* "You're already late and the movie starts at eight. We just have time for a quick bite to eat, and then we have to leave."
>
> **>>John:** "There was nothing I could do to avoid being late. First, my appointment didn't show up, and when he finally did we still had to go over all the points, and that ran over time. *(A detailed description of everything he discussed with that colleague follows.)*
>
> **>>Therapist:** "That's already very annoying to hear, because you could have told him just to come back another time. Isn't our date important?"
>
> **>>John:** "That's the wrong question. If I hadn't dealt with things today at work, it would have been a big mess tomorrow." *(Another detailed explanation follows.)*
>
> **>>Therapist:** "What nonsense, and now you want to start making calls, too? We won't make it to the movie in time."
>
> **>>John:** "Yes, but I'm responsible for that project." *(Wants to embark on a long explanation again.)*
>
> **>>Therapist:** *(angrily)* "So everything is more important than me. I don't even feel like going to see the movie with you anymore. Figure it out." *(Walks away.)*
>
> *The therapist suggests stepping out of the roleplay for a moment and sitting back on the other chairs. There, the therapist and John briefly go over whether that was approximately how it really went..*

Once you have established that the way the initial roleplay went was approximately how things transpired in reality, it is time to reverse the roles in order to give the client an opportunity to experience how their conduct comes across to others. For John in the example, the goal is not only for him to realize that he handled the situation wrongly, but also for him to get a sense of why his wife became so angry with him.

> ### Example of roleplay with role reversal – continued
>
> *The therapist suggests reversing the roles so John can experience how he comes across to others. John will now play his wife, and the therapist will act out what John just said.*
>
> **>>John:** (*in the role of his wife*) "You're already late and the movie starts at eight. We just have time for a quick bite to eat, and then we have to leave."
>
> **>>Therapist:** (*delivers the whole story as told by John, and then pauses the roleplay for a moment*) "How do you feel when you're faced with this reaction?"
>
> **>>John:** (*in the role of his wife*) "That really is quite a long answer, and what I hear is that you're only concerned with yourself and your work."
>
> **>>Therapist:** "Okay, just say what Laura said, that I should have been able to send him away, and so on."
>
> **>>John:** (*in the role of his wife*): "That's already very annoying to hear, because you could have told him just to come back another time. Isn't our date important?"
>
> **>>Therapist:** "That's the wrong question." (*Another detailed explanation follows.*)
>
> **>>John:** (*in the role of his wife*): "Yes, but you can't also start making calls now."
>
> **>>Therapist:** "Yeah, but I really need to!"
>
> (*The therapist in the role of John wants to start telling another long story, but now he pauses the roleplay again and asks John what it's like to be his wife who has to listen to all these elaborate stories without any understanding for what she is saying. The therapist then suggests ending the roleplay and sitting back on the other chairs.*)

In the example, as John and the therapist reflect on the roleplay together, John will begin to understand why Laura became so angry – not only did he get home too late due to his Perfectionistic Overcontroller, but he is also explained what happened in far too much detail without listening to his wife's point of view. Seeing things from the other person's perspective like this does take effort, because from time to time the Demanding Mode still wants to take over from the Healthy Adult. However, once the client gains confidence with it, they can see how different responses might improve situations. In the example, John might be more understanding of Laura's needs and her point of view, and make sure that they can still get to the cinema on time despite his work commitments.

9.6 Empathic confrontation in the final phase

Over the course of the therapy, you have used empathic confrontation many times. In the initial phase, the focus was on empathy, and when you confronted the client with their patterns you did so with a lot of understanding – explaining that you clearly understood the background to those patterns and that in many ways those patterns had served a useful function in the client's life. The most important objective of the empathic confrontation in the initial phase is for the client to gain greater insight into their different modes and how they are intertwined with their life history.

As therapy moves into the final phase, more explicit work needs to be done to actively change those patterns. This means that the emphasis in empathic confrontation moves increasingly away from empathy and towards confrontation. After all the understanding and insights, now it is important for the client to actually do something with the knowledge they have gained. Much like the parent of a growing child, you are likely to be frustrated at times when confronted by the persistent nature of the client's Coping Modes. You can try to make use of those natural frustrations by using them to fuel your confrontations.

> **Example of empathic confrontation in the final phase**
>
> **>>John:** "It was a particularly busy week, and I really had to work very hard. Sorry, I didn't get to the homework because of that. I know I'd said I would take my wife out for dinner before the next session, but there really was no chance of that this week."
>
> **>>Therapist:** "No? Why wasn't it possible?"
>
> **>>John:** "Well, like I said, it was just very busy with deadlines and the usual amount of work on top of that. And yes, it really does have to be done. I can't ignore it. And if I do it now, it won't keep piling up."
>
> **>>Therapist:** "So your plan was to pay some extra attention to your relationship with your wife, but work made that impossible… again."
>
> **>>John:** "Yes. I really would have liked it to be different, but it is what it is."

Possibly you may feel that there is still room to actively help your client recognize their old behaviour patterns, but by now you have probably heard the client say that they were too busy for other things far too often. Maybe you feel a sense of impatience or frustration. In this final stage, it might be better to show that impatience or frustration to your client. In fact, your impatience can be an extra motivation for the client to actually start breaking behavioural patterns. Hiding your impatience might make the session less confrontational, but it will not help the client's process of change.

> ### Example of empathic confrontation in the final phase – continued
>
> **>>Therapist:** (*sighing from a rising sense of frustration and fatigue*) "Yes, but John, if you're talking again about being busy and work taking priority, who am I listening to?"
>
> **>>John:** "To me… but that's not what you mean?"
>
> **>>Therapist:** (*sighing again*) "No, that's not what I mean. Sorry to sigh like that, John, but to be honest, I'm getting a bit tired of you always telling me that you're just busy and you have no control over it. We've obviously talked about this many times."
>
> **>>John:** "Yes, but it really is true that it was busy, I'm not making that up or anything."
>
> **>>Therapist:** "I'm not saying you're making it up, but I am saying that I'm tired of you not changing your behaviour, and not taking more time out from your work so you can go and do fun things. How do you feel when I say this?"
>
> **>>John:** (*remains silent for a moment*) "It's frustrating, but I'm not sure how else to do it."
>
> **>>Therapist:** "I do believe you, that it's your reality. But it's always been the reality that there was a lot of work. I guess with all that pressure, you've slipped back into the Hard Worker after all. And to be honest, I'm a bit frustrated that he still has so much room to take over. I'd like to explain what that frustration is. When the Hard Worker is in charge, everything we've discussed together here, all the arguments I've made, don't seem to matter anymore. It feels like all that just gets pushed aside, and you just go your own way. Meanwhile, I'm very aware that this also has an impact on Laura. So I've been asked to help you change, but when I do my efforts are pushed aside whenever there's a bit of pressure at work. Can you imagine how that doesn't feel too great for me?"

In this way, you confront the client more firmly than you have done up to now. Not only do you spend more time and attention on the adverse effects of the Coping Mode, but you are also firmer in your wording with terms like 'frustrating'. Such clear confrontation can help your client to become more aware of what has been happening. However, behavioural patterns can be so stubborn that this confrontation may still be ineffective, and the client may still remain stuck in them. You will then have to repeat your confrontation more often, and in different terms, in order to make yourself heard.

> ### Example of empathic confrontation in the final phase – continued
>
> **>>John:** "Yeah, but wow, you don't have to take it personally. I'm just busy at work, that doesn't have much to do with you."
>
> **>>Therapist:** "So, when I say it bothers me, you seem to be suggesting that maybe it's my own interpretation and I just shouldn't see it or feel it that way?"
>
> **>>John:** "Well, maybe a not as sharply as you say it now. But yes, it doesn't have that much to do with you."
>
> **>>Therapist:** "And that's exactly my point, John, because once again what I think or feel doesn't seem to matter all that much. Once again, that seems to get pushed aside because there are more important things going on – and for you that is mainly work. My point, John, is that it bothers me and I need you to realize that, because otherwise the Hard Worker can take over without any problem."

Reaching this point, you can relate the pattern that has occurred in the therapy session to a pattern that occurs in the client's broader life. Indeed, the core purpose of empathic confrontation is to address something in a personal and specific way, in order to make the client aware of what is constantly going on in their broader lives.

> ### Example of empathic confrontation in the final phase – continued
>
> **>>Therapist:** "My point, John, is that it bothers me. And don't worry, I can handle that. It's not like I'm really upset about it or anything. But my concern is not so much my own peace of mind – it's much more that this is a pattern that keeps playing out in your life. And now it's also playing out between us. My concern is that your wife, and other people too, keep running into the Hard Worker. And if I can already feel how frustrating it is to be pushed aside, they must feel the same. I wouldn't say it so emphatically if this was the first time. And I didn't do that earlier in the therapy either. I've often spoken to you about this with a lot of understanding. I told you then that I understand the background of that Hard Worker, and why you needed it. But we're a long way on now, and your Hard Worker still keeps taking over. And I really want you to realize that the Hard Worker is a dead end. It will lead to people feeling uncomfortable and perhaps even leaving you, as your wife has indicated. So, this really is a message for you, John, →

as the captain of your ship: the Hard Worker is running things again. I don't like being faced with that, and other people don't like it either. If you want life to be more than just hard work and becoming competent, you really need to step in now and push the Hard Worker aside for a while, instead of pushing other people aside."

\>\>**John:** "…

\>\>**Therapist:** "How do you feel now, when you hear me say that?"

\>\>**John:** "It feels like… I don't know, like pressure."

\>\>**Therapist:** "Pressure from me, or pressure to change?"

\>\>**John:** "Pressure to change, I guess. I do understand, and I do think you're right that I've been going back to the old way a bit."

\>\>**Therapist:** "It's great that you see that, and good that you say so, John. It feels very different talking to each other like this than when I'm talking to the Hard Worker. Shall we take another look at why taking your wife out for dinner seemed like a good idea?

(John nods).

9.7 Ending the therapy

In the last sessions of the treatment, pay explicit attention to the end of the therapy. First of all, it is important that you stick to the agreed ending. There may well still be all kinds of reasons why it seems necessary to continue therapy. However, as we have mentioned, the effects of therapy do not stop at the end of the last session. Research has shown that these changes continue, even after the last session (Bamelis *et al*, 2014), and this is an important reason to stick to your original treatment plan.

Of course, there may be situations in which you do choose to deviate from that plan. For example, perhaps John's wife still wants a divorce, and he is struggling so much emotionally that therapy may still be necessary. Or maybe Jenny loses her job in the final phase of treatment and risks falling into a hole where she isolates herself and starts to drink heavily. However, such situations are exceptions, and in all other cases it is important to keep to the original treatment plan and end at the agreed time.

That is not to say that this is always easy. You and your client will probably have doubts about whether it is feasible to put everything that has been learned into practice. Many therapists have such doubts, even toward the end of what seems to have been successful therapy. Perhaps these doubts can be compared to the worries that parents have when their children leave home. These worries are not pure fictions, because there usually are all sorts of real indications that children are not yet able to take care of themselves as well as you would like! However, it might help to think back to your own early adulthood, when you probably struggled at time but did well in the end and became a Healthy Adult through trial and error. And that is the process your clients will also have to go through.

Ending treatment may not always be easy for your client, but you can make sure it is a healthy, and therefore positive, experience. By structuring the farewell properly, with care and attention for the different aspects of it, your client learns that the leap to independence does not have to be a traumatic experience. You can create a relapse prevention plan together, and some guidelines you can use for this are given below. They can help you shape the farewell in a healthy way.

- **Look back at the therapy process and take stock of all the learning experiences.**

  By summarizing everything that took place in therapy, you make the client aware of the process they have gone through. Summarizing the most important learning experiences is a good way to remember them.

- **Consolidate these learning experiences, for example by using transitional objects.**

  Evaluate the most important messages the client has learned that they would like to take with them into the future. Remember that explicitly complimenting those learning experiences is a form of consolidation. Other forms of consolidation are:
  - Recording audio flashcards.
  - Writing down (or dictating) those key learning experiences, for example in the form of a warm letter to the Vulnerable Child or to the Healthy Adult.
  - Asking your client to make or buy a gift for themselves to symbolize the growth process they have gone through (for example a bracelet, book or gemstone).

- **Discuss the therapeutic relationship.**

  Evaluate what your client liked about you and what they will miss about you as a therapist. Also ask what they didn't like that much! As the therapist, don't forget to say all the things you liked about your client and what you will miss.

- **Discuss future pitfall moments.**
  Discuss the near and distant future, and identify potential pitfalls. Discuss how your client intends to handle those pitfalls.

9.8 Chapter summary

This chapter has described how to use methods and techniques in the final phase of therapy to break the client's behavioural patterns. When the final phase begins, it is wise to take a fresh look at these behavioural patterns. People from your client's environment, such as friends and family members, can serve as useful sources of information about them, to help you assess what changes the client has not yet made.

The final phase brings a new level of independence for the client within the experiential exercises. In a historical roleplay, they practice standing up for their own needs, and in future-oriented imagery work they can mentally prepare for future situations in which schemas are activated. By performing healthy behaviour in the exercise, your client will be better able to respond in healthy ways when such situations arise in the future.

Behavioural patterns are persistent, and even towards the end of therapy the chances are very high that the client will be prone to fall back into them. You will need to confront the client with those behavioural patterns more clearly at this stage. You no longer have the role of a guiding parent, but much more that of an encouraging coach on the sidelines. In the limited time left in treatment, you can help the client to remain aware of the need to constantly resist those old patterns by doing roleplays with role reversal.

Finally, this chapter has described how to complete the therapy, ensuring that the corrective emotional experiences from therapy are consolidated as well as possible.

Conclusion

Research has shown that schema therapy can be an effective form of treatment for cluster C personality disorders (Bamelis *et al*, 2014). In this book, we have described how this treatment can be set up and implemented in practice, from the case conceptualization to the end of a fifty-session course of therapy. Dependent, Avoidant and Obsessive-Compulsive personality disorders are characterized by specific basic needs, schemas and modes. The treatment of the three disorders therefore varies, using different forms of limited reparenting and applying a range of methods and techniques.

For example, the style of limited reparenting in clients with Dependent Personality Disorder is focused on encouraging and developing autonomy, while for clients with Obsessive-Compulsive Personality Disorder the focus is more on developing the Happy Child. The methods and techniques that characterize schema therapy, such as imagery rescripting and chairwork, are adapted and applied for cluster C personality disorders. With these techniques, different Critical Modes are worked on differently. For instance, you take a firm stand against the Punitive Mode, argue more with a Demanding Mode, and first make the implicit messages of the Blaming Mode explicit before contradicting them. We also provide guidance on how to help the client develop a Healthy Adult.

Further, the application of the various methods and techniques differs across the three phases of treatment. You have a bigger role as a therapist in the early stages than in the later stages. In the initial phase, as the therapist you will negotiate directly with Coping Modes, contradict Critical Modes, and fulfil the needs of the Vulnerable Child. By the final phase, if all has gone well, your client will have learned to do that for themselves.

References

Alden, L. (1989). Short-term structured treatment for avoidant personality disorder. *Journal of Consulting and Clinical Psychology, 57*(6), 756.

Arntz, A. (2012). Schema therapy for cluster C personality disorders. In: M. Van Vreeswijk, J. Broersen, M. Nadort (Red.), *The Wiley-Blackwell handbook of schema therapy: Theory, research and practice* (pag. 397–414). Wiley-Blackwell.

Arntz, A., & Jacob, G. (2012). *Schematherapie: een praktische handleiding* (translation by Guido Sijbers). Uitgeverij Nieuwezijds.

Arntz, A., Rijkeboer, M., Chan, E., Fassbinder, E., Karaosmanoglu, A., Lee, C. W., & Panzeri, M. (2021). Towards a reformulated theory underlying schema therapy: Position paper of an international workgroup. *Cognitive Therapy and Research, 45*, 1007–1020.

Baljé, A., Greeven, A., Van Giezen, A., Korrelboom, K., Arntz, A., & Spinhoven, P. (2016). Group schema therapy versus group cognitive behavioral therapy for social anxiety disorder with comorbid avoidant personality disorder: Study protocol for a randomized controlled trial. *Trials, 17*, 487. DOI 10.1186/s13063-016-1605-9

Bamelis, L. L. M., Renner, F., Heidkamp, D., & Arntz, A. (2011). Extended schema mode conceptualizations for specific personality disorders: An empirical study. *Journal of Personality Disorders, 25*, 41–58.

Bamelis, L. L. M., Evers, S. M. A. A., & Arntz, A. (2012). Design of a multi-centered randomized controlled trial on the clinical and cost effectiveness of schema therapy for personality disorders. *BMC Public Health, 12*, 75. doi:10.1186/1471-2458-12-75

Bamelis, L. L. M., Evers, S. M. A. A., Spinhoven, P., & Arntz, A. (2014). Results of a multicentered randomised controlled trial of the clinical effectiveness of schema therapy for personality disorders. *American Journal of Psychiatry, 171*(3), 305–322. doi: 10.1176/appi.ajp.2013.12040518.

Bamelis, L. L. M., Arntz, A., Wetzelaer, P., Verdoorn, R., & Evers, S. M. A. A. (2015). Economic evaluation of schema therapy and clarification-oriented psychotherapy for personality disorders: A multicenter, randomized controlled trial. *Journal of Clinical Psychiatry, 76*(11), 1432–1440. dx.doi.org/10.4088/JCP.14m09412

Bögels, S. M., & Van Oppen, P. (2019). *Cognitieve therapie: Theorie en praktijk*. Bohn Stafleu van Loghum.

Brockman, R., Simpson, S., Hayes, C., Van der Wijngaart, R., & Smout, M. (2023). *Cambridge Guide to Schema Therapy* (Cambridge Guides to the Psychological Therapies). Cambridge University Press. doi:10.1017/9781108918145

Taylor, C. T., Laposa, J. M., & Alden, L. E. (2004). Is avoidant personality disorder more than just social avoidance? *Journal of Personality Disorders, 18*(6),571–594.

De Klerk, N., Abma, T. A., Bamelis, L. L., & Arntz, A. (2017). Schema therapy for personality disorders: A qualitative study of patients' and therapists' perspectives. *Behavioural and Cognitive Psychotherapy, 45*(1), 31–45. doi:10.1017/S1352465816000357

Dibbets, P., & Arntz, A. (2016). Imagery rescripting Is incorporation of the most aversive scenes necessary? *Memory (Hove, England), 24*(5), 683–695. https://doi.org/10.1080/09658211.2015.1043307

Dweck, C. S. (2017). From needs to goals and representations: Foundations for a unified theory of motivation, personality and development. *Psychological Review, 124*, 689–719. https://doi.org/10.1037/rev00 00082

Farrell, J. M., Reiss, N., & Shaw, I. A. (2014). *The schema therapy clinician's guide: A complete resource for building and delivering individual, group and integrated schema mode treatment programs* (B. Finkelmeier, Illustrator). Wiley. https://doi.org/10.1002/9781118510018

Farrell, J., Reiss, N., & Shaw, I. (2016). *Schematherapie in de klinische praktijk: Een complete gids voor individuele, groeps-en geïntegreerde behandeling met schemamodi* (translation by T. Meynen). Uitgeverij Nieuwezijds.

Friborg, O., Martinsen, E. W., Martinussen, M., Kaiser, S., Øvergård, K. T., Rosenvinge, J. H. (2013). Comorbidity of personality disorders in anxiety disorders: A meta-analysis of 30 years of research. *Journal of Affective Disorders, 145*(2), 143–155. https://doi.org/10.1016/j.jad.2012.07.004.

Friborg, O., Martinsen, E. W., Martinussen, M., Kaiser, S., Øvergård, K. T., Rosenvinge, J. H. (2014). Comorbidity of personality disorders in mood disorders: A meta-analytic review of 122 studies from 1988 to 2010. *Journal of Affective Disorders, 152–154*, 1–11. https://doi.org/10.1016/j.jad.2013.08.023

Van Genderen, H., & Arntz, A. (2021). *Schematherapie bij borderline-persoonlijkheidsstoornis* (second, fully revised edition). Uitgeverij Nieuwezijds. ISBN 9789057124853.

Van Genderen, H. (2023). *Doorbreek je patronen in vijf stappen*. Uitgeverij Nieuwezijds.

Giesen-Bloo, J., Van Dyck, R., Spinhoven, P., Van Tilburg, W., Dirksen, C., Van Asselt, T., Kremers, I., Nadort, M., & Arntz, A. (2006). Outpatient psychotherapy for Borderline Personality Disorder: A randomized controlled trial of schema-focused therapy versus transference focused psychotherapy. *Archives of General Psychiatry, 63*, 649–658.

Groot, I. Z., Venhuizen, A. S. S., Bachrach, N., Walhout, S., De Moor, B., Nikkels, K., ..., & Arntz, A. (2022). Design of an RCT on cost-effectiveness of group schema therapy versus individual schema therapy for patients with Cluster-C personality disorder: The QUEST-CLC study protocol. *BMC Psychiatry, 22*, 637. https://doi.org/10.1186/s12888-022-04248-9

Holmes, E. A., & Mathews, A. (2010). Mental imagery in emotion and emotional disorders. *Clinical Psychology Review, 30*(3), 349–362. http://dx.doi.org/10.1016/j.cpr.2010.01.001

Heimberg, R. G., Dodge, C. S., Hope, D. A., Kennedy, C. R., Zollo, L. J., & Becker, R. E. (1990). Cognitive behavioral group treatment for social phobia: Comparison with a credible placebo control. *Cognitive Therapy and Research, 14*(1), 1–23.

Kaeding, A., Sougleris, C., Reid, C., Van Vreeswijk, M., Hayes, C., Dorrian, J., & Simpson, S. (2017). Professional burnout, early maladaptive schemas and the effect on physical health in clinical and counseling trainees. *Journal of Clinical Psychology, 73*(12), 1782–1796. DOI: https://doi.org/10.1002/jclp.22485.

Krans, J. (2022). Personal communication. Radboud University & Pro Persona Deputy director of BSI, assistant professor, senior researcher.

Krans, J., & Van der Wijngaart, R. (2022). In Van der Wijngaart, R. (Ed.), *Stoelentechniek, theorie en praktijk* (Chapter 1 Introduction). Bohn Stafleu van Loghum. ISBN 978-90-368-2796-6

Libby, L. K., Shaeffer, E. M., Eibach, R. P., & Slemmer, J. A. (2007). Picture yourself at the polls: Visual perspective in mental imagery affects self-perception and behavior. *Psychological Science, 18*(3), 199–203.

Nadort, M., Arntz, A., Smit, J. H., Giesen-Bloo, J., Eikelenboom, M., Spinhoven, P., Van Asselt, T., Wensing, M., & Van Dyck, R. (2009). Implementation of outpatient schema therapy for borderline personality disorder with versus without crisis support by the therapist outside office hours: A randomized trial. *Behaviour research and therapy, 47*(11), 961–973. https://doi.org/10.1016/j.brat.2009.07.013

Nijenhuis M & Krans, J. (2024, in preparation). *Schematherapeutische exposure voor angst- en dwangstoornissen*. Bohn Stafleu van Loghum.

Panagiotopoulos, A., Despoti, A., Varveri, C. et al (2023). The relationship between early maladaptive schemas and cluster C personality disorder traits: A systematic review and meta-analysis. *Current Psychiatry Reports, 25*, 439–453. https://doi.org/10.1007/s11920-023-01439-3

Peeters, N., Van Passel, B., & Krans, J. (2021). The effectiveness of schema therapy for patients with anxiety disorders, OCD, or PTSD: A systematic review and research agenda. *The British Journal of Clinical Psychology, 61*(3), 579–597. https://doi.org/10.1111/bjc.12324

Renner, F., Arntz, A., Leeuw, I., & Huibers, M. (2013). Treatment for chronic depression using schema therapy. *Clinical Psychology Science and Practice, 20*, 166–180. http://dx.doi.org/10.1111/cpsp.12032

Renner, F., Arntz, A., Peeters, F. P., Lobbestael, J., & Huibers, M. J. (2016). Schema therapy for chronic depression: Results of a multiple single case series. *Journal of Behavior Therapy and Experimental Psychiatry, 51*, 66–73. http://dx.doi.org/10.1016/j.jbtep.2015.12.001

Reubsaet, R. J. (2018). *Schema therapy Werken met fases in de klinische praktijk*. Bohn Stafleu van Loghum. 10.1007/978-90-368-2115-5.

Rijkeboer, M. M., & Lobbestael, J. (2012). *The relationships between early maladaptive schemas, schema modes and coping styles*. Paper presented at the 5th World Conference of Schema Therapy, May 17th-19th, New York, USA.

Sachse, R. (2001). *Psychologische Psychotherapie der Persönlichkeitsstörungen*. Hogrefe.

Schacter, D. L., & Addis, D. R. (2007). The cognitive neuroscience of constructive memory: Remembering the past and imagining the future. *Philosophical Transactions of the Royal Society of London. Series B, Biological sciences, 362*(1481), 773–786. doi:10.1098/rstb.2007.2087

Schacter, D. L., Addis, D. R., & Buckner, R. L. (2008). Episodic simulation of future events concepts, data, and applications. *New York Academy of Sciences, 1124*, 39–60.

Simon, W. (2009). Follow-up psychotherapy outcome of patients with dependent, avoidant and obsessive-compulsive personality disorders: A meta-analytic review. *International Journal of Psychiatry in Clinical Practice, 13*(2), 153–165.

Simpson, S., Simionato, G., Smout, M., Van Vreeswijk, M. F., Hayes, C., Sougleris, C., & Reid, C. (2019). Burnout amongst clinical and counselling psychologist: The role of early maladaptive schemas and coping modes as vulnerability factors. *Clinical Psychology & Psychotherapy, 26*(1), 35–46. https://doi.org/10.1002/cpp.2328

Skewes, S. A., Samson, R. A., Simpson, S. G., & Van Vreeswijk, M. (2015). Short-term group schema therapy for mixed personality disorders: A pilot study. *Frontiers in Psychology, 5*, 1592 https://doi.org/10.3389/fpsyg.2014.01592

Ten Napel-Schutz, M. C., Abma, T. A., Bamelis, L. & Arntz, A. (2011). Personality disorder patients' perspectives on the introduction of imagery within schema therapy: A qualitative study of patients' experiences. *Cognitive and Behavioral Practice, 18*, 482–490. doi:10.1016/j.cbpra.2011.04.005.

Ten Have, M., Tuithof, M., Van Dorsselaer, S., Schouten, F., & De Graaf, R. (2023). The Netherlands Mental Health Survey and Incidence Study-3 (NEMESIS-3): Objectives, methods and baseline characteristics of the sample. *International Journal of Methods in Psychiatric Research, 32*(1), e1942. https://doi.org/10.1002/mpr.1942

Ten Napel-Schutz, M. C., Abma, T. A., Bamelis, L. L., & Arntz, A. (2017). How to train experienced therapists in a new method: A qualitative study into therapists' views. *Psychotherapy, 24*(2), 359–372. 10.1002/cpp.2004

Spek, A., Fernandes Pinto, L., Grevers, R., Kiep, M., Snouckaert, V., Ten Barge, L., De Boer, F., Metten, D., & Curiël, Y. (n.d.). *Whitepaper ASS en / of Dwangmatige persoonlijkheidsstoornis*. Autisme Expertisecentrum (Eemnes).

Tjoa, E. E. M. L., & Muste, E. H. (2021). *Handleiding groepsschematherapie voor cluster C-persoonlijkheidsstoornissen*. Bohn Stafleu van Loghum.

Van der Wijngaart, R. (2020). *Imagery rescripting: Theory and Practice*. Pavilion Publishing.

Van der Wijngaart, R. (2020). *Chairwork: Theory and Practice*. Pavilion Publishing.

Van der Wijngaart, R., & Sijbers, G. (2018). *Schema therapy for the Avoidant-, Dependent-, and Obsessive-Compulsive personality disorder*. USB-stick.

Videler, A. C., Van Alphen, S. P. J., Van Royen, R. J. J., Van der Feltz-Cornelis, C. M., Rossi, G., & Arntz, A. (2018). Schema therapy for personality disorders in older adults: A multiple-baseline study. *Aging and Mental Health, 22*(6), 738–747. http://dx.doi.org/10.1080/13607863.2017.1318260

Vuijk, R., Deen, M., Sizoo, B., & Arntz, A. (2018). Temperament, character, and personality disorders in adults with autism spectrum disorder: A systematic literature review and meta-analysis. *Review Journal of Autism and Developmental Disorders, 5*, 176–197. https://doi.org/10.1007/s40489-018-0131-y

References

Vuijk, R., Deen, M., Geurts, H. M., & Arntz, A. (2023). Schema therapy for personality disorders in adults with autism spectrum disorder: Results of a multiple case series study. *Clinical Psychology & Psychotherapy, 30*, 458–472. https://doi.org/10.1002/cpp.2817

Wibbelink, C. J. M., Venhuizen, A. S. S. M., Grasman, R. P. P. P., Bachrach, N., Van den Hengel, C., Hudepohl, S., Kunst, L., De Lange, H., Louter, M. A., Matthijssen, S. J. M. A., Schaling, A., Walhout, S., Wichers, K. (R.), & Arntz, A. (2023). Group schema therapy for cluster-C personality disorders: A multicentre open pilot study. *Clinical Psychology & Psychotherapy, 1–24.* https://doi.org/10.1002/cpp.2903

Yakin, D. Grasman, R., & Arntz, A. (2020). Schema modes as a common mechanism of change in personality pathology and functioning: Results from a randomized controlled trial. *Behaviour Research and Therapy, 126*, 103553. 10.1016/j.brat.2020.103553.

Young, J. E. (1990). *Cognitive therapy for personality disorders: A schema-focused approach*. Professional Resource Exchange.

Young, J. E., Klosko J. S., & Weishaar, M. E (2020 or 2005). *Schemagerichte therapie: Handboek voor therapeuten*. Bohn Stafleu van Loghum.

Appendix: Modes

In this Appendix, we provide the names and forms of expression of all the modes, along with their relationship to the specific schemas, as proposed by Arntz and colleagues (Arntz et al, 2021). Where possible, we have adopted the existing names as used in the current literature and questionnaires (with a name you could use with clients in brackets). For the Child Modes, we describe which is relevant for each schema. For the Critical Modes, only a limited number of schemas are relevant. For the Avoidant and Inverted Coping Modes, we explain which schema's activation could be avoided or inverted.

In Chapter 2, we explained only the modes that are relevant for clients with a cluster C personality disorder. This more comprehensive table lists all the modes. The other modes that are relevant to other personality disorders are given in italics. The Blaming Mode has been added by the authors (see 2.4.3. Modes). Arntz *et al*'s research group is still investigating this model, so this list may change in the future.

Appendix: Modes

Vulnerable and Angry Child Modes with the related schemas and experience

Schema	Vulnerable Child	Angry, Sulking, Rebellious child	Expression
Acceptance, connection, security and predictability			
Emotional Deprivation	Lonely and Unloved Child		You feel like no one really understands you, knows how you feel or cares about you. There can also be the sense that your feelings are too much for others.
		Angry Child	You get angry at others when they don't consider your feelings, even if you haven't expressed them.
		Impulsive Child	You impulsively seek attention and love. You seek attention through short-term relationships.
Mistrust/Abuse	Abused Child		You experience intense fear of being abused and expect that no one will help you. You think that other people are not trustworthy.
		Angry Child	You react angrily when you think someone wants to abuse you or you suspect them of bad intentions. You can be obsessed with thoughts of revenge.
		Impulsive Child	You react impulsively when you think you could be abused. You are ready to attack if you think the other person wants to harm you.
Abandonment/ Instability	Abandoned Child		You feel intense despair because you think you won't get love, security or acceptance. You feel easily let down. Because of this, you cling to people.
		Angry Child	You react angrily to the (perceived) threat of abandonment or actual abandonment. Sometimes you angrily break up a relationship so that the other person cannot leave you.
		Impulsive Child	You transgress boundaries in the way you check whether someone else might leave you.

Schema	Vulnerable Child	Angry, Sulking, Rebellious child	Expression
Social Isolation / Alienation	Alienated and Misunderstood Child		You feel like you are very different from other people. You feel like you don't fit in or belong to a group.
		Angry Child	You react angrily to the (perceived) threat that you don't belong, or when someone does not understand what is going on within you.
		Impulsive Child	*You do impulsive things to achieve belonging.*
Defectiveness / Shame	Inferior and Ashamed Child		You feel inadequate and bad. This can be accompanied by feelings of shame.
		Angry Child	You are angry at others who give you the impression that you are inferior and that they think you should be ashamed of yourself
		Impulsive Child	*You act impulsively in a defective, shameful way when you believe others think you are inferior.*
Competence and autonomy			
Dependence / Incompetence	Dependent and Incompetent Child		You feel anxious and unable to handle everyday responsibilities. You can't do anything without help from others.
		Angry Child	You get angry at the impression that too much responsibility is placed on your shoulders.
Failure	Failing Child		You believe you will fail at your tasks. You believe that your own skills, knowledge and ideas are worse than those of others.
		Angry Child	You get angry when others criticize your behaviour or when others do better, and also when others put you in a situation where you fail.

Schema	Vulnerable Child	Angry, Sulking, Rebellious child	Expression
Vulnerability to Harm or Illness	Anxious Child		You feel anxious and unsafe. You feel overwhelmed by perceived dangers. You are constantly worried that you are not safe and seek reassurance from others.
		Angry Child	You get angry when others don't take your fears and concerns seriously.
Enmeshment / Undeveloped Self	Non-individualized Child		You think that one or several significant others cannot survive if you separate from them. You experience a duty to stay connected to these others and feel guilty if you try to do something independently of them.
		Angry Child	You get angry when others put pressure on you to individualize more.
		Sulking Child	You passively-aggressively resist the duty of always having to be connected to others.
		Rebellious Child	You rebel against the suffocating atmosphere of enmeshment by acting defiantly.
Self-expression; expressing your needs, opinions and feelings			
Subjugation	Intimidated Child (Subordinate Child)		You feel intimidated by others and believe that expressing your own needs will have negative consequences. You feel small and powerless.
		Angry Child	You get angry at the feeling of not getting a chance to express your own wants and needs, or when you think others do not take them seriously.
		Rebellious Child	You act defiantly and do forbidden things in protest. You refuse to follow the rules and do not consider the consequences.

Schema	Vulnerable Child		Expression
	Angry, Sulking, Rebellious child		
Self-sacrifice		Parentified Child	You firmly believe that you need to care for others, ignoring whether this is needed or refused.
		Angry Child	You have outbursts of angry accusations because you have to constantly sacrifice yourself and others do not recognize your concern.
		Victimized Child	You experience the imbalance between giving and receiving care as unfair. You feel you have been wronged and that you are being treated unfairly.
Approval-seeking/ Recognition-seeking		Attention-Demanding Child	You cannot manage without attention and recognition from others. And you put a lot of effort into getting it. You become insecure when others get more attention.
		Sulking Child	You have a passive-aggressive way of showing your displeasure when you do not get attention or approval.
		Impulsive Child	You behave seductively or try to please others to get attention.
Realistic limits and self-control (overconfidence)			
Entitlement/ Grandiosity		Spoiled Child	You think you are entitled to get and do what you want without regard for others. You impose your will to force instant gratification of your needs. You cannot handle frustrations.
		Superior Child (Grandiose Child)	You think you are better and more important than others. You feel superior to most people and expect them to admire you. You like to have power and control over others.
		Angry Child	You get angry when you don't get your way or receive enough admiration. Or you get angry when others disobey you and you blame others for your own mistakes.

343

Appendix: Modes

Schema	Vulnerable Child		Expression
	Angry, Sulking, Rebellious child		
Entitlement/ Grandiosity (Continued)		Enraged Child	You become enraged and aggressive and lose control of yourself when the Angry Child does not get his way.
		Impulsive Child	You behave impulsively to gain admiration, attention or obedience. You don't care about the consequences because you think you deserve them, disregarding others.
Insufficient Self-Control/Self-Discipline		Undisciplined Child	You have not developed sufficient self-control and do not feel motivated to do boring or hard tasks. You are easily distracted, act chaotically, and express your feelings and needs in an uncontrolled way.
		Angry Child	You get angry when you have to do things that require self-control or self-discipline to achieve your goals.
		Sulking Child	You resist boring difficult or frustrating tasks in a passive way and by remaining silent because you fear the negative consequences if you get really angry.
Spontaneity and play (excessive vigilance and control)			
Negativity / Pessimism		Pessimistic Child	You tend to interpret situations in a negative, pessimistic way. You expect that things will go wrong. The future is dark and disasters are likely. You usually feel hopeless and dejected. You don't let others cheer you up.
		Angry Child	You get very angry when others are optimistic, or even realistic, because you really believe in your pessimistic and gloomy expectations.
Emotional Inhibition		Inhibited Child	You don't dare to express emotional needs. You are easily embarrassed and lack spontaneity and playfulness. This is perceived by others as cold, stiff and overly formal.

Appendix: Modes

Schema	Vulnerable Child	Angry, Sulking, Rebellious child	Expression
Emotional Inhibition (Continued)		Frightened and Panicking Child	You are afraid of losing control over negative feelings, including anger, sadness and fear.
Unrelenting Standards	Disappointing and Underperforming Child*		You are disappointed in yourself with regard to your own performance and standards.
	Over-diligent Child*		You work hard, are obedient and behave well and nicely.
		Angry Child	You get angry because of unrealistic or unreasonable demands. You are often angry at others or organizations and you don't realize that you are actually angry at your own unrelenting standards. You feel angry because you think that others demand too much of you.
		Rebellious Child	You are not overtly angry, but you deliberately do things badly in protest against the high demands.
		Sulking Child	You protest in a passive, indirect, non-verbal way against excessive demands and expectations.
Punitiveness	Bad Child		You feel bad and guilty, and think you deserve punishment.
		Angry variant: Protesting Child	You protest emotionally against the punishment you are experiencing. Usually, you direct your anger at others, who are perceived as critical.

* There is discussion as to whether the *Unrelenting Standards* schema has Vulnerable Child Modes. On the one hand, surrendering to this schema would only involve the Demanding Mode. On the other, in addition to the Demanding Mode, there could also be two Vulnerable Child Modes, namely the Disappointing/Underperforming Child and the Over-diligent Child. Research on this is still underway.

Schema	Vulnerable Child	Angry, Sulking, Rebellious child	Expression
Punitiveness (Continued)		Sulking Child	You protest passive aggressively, indirectly, and non-verbally against excessive punishments, accusations and restrictions.
		Impulsive Child	You impulsively do pleasurable things to protest against the restrictions and punishment, but do this excessively (impulsive purchases, sex or substance abuse).
Self-coherence (coherent self-image and clear picture of the world)			
Lack of self-coherence	Confused Child		You perceive yourself not as a coherent whole, but as chaotic and as if you are falling apart. This makes you feel anxious and confused, and you feel empty.
(Confusion about who you are)		Angry Child	You perceive yourself not as a coherent whole, but as chaotic and as if you are falling apart, and this makes you uncontrollably angry.
Lack of a meaningful world	Alienated Child		You experience the world as meaningless and fragmented. This makes you feel scared, confused and lost, and you feel like everything is meaningless.
		Angry Child	You experience the world as meaningless and fragmented. This makes you angry.
Fairness			
Unfairness	Victimized Child		You constantly feel aggrieved and unfairly treated. You magnify bad luck or something unfair to excessive proportions.
		Angry Child	You protest against (perceived) unfair treatment with uncontrolled anger. You misinterpret the reason and why something might be unfair.
		Impulsive Child	You act impulsively because of expected unfairness.

Van Genderen (2023) and Arntz et al (2021)

Critical Modes		
Critical Mode	**Schema**	**Expression**
Demanding Mode	■ Emotional Inhibition ■ Unrelenting Standards	You have to keep going until things are finished and perfect. It can always be better. You can only relax once everything is finished.
Punitive Mode	■ Punitiveness	You are bad, stupid and ugly. If something goes wrong, it is your own fault and you shouldn't complain.
Blaming Mode	■ Punitiveness ■ Subjugation	You should always be there for others. You are a burden to others when you think of yourself. It is your fault if family or friends are unhappy.

Van Genderen (2023) and Arntz *et al* (2021)

Appendix: Modes

Avoidant Coping Modes*		
Avoidant Coping Mode	**Schema**	**Expression**
The Detached Protector (The Feeling Blocker)	All schemas, except: - Entitlement/Grandiosity - Insufficient Self-control/Self-discipline	*Shutting off feelings* You ignore your feelings, do not react, dissociate or abuse numbing drugs.
The Funny Protector	- Mistrust/Abuse - Abandonment/Instability - Social Isolation/Alienation - Emotional Deprivation - Defectiveness/Shame - Dependence/Incompetence - Failure - Vulnerability to Harm or Illness - Enmeshment - Subjugation	*Making jokes* When something unpleasant happens, you make jokes about it.
The Angry Protector (The Angry Cynic)	- Mistrust/Abuse - Social Isolation - Defectiveness/Shame - Emotional Inhibition	*Getting cynical or angry* When someone does something annoying or is critical, you react angrily or cynically.
The Avoidant Protector	- All schemas	*Avoiding situations* You literally avoid situations, awkward contacts or difficult tasks.
The Detached Self-Soother (The Stupefier)	- All schemas except Subjugation	*Seeking distraction* You avoid lingering on your feelings by constantly engaging in activities that distract you from your feelings.

* The second column shows which schema avoids activation by this Coping Mode. The third column explains the behaviour by which that mode can be recognized.

Avoidant Coping Mode	Schema	Expression
The Compliant Surrenderer (The Subordinate)	■ Abandonment/Instability ■ Emotional Deprivation ■ Dependence/Incompetence ■ Enmeshment/Undeveloped Self ■ Subjugation	*Making yourself subordinate* You always do what others want and deny your own needs or allow yourself to be abused.
The Reassurance Seeker	■ Abandonment/Instability ■ Dependence/Incompetence ■ Failure ■ Vulnerability to Harm or Illness	*Seeking reassurance* You constantly seek advice and reassurance with concerns both large and small, so you don't have to feel or endure your fears and insecurities.
The Suspicious Overcontroller (The suspicious person)	■ Mistrust/Abuse ■ Abandonment/Instability	*Paranoid need for control* You are constantly alert and watch others to prevent them from taking advantage of you or letting you down.

* The second column shows which schema avoids activation by this Coping Mode. The third column explains the behaviour by which that mode can be recognized.

Van Genderen (2023) and Arntz *et al* (2021)

Inversion Coping Modes **		
Inverted Coping Mode	**Schema**	**Expression**
The Independent	<ul><li>Abandonment/Instability</li><li>Dependence/Incompetence</li><li>Enmeshment/Undeveloped Self</li><li>Subjugation</li><li>Self-sacrifice</li><li>Approval-seeking/Recognition-seeking</li></ul>	*Extreme independent behaviour:* You act like you don't need anyone. But you're really afraid of being abandoned or forced into doing something you don't want.
The Clown	<ul><li>Mistrust/Abuse</li><li>Abandonment/Instability</li><li>Emotional Deprivation</li><li>Social Isolation/Alienation</li><li>Defectiveness/Shame</li><li>Dependence/Incompetence</li><li>Failure</li><li>Fear of Harm or Illness</li><li>Enmeshment/Undeveloped Self</li><li>Subjugation</li><li>Self-sacrifice</li><li>Negativity/Pessimism</li><li>Emotional Inhibition</li></ul>	*Ridiculing needs:* You deny your needs by calling them ridiculous, petty or excessive. You pretend that your experiences or shortfalls are no big deal to avoid feeling the pain about them.
The Attention and Approval Seeker (The Attention-Getter)	<ul><li>Emotional Deprivation</li><li>Defectiveness/Shame</li><li>Social Isolation/Alienation</li><li>Emotional Inhibition</li><li>Vulnerability to Harm or Illness</li></ul>	*Drawing attention to yourself:* You can invert your insecurity and sense of not belonging by attracting attention to what you can do or have experienced.
* The second column shows which schema activation is avoided by this Coping Mode by inverting what the schema dictates. The third column explains the behaviour by which that mode can be recognized.		

Appendix: Modes

Inverted Coping Mode	Schema	Expression
The Daredevil	■ Vulnerability to Harm or Illness	*Seeking danger* While you are actually afraid, you suppress that feeling precisely by seeking out danger.
The Perfectionistic Overcontroller (The Perfectionist)	■ Emotional Deprivation ■ Failure ■ Insufficient Self-control/Self-discipline	*Continuing until it is perfect* To avoid the feeling of failure or sloppiness, you try extremely hard.
The Slacker	■ Unrelenting Standards	*Deliberately being lazy and inactive* You do little or nothing, you cut corners, you don't try at all.
The Over-Optimist	■ Negativity/Pessimism ■ Unfairness	*Being excessively optimistic:* You close your eyes to unfairness or abuse by pretending that everyone always has good intentions.
The Merciful	■ Punitiveness ■ Entitlement / Grandiosity	*Acting overly humble and forgiving:* You do feel superior, but out of fear that people will think you are arrogant, you act very humble.
The Self-Aggrandizer (The Braggart)	■ Defectiveness / Shame ■ Social Isolation / Alienation ■ Subjugation ■ Self-sacrifice ■ Approval-seeking / Recognition-seeking	*Bragging:* You pretend to be very special and brag about who you are and what you do.

* The second column shows which schema activation is avoided by this Coping Mode by inverting what the schema dictates. The third column explains the behaviour by which that mode can be recognized.

Appendix: Modes

Inverted Coping Mode	Schema	Expression
The Bully and Attack Mode (The Attacker)	■ Mistrust / Abuse ■ Abandonment / Instability ■ Subjugation ■ Unfairness	*Attacking and intimidating:* You think that offence is the best defence to avoid being deceived, abused or suppressed.
The Conning and Manipulation Mode (The Pretender)	■ Abandonment / Instability ■ Unfairness	*Lying and cheating:* You manipulate others to avoid being cheated or abandoned.
The Predator	■ Unfairness	*Threat:* You take out potential threats, rivals or enemies in a cold, calculated way.

* The second column shows which schema activation is avoided by this Coping Mode by inverting what the schema dictates. The third column explains the behaviour by which that mode can be recognized.

Van Genderen (2023) and Arntz *et al* (2021)